INVERTEBRATE
ENDOCRINOLOGY
and HORMONAL
HETEROPHYLLY

INVERTEBRATE
ENDOCRINOLOGY and
HORMONAL HETEROPHYLLY

Edited by
Walter J. Burdette

SPRINGER-VERLAG New York · Heidelberg · Berlin

WALTER J. BURDETTE, Ph.D., M.D., Professor of Surgery,
The University of Texas, Houston, Texas 77025/U.S.A.

Sponsored by

The National Biomedical Foundation

Library of Congress Cataloging in Publication Data

Burdette, Walter J.
  Invertebrate endocrinology and hormonal heterophylly.

  1. Endocrinology. 2. Hormones. 3. Invertebrates
—Physiology. I. Title. [DNLM: 1. Invertebrate
hormones. QL364 B95li 1973]
QP187.B79   595.7'01'927   73-20188

© 1974 by Springer-Verlag New York Inc.

Printed in the United States of America.

ISBN 0-387-06594-6 Springer-Verlag New York · Heidelberg · Berlin
ISBN 3-540-06594-6 Springer-Verlag Berlin · Heidelberg · New York

Contributors

John S. Bjerke, Ph.D.
Harvard University
Cambridge, Massachusetts

Dianne D. Black, M.S.
The University of Texas at Houston
M. D. Anderson Hospital and Tumor Institute
Houston, Texas

Walter J. Burdette, Ph.D., M.D.
The University of Texas
Medical School at Houston

James E. Carver, Jr., Ph.D.
The University of Texas at Houston
M. D. Anderson Hospital and Tumor Institute
Houston, Texas

Karl H. Dahm, Ph.D.
Texas A & M University
College Station, Texas

S. R. Dutky, Ph.D.
Insect Physiology Laboratory
Agricultural Research Service
United States Department of Agriculture
Beltsville, Maryland

N. Burr Furlong, Ph.D.
The University of Texas at Houston
M. D. Anderson Hospital and Tumor Institute
Houston, Texas

M. N. Galbraith, Ph.D.
Division of Applied Chemistry
Commonwealth Scientific & Industrial Research Organization
Melbourne, Australia

A. Clark Griffin, Ph.D.
The University of Texas at Houston
M. D. Anderson Hospital and Tumor Institute
Houston, Texas

Hiroshi Hikino, Ph.D.
Pharmaceutical Institute
Tohoku University
Sendai, Japan

L. S. Hnilica, Ph.D.
The University of Texas at Houston
M. D. Anderson Hospital and Tumor Institute
Houston, Texas

D. H. S. Horn, Ph.D.
Division of Applied Chemistry
Commonwealth Scientific & Industrial Research Organization
Melbourne, Australia

R. B. Hurlbert, Ph.D.
The University of Texas at Houston
M. D. Anderson Hospital and Tumor Institute
Houston, Texas

Kenneth J. Judy, Ph.D.
Zoecon Corporation
Palo Alto, California

John N. Kaplanis, Ph.D.
Insect Physiology Laboratory
Agricultural Research Service
United States Department of Agriculture
Beltsville, Maryland

Peter Karlson, Ph.D.
Physiologisch-chemisches Institut der Philipps-Universität
Marburg (Lahn), Germany

David Shaw King, Ph.D.
Zoecon Corporation
Palo Alto, California

Masatoshi Kobayashi, Ph.D.
Sericultural Experiment Station
Tokyo, Japan

M. Koreeda, Ph.D.
Columbia University
New York, New York

Hiroyuki Matsuda, M.D.
Rohto Pharmaceutical Co., Ltd.
Osaka, Japan

Manfred Metzler, Ph.D.
Texas A & M University
College Station, Texas

Dietrich Meyer, Ph.D.
Texas A & M University
College Station, Texas

E. J. Middleton, Ph.D.
Division of Applied Chemistry
Commonwealth Scientific & Industrial Research Organization
Melbourne, Australia

Koji Nakanishi, Ph.D.
Columbia University
New York, New York

Nobushige Nishimoto, Ph.D.
Rohto Pharmaceutical Co., Ltd.
Osaka, Japan

Shuntaro Ogawa, Ph.D.
Rohto Pharmaceutical Co., Ltd.
Osaka, Japan

Antonio Orengo, M.D.
The University of Texas at Houston
M. D. Anderson Hospital and Tumor Institute
Houston, Texas

Tadahiko Otaka, Ph.D.
Pharmaceutical Institute
Tohoku University
Sendai, Japan

W. E. Robbins, Ph.D.
Insect Physiology Laboratory
Agricultural Research Service
United States Department of Agriculture
Beltsville, Maryland

Herbert Röller, Ph.D.
Texas A & M University
College Station, Texas

D. A. Schooley, Ph.D.
Zoecon Corporation
Palo Alto, California

Constantin E. Sekeris, M.D.
Physiologisch-chemisches Institut der Philipps-Universität
Marburg (Lahn), Germany

John B. Siddall, Ph.D.
Zoecon Corporation
Palo Alto, California

Michael Slade, Ph.D.
Zoecon Corporation
Palo Alto, California

T. C. Spelsberg, Ph.D.
Vanderbilt University School of Medicine
Nashville, Tennessee

Tsunematsu Takemoto, Ph.D.
Pharmaceutical Institute
Tohoku University
Sendai, Japan

M. J. Thompson, M.S.
Insect Physiology Laboratory
Agricultural Research Service
United States Department of Agriculture
Beltsville, Maryland

John A. Thomson, Ph.D.
University of Melbourne
Victoria, Australia

Y. H. Tsai, Ph.D.
The University of Texas at Houston
M. D. Anderson Hospital and Tumor Institute
Houston, Texas

Mitsuru Uchiyama, Ph.D.
Pharmaceutical Institute
Tohoku University
Sendai, Japan

Earl F. Walborg, Jr., Ph.D.
The University of Texas at Houston
M. D. Anderson Hospital and Tumor Institute
Houston, Texas

Darrell N. Ward, Ph.D.
The University of Texas at Houston
M. D. Anderson Hospital and Tumor Institute
Houston, Texas

Sir Vincent B. Wigglesworth, Sc.D., M.D.
Department of Zoology
University of Cambridge
Cambridge, England

Masayoshi Yamazaki, Ph.D.
Sericultural Experiment Station
Tokyo, Japan

Takemi Yoshida, M.S.
Pharmaceutical Institute
Tohoku University
Sendai, Japan

Table of Contents

Part I

Invertebrate Endocrinology

Hormonal Control of Metamorphosis

Chapter

Assays

Part II

Isolation, Distribution, and Supply of Invertebrate Hormones, Phytohormones, and Analogs

Ecdysones

Part III

Hormones and Protein Synthesis in Mammals

Part IV

Hormonal Heterophylly

The Concept

Pharmacology

Effect of Invertebrate Hormones and Analogs on Tumors

Action of Invertebrate Hormones on Vertebrate Tissues

Preface

Full recognition of the important role that hormones play in the growth, differentiation, and function of insects was preceded by rather advanced information about identity and action of mammalian hormones. However, extirpation and transplantation of endocrine glands in insects and segmental ligation of larvae gradually yielded knowledge about the location of endocrine cells in insects and led to labeling their hormonal product with appropriate names. The development of relatively sensitive assays permitted the separation of active extracts of the hormones associated with metamorphosis and quickened the pace of discovery. Finally, identification of structural formulae of natural hormones now has provided the means for detailed study of biochemical events with which they are associated. In the meantime, better interpretation of the mechanism for morphologic and functional effects of hormones in vertebrates has come about through knowledge of binding of hormones in target tissues, feed-back, and other mechanisms.

There has been a prodigious increase in information recently, not only about the structure of molting and juvenile hormones, but also about their molecular action, as well as recognition of problems still posed by their biosynthesis, interactions, sites of origin, and relation to genic derepression. Discovery and study of phytohormones and analogs has added interest and amplified techniques for investigation.

Brain hormones have not been identified structurally, but the ecdysones are proving to be particularly useful steroidal compounds because of their biological activity, water solubility, and the opportunity they and juvenile hormones offer for relating molecular structure to biological function. Also the potential use of juvenile hormones, and perhaps ecdysones, as insecticides and chemosterilants implies that the human population will be exposed to them and/or their analogs in large quantities when they are released in the global environment. For this reason alone, the pharmacology of these compounds related to mammalian tissues should be clarified. In addition, the possible action of invertebrate hormones on vertebrate tissues is an intriguing biological and evolutionary possibility that justifies careful study.

Since so much information has accumulated about invertebrate hormones related to metamorphosis, it seems profitable to focus attention on brain hormone(s), ecdysones, and juvenile hormones in a treatise embracing such a broad spectrum of biological targets. Encouragement for the view that transphylar effects of these hormones occur comes from more recent confirmation of earlier work a decade ago suggesting that ecdysones can alter the metabolism of mammalian tissues. Obviously it is not possible to bring together in one volume the entire body of information now in existence about both vertebrate and invertebrate endocrinology limited even in this way, but it does seem appropriate to select information and concepts that are currently most useful in understanding the action of invertebrate hormones important in metamorphosis along with information about their possible application to studies on mammalian metabolism and pharmacology.

This material has been divided into four sections. The chapters devoted to invertebrate endocrinology include the hormonal control of metamorphosis in insects, biosynthesis and degradation of the hormones, assays for their detection, and effects of hormones on chromosomes. Chapters follow on the isolation, distribution, and supply of ecdysones, juvenile hormones, their analogs, and phytohormones. Since so much attention justifiably has been devoted to molecular events, a section is included on protein synthesis and genic derepression in relation to hormones, with emphasis on current ideas about possible roles of hormones in mammalian protein synthesis. Finally, the concept and evidence for hormonal heterophylly (the action of invertebrate hormones on vertebrate normal and neoplastic tissue) is presented with inclusion of data on the pharmacology of ecdysones and juvenile hormones.

This information is recorded to encourage exploration of the view that these invertebrate hormones and analogs may be useful in the investigation of responses to hormones in vertebrate as well as invertebrate systems and that such studies thus may widen the scope of knowledge about the initiation of genic action and regulation of sequellae. Whether a role for them in therapy will be found remains for the future to disclose.

Walter J. Burdette

INVERTEBRATE ENDOCRINOLOGY AND
HORMONAL HETEROPHYLLY

PART I
INVERTEBRATE ENDOCRINOLOGY

Hormonal Control of Metamorphosis

INTRODUCTION

Vincent B. Wigglesworth, Kt.

Ideas derived from the study of hormones in invertebrates have been and will continue to be of undoubted value in understanding the regulation of growth and metabolism in general. The investigation of the eye-color 'hormones' of Drosophila and Ephestia in the 1930's, by Ephrussi and Beadle and by Kühn and Butenandt, led to the first clear demonstration of the one gene-one enzyme principle; to be followed by the even more illuminating studies by Beadle and Tatum on Neurospora and its enzyme mutants.

No one would now speak of eye-color hormones in referring to the metabolic intermediates in the derivation of eye pigments from excess tryptophan. But the undoubted hormones of insects have also made a certain impact on general endocrinology. By 1933 it was recognized that the first stage in the initiation of growth under the action of the molting hormone consisted in activation of the epidermal cells: enlargement of the nucleolus and increase in volume and in the density of basophilic staining of the cytoplasm. By 1956 this change could be seen occurring within an hour or two of exposure of cells to ecdysone and the visible changes were recognized as an increase in ribonucleic-acid formation and the initiation of active protein synthesis. The same interpretation was soon adopted for the effects of growth hormone in vertebrates. In the insect this hormonal action was regarded as the result of facilitating the interaction between substrates and enzymes. The key site at which this change occurs is still being sought; but the striking effects of ecdysone in the puffing of the polytene chromosomes in Diptera has suggested that it may lie very close to the genes themselves.

The cytological changes in the epidermal cells during the healing of wounds are identical with those appearing during normal growth induced by ecdysone. Can one suppose that the same active factor is operating in the two cases: centrally produced by endocrine glands during molting; produced peripherally and locally in response to injury? Ecdysone seems to be extractable from various tissues in the abdomen, quite apart from the prothoracic glands, and to be extractable from adult Lepidoptera in which growth and molting do not occur.

Experimental interference with the cuticular pattern of insects has shown quite clearly that at the time when the larval pattern is visible in the cuticle, a totally different adult pattern is also present—although it is latent and cannot be seen unless metamorphosis to the adult stage is induced by manipulating the hormonal stimulus; the adult pattern remains latent so long as the juvenile hormone is present.

I remember Ephrussi's remarking to me, at a very early demonstration of the effects of the juvenile hormone in the 1930's, that this was the first clear-cut example of a morphogenetic hormone. What is a morphogenetic hormone? It was early realized that the action of the juvenile hormone was a gradual one operating over a considerable period of growth. By 1940 it had been established that the various faculties of a given cell could be controlled by the presence or absence of the juvenile hormone to some extent independently of one another. That led to the suggestion that each cell contained a metabolic system responsible for larval syntheses and a metabolic system responsible for adult syntheses; and that the larval system was brought into action by the juvenile hormone.

Since it was still possible to switch development of some characters from adult to larval long after mitosis in the epidermis had ceased, and therefore when presumably DNA synthesis was no longer occurring, it was concluded that these postulated metabolic systems were located in the cytoplasm. In modern terms one would suggest that we are observing here the action of persistent messenger RNAs and that the juvenile hormone is exerting its action on the gene system at the level of translation.

The same applies to the interpretation of other experiments going back to 1940 in which it was shown that certain of the characters of the cuticle of the adult could be caused to revert to those of the larva if renewed molting of the adult were induced in the presence of the juvenile hormone. Many of the epidermal cells involved do not undergo mitosis and that again suggests that the action of the hormone is at the translational level.

On the other hand, it seems likely that many of the changes of metamorphosis are taking place farther back, at the level of transcription. Epidermal cells in different areas of the body surface are committed to form specific elements in the pattern of cuticular pigmentation or structure. When the cells multiply and migrate during the repair of a burn, the daughter cells carry with them their specific properties. Twenty years ago this phenomenon was compared with "the 'transformation principle' of Avery *et al.*, apparently a desoxyribose nucleic acid, which will induce a permanent inheritable transformation of unencapsulated variants of Type II pneumococci into the fully encapsulated type."

Since the juvenile hormone may produce diametrically opposed effects upon the pattern in different parts of the body, it was recognized from the time of its discovery that it must be acting in some very general way—which we are still hoping to define in terms of molecular biology.

Graded concentrations of insect hormones may produce qualitatively different effects. In certain caterpillars a low concentration of ecdysone will affect tryptophan metabolism and evoke the color changes that precede pupation; a high concentration will induce molting before changes in color can take place. In the case of the juvenile hormone: a high concentration in Lepidoptera maintains the formation of larval characters; a low concentration evokes pupal characters; whereas in the presence of ecdysone alone but no juvenile hormone, adult characters appear.

Such qualitative differences produced by quantitative changes are familiar in gradients. For many years C. M. Child battled for his conviction that gradients of single factors were important in differentiation; but only in recent years has this theory been taken seriously. Recent work strongly suggests the graded distribution of chemical factors in the insect epidermis, each level in the gradient evoking a characteristic response by the cells. Here again we are faced with the problem of what is the nature of the substrate on which the chemical determinants operate. Almost certainly they act on the gene system; but at which point in the operative chain from gene to final enzyme protein, or integrated group of enzyme proteins, we do not know.

In winding up a symposium on embryonic differentiation in 1934, T. H. Morgan hazarded the suggestion that the initial differentiation of cells in the germ band of the early embryo might be the result of localized chemical factors which evoked specific genetic activities in the cell nuclei which came within their sphere of influence. This idea still provides a guide-line for the understanding of differentiation.

All these effects are of equal interest in understanding the basic principles in the regulation of growth and differentiation, whether in insects or in vertebrates. The details are special to the organism or groups of organisms under investigation. This specificity presumably reflects genetic specificity. But is it not possible that hormones have other effects which are sufficiently general to influence a wide range of unrelated organisms?

Acetyl choline was used as a pharmacological tool for the study of synaptic transmission for nearly half a century before its normal utilization by the vertebrate was recognized. We now know that, although acetyl choline seems not to be concerned in neuromuscular transmission in the insect, it is of prime importance in the synapses of the central nervous system. The same story can be told about dopamine and others of the queerly named 'biogenic' (that is, 'life-producing') amines. These widely distributed substances turn up with different functions in different groups. For the entomologist, derivatives of pterine are seen as alternatives to purines as vehicles for the elimination of excess nitrogen; for the enzyme biochemist they are regulators of key processes in metabolism. Amino acids, which we used to think of solely as building blocks for protein synthesis, are discovering all sorts of functions as metabolic regulators. Terpenoids closely related to the juvenile hormone are widely dispersed in nature. Steroids of many kinds, including ecdysone and its close relatives, are widespread in animals and plants. Do they have general functions of importance quite apart from their special uses as hormones that we know; or are they merely useless by-products of metabolism?

We are on uncertain ground here; but in the later chapters of this book a number of suggestive examples give ground for the hope that something of great interest may turn up in this field—something perhaps which at this moment cannot be foreseen. After all, the search for the Philosopher's Stone and the Elixir of Life led the way to the foundation of chemistry, which was by no means an unprofitable outcome.

HORMONAL CONTROL of
INSECT DEVELOPMENT

Kenneth J. Judy

The field of insect endocrinology has developed very rapidly from inauspicious beginnings a half century ago when Kopeč laid the foundation with innovative experiments showing that the insect brain produced an humoral factor indispensable for initiating the process of molting. Subsequent investigators demonstrated the existence of other morphogenetic hormones and identified the glands that produced them. As more data were obtained, patterns appeared suggesting that there were certain homologies even among extremely diverse insect groups. Eventually these patterns were synthesized into a unified scheme of endocrine regulation for all insects. Supportive evidence came from many sources, although an inordinate amount came from investigations of only a dozen or so species representing three or four insect orders. Now this basic classical scheme has rightfully been accepted as a milestone in biology.

Nevertheless, the full story of insect endocrinology is still unfolding. New glands, hormones, effects, and interactions are continually being reported as more refined techniques are applied to increasing numbers of species. Some of the basic assumptions that supported earlier studies have been challenged recently. It is not at all imprudent to suggest that one or more basic tenets for the classical scheme will be substantially modified in the near future.

The intention of this chapter, then, is to provide a limited overview of the current status of insect endocrinology along with some of the salient problems presently under investigation. The limitations of space preclude more than a brief mention of certain critical issues related to the three major hormones controlling growth and development. Other chapters in this volume provide more details. Furthermore, the subject of insect hormones has been reviewed a number of times, most recently and comprehensively by Wigglesworth (1970), Wyatt (1972), and Gilbert and King (1973).

THE CLASSICAL SCHEME

The typical insect emerges from the egg as a sexually immature larva encased in a protective exoskeleton and predisposed to a career of feeding. As growth ensues, the exoskeleton becomes restrictive and, by the process of molting, is shed and replaced by a new, larger covering. At each larval molt, the insect may undergo some slight changes in external and internal morphology but the resultant form and behavior generally conserve larval characteristics. At some point in its development, the larva completes sufficient growth to permit sexual maturation and the ensuing molt permits final expression of the adult phenotype appropriate for that species. The metamorphic changes that occur between larva and adult may be modest, as in hemimetabolous insects such as a grasshopper or cockroach. Changes in appearance, both internal and external, may be virtually total as in holometabolous insects such as a beetle or butterfly. Those insects undergoing complete metamorphosis often include an intermediate stage, the pupa, in which to bridge the differences between the larva, highly specialized for feeding, and the adult, highly specialized for reproduction.

The endocrine processes underlying insect growth and development are currently understood as follows. As a larva feeds and grows, unknown stimuli, probably both extrinsic and intrinsic, influence the synthesis and eventual release of secretions by specialized neurons of the brain. A neurosecretion, termed brain hormone (BH), is released into the blood and acts on the prothoracic glands in the thorax. The prothoracic glands are stimulated to produce ecdysone, a hormone whose accumulation in the blood triggers a series of events culminating in a molt. Another pair of glands, the corpora allata, are located near the brain and are attached to it by several nerves (Figure 1). The corpora allata are capable of secreting a hormone, the juvenile hormone (JH), which directs the qualitative expression of each molt. When a relatively high titer of JH is present in the insect's blood, the ensuing molt will be larval in nature. When JH is absent, the succeeding molt will be to the adult. In holometabolous insects, a diminished titer of JH occurs at the end of

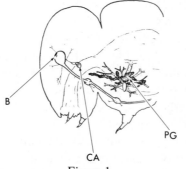

B

PG

CA

Figure 1

Section of the head and prothorax of a typical lepidopterous larva showing the location of the major endocrine organs. The brain (B) contains neurosecretory cells, some of which produce the brain hormone (prothoracotropic). The corpora allata (CA), adjacent to the corpora cardiaca and attached by nerves to the brain, produce juvenile hormone. The prothoracic glands (PG) are diffuse organs entwined in tracheae near the lateral body wall and are involved in molting-hormone (ecdysone) production.

larval life, and the subsequent molt is to a pupa rather than directly to an adult. After appropriate development occurs, the pupa initiates a final molting process in the total absence of JH to form the "perfect" or adult insect.

In the adult insect, the prothoracic glands degenerate and no further molting occurs. The corpora allata, on the other hand, are reactivated, and, at least in many species, provide a stimulus (JH) essential for the process of egg maturation. In certain insects, growth is interrupted by a period of quiescence or diapause. Diapause in the larva or pupa, characterized by a reduced metabolic rate and the lack of molting, is attributable to the cessation in the production or release of brain hormone. Adult diapause, also referred to as reproductive diapause, need not be accompanied by depressed metabolic rates and is caused by the failure of JH production leading to a cessation in the process of oogenesis.

Despite the fact that the three major hormones controlling growth and development interact with one another, each shall be considered separately in order to describe certain exceptional observations and how these may affect interpretations of the classical scheme.

BRAIN HORMONE

The present state of knowledge concerning the brain hormone of insects is seriously incomplete. At least three critical questions remain unresolved. What is the chemical identity of BH? Precisely where is it made? How are its synthesis and release regulated? Investigations into these areas have proceeded slowly, but some of the more recent findings have proved encouraging.

Concerning the chemical identity of BH, Kobayashi *et al.* (1962) first reported it to be cholesterol. For a number of reasons, this identification is most unlikely (Schneiderman and Gilbert, 1964) and was due to the rather nonspecific nature of the bioassay used. Subsequent studies (Ichikawa and Ishizaki, 1963; Kobayashi and Yamazaki, 1966) suggest that the active agent is a protein or a polypeptide, a view that is more consistent with the known secretory products of other neurosecretory cells. Although BH is water soluble, nondialyzable, and inactivated by certain bacterial proteinases, it is resistant to trypsin, pepsin, and chymotrypsin, stable at 90° C. for 90 minutes (pH 6.0), and fails to show the characteristic ultraviolet absorption of proteins (Williams, 1967a). For these reasons, Williams (1969) suggests it may well be a mucopolysaccharide or mucoprotein.

Definitive answers to corollary questions on the biosynthesis, degradation, and mode of action of BH must await its eventual identification.

Regarding the source of BH, it would appear that the early investigations are somewhat misleading. Even the name, brain hormone, suggests that its site of production is well established. However, histological examination of the brain reveals at least four major neurosecretory types of cells with numerous possible subdivisions. Several regulatory functions have been attributed to secretory products of the brain (see reviews by Wyatt, 1972, and Gilbert and King, 1973), and these are probably not related to the hormone designated BH.

A number of investigations have pointed to the conclusion that the brain is not absolutely essential to activate the molting or metamorphic processes. Gilbert (1958) observed that some chilled, brainless Polyphemus pupae develop normally into adults, and Marks (personal communication) has observed molting in larval cockroaches several days or weeks after brain extirpation. Kobayashi *et al.* (1960) induced an artificial diapause by debraining newly pupated Bombyx but observed the spontaneous initiation of adult development as much as three months later. McDaniel and Berry (1967) found that diapausing, brainless Polyphemus pupae could be stimulated to develop by either exposure to low temperature or injury.

Most recently, I have reported (Judy, 1972) termination of spontaneous diapause and adult development in tobacco hornworms debrained as diapausing pupae. Some of these remained in diapause for almost a year before developing. In a few cases, individuals debrained as one- or two-day-old fifth-instar larvae molted to pupae, entered an apparent state of diapause, and, more than 30 days later, initiated adult development.

The most reasonable explanation for these diverse and exceptional findings may lie in the discovery of Gersch and Stürzebecher (1968) that substances with BH activity are present in extracts of the ventral nerve cord of roaches. It is well known (see, for example, Delphin, 1965) that the ganglia of the ventral nerve cord contain numerous neurosecretory cells, including types that stain in the same manner as several types of neurosecretory cells in the brain. Since the brain of insects is believed to be derived from the fusion of several ganglia in the primitive ancestral insect, it seems reasonable that some redundancy of function may persist even in present-day forms. Sources of BH in the ventral nerve cord may serve to supplement the sources in the brain or may be activated only if an inhibitory factor from the brain is removed. It is even conceivable that different sets of stimuli may activate the neurosecretory cells in the two different regions of the nervous system.

More conclusive studies on the sources of BH are sorely needed and will very likely lead to the expansion of the classical scheme in the near future.

Little is known concerning the regulation of BH production. The majority of studies bearing on this point have been restricted to indirect techniques frequently employing whole animals, which allow for a variety of indirect interactions between stimulus and response. Numerous histological investigations have been reported, but these are of only limited value until the precise source of the active principle is determined and definitive correlations between cytological changes and BH titer in the blood are established. Adding to the complexity of the problem is the possibility that the processes of BH synthesis and release are controlled separately, and that more than one type of stimulus can affect either response (Highnam, 1967).

Allowing for the indirect nature of most tests, a number of different types of stimuli have been implicated in the control of molting *via* the brain. Light (photoperiod) and temperature have long been known to affect the timing of molting and metamorphosis. These external stimuli probably act through sensory-nerve pathways, but both may be capable of stimulating the brain directly (Highnam, 1967). Recently, Pipa (1971) demonstrated that deprivation of space results in delayed pupation in Galleria, apparently by inhibiting BH secretion. Proprioceptive stimuli can also influence the activation of the brain. Abdominal distension, such as that caused by feeding, is an essential stimulus for molting in Rhodnius (Wigglesworth, 1934) as well as several other insects. Body constraint was shown by Edwards (1966) to inhibit the metamorphosis of Galleria. This effect was negated by ecdysone injection, suggesting that inhibition was mediated through a higher center. Krishnakumaran (1972), also using Galleria, reported that injury acting *via* the brain affects the timing of pupation and may even induce supernumerary larval molts.

Endocrine agents have also been implicated in regulating BH secretion. Beck and Alexander (1964) described a new hormone, proctodone, which is produced by specialized cells of the hind gut of the European corn borer. Proctodone supposedly regulates the processes of larval diapause development, including the eventual activation of the brain. The chemical nature of this hormone, its mode of action, and its significance in the general scheme of regulation in insects remain to be investigated.

An interesting interaction between the brain and JH was demonstrated by Riddiford (1972). Application of JH to Cecropia prepupae at an appropriate time prevented the termination of prothoracotropic activity. The resulting pupae skipped the period of obligatory diapause and promptly initiated adult development. More direct support for the hypothesis was obtained by showing that brains transplanted from JH-treated to brainless, untreated animals were active whereas controls from untreated donors were not.

One last example of possible humoral control of brain-hormone production comes from a recent report by Marks *et al.* (1972) in which β-ecdysone applied to brains of cockroaches *in vitro* stimulated the release of accumulated neurosecretions. The neurosecretory products in this case were not specifically identified, but the effect seemed to be somewhat specific since 22-isoecdysone, a compound without molting-hormone activity, failed to evoke the response.

In summary, there seem to be many more real or potential systems of control described than any individual insect might require. It is certainly possible that some of the stimulatory mechanisms described above are nonspecific, experimental artifacts; yet until the normal system or systems of control are uncovered, the possible significance of each newly described interaction should be considered carefully. It would not be surprising to find considerable divergence between the many insect species in the mechanisms chosen to regulate the timing of a molt, since each environmental niche would provide a different set of stimuli to which insects must relate.

ECDYSONE

The number of authoritative papers in this volume dealing with various aspects of ecdysone biochemistry and physiology attests to the advanced state of research concerning the molting hormone of insects. Investigations have proceeded even to the molecular level of hormonal action. In light of the coverage provided by other contributors, this section shall be restricted to a consideration of only a few general concepts which may be regarded as departures from the classical view of ecdysone action.

The classical scheme holds that ecdysone is produced by the prothoracic glands in response to stimulation by brain hormone. The titer of ecdysone in the blood builds until a threshold is surpassed and the molting process is initiated. The glands then become inactive or reduce their activity and inter-molt activities commence.

However, significant evidence has accumulated to suggest that the actual events in an insect are not nearly so simple or straightforward. Ecdysone (*a*-ecdysone) may not be the actual hormonal agent (Figure 2). The prothoracic glands may not synthesize the active hormone *per se*; other tissues may also be involved. Even the regulation of ecdysone production seems to be under the control of more than just the brain hormone. Support for these various contentions come from a variety of investigations.

King and others (see chapter 12) have shown clearly that *a*-ecdysone is converted to *β*-ecdysone by a number of tissues. Since *β*-ecdysone is far more effective than *a*-ecdysone in many *in-vitro* test systems, it has been suggested that *β*-ecdysone is the true hormone, *a*-ecdysone serving only as a prohor-mone. Under this view, peripheral target tissues more properly should be considered para-endocrine organs (King, 1972).

On the other hand, Oberlander (1969) presents evidence that *a*-ecdysone

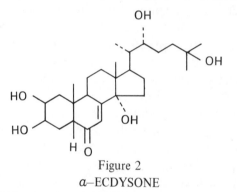

Figure 2

a–ECDYSONE

(20S)–2*β*, 3*β*, 14*a*, 22R, 25 PENTAHYDROXY–5*β*–CHOLEST–7–EN–6–ONE [*β*–ECDYSONE = 20–HYDROXYECDYSONE, ECDYSTERONE, CRUSTECDYSONE .]

has a specific function in sustaining DNA synthesis in Galleria wing discs that cannot be duplicated by *β*-ecdysone. Thus, the possibility remains that *a*-ecdysone is at least one of the active molting hormones.

A radically different view has been presented recently by Kambysellis and Williams (1971a, b). These investigators reported that spermatogenesis *in vitro* required not only ecdysone but a macromolecular factor (MF) which is unidentified as yet. They believe that the stimulatory factor for sperm differentiation is MF, and ecdysone serves only to open gates in the testi-cular sheath to allow MF to enter; on naked spermatocysts, ecdysone has no effect while MF is fully effective. This might explain the earlier obser-vation of Yagi *et al.* (1969) that spermatocysts within intact testes of Chilo elongated *in vitro* only when ecdysterone was added to the medium, but would also elongate in medium devoid of ecdysterone if they were liberated from the testes.

MF is believed to be synthesized by hemocytes and is present in the blood at all stages except for a brief period during pupal diapause. To complicate matters further, substances with MF activity are present in fetal calf serum and possibly other serum constituents of culture media, making it nearly impossible to exclude from conventional *in-vitro* test systems. Kambysellis and Williams speculate that MF may be the functional agent in all ecdysone-responding systems; however, Takeda (1972) has demonstrated that moth-sperm maturation *in vitro* is most efficiently stimulated by rubrosterone, a substance with little or no molt-stimulating activity. Thus, MF may be a factor specific for spermatogenesis alone.

Questions concerning the exact role of the prothoracic glands in production of ecdysones were raised by Piepho (1948), Bodenstein (1955), and Chadwick (1955; 1956). They observed molting in insects from which the prothoracic glands had supposedly been removed. These findings could not be explained by the classical scheme, and, considering the surgical difficulties which the authors themselves admitted, it was supposed that either the glands were not completely extirpated or that perhaps the operation was performed after (or caused) the activation of the glands.

A similar unexpected result was reported by Ichikawa and Nishiitsutsuji-Uwo (1960). They found that isolated pupal abdomens of *S. cynthia*, preparations devoid of prothoracic glands, were induced to molt by implantations of brains from larvae, pupae, or adults; and they suggested tentatively that brain hormone may serve as a precursor for synthesis of molting hormone. The customary organs for converting brain hormone would be the prothoracic glands, but other organs may also be adequate in their absence. Recent events have led to a reëvaluation of these observations.

Moriyama *et al.* (1970) reported α-ecdysone is synthesized from cholesterol in isolated Bombyx abdomens. Gersch and Stürzebecher (1971) made a similar discovery using the moth, Mamestra. Weir (1970) showed that Calpodes larvae were unable to molt anterior to a ligature if that ligature excluded portions of the abdomen, even though active prothoracic glands were present. Such isolated thoraces could still respond to injected ecdysone, indicating that they were not incompetent or inhibited. Weir suggested that the oenocytes of the abdomen may function in some way in the production of molting hormone; Locke (1969) suggested the same possibility from ultrastructural studies; and Romer (1971) was able to obtain active molting-hormone extracts from oenocytes of Tenebrio.

As evidence of this sort accumulates, it becomes increasingly apparent that the prothoracic glands may not be the only organs capable of secreting molting hormone or its prohormone.

The classical scheme holds that production of ecdysone is under the firm control of brain hormone. Considering the aforementioned uncertainties regarding possible alternate sources of both ecdysone and BH, experimental evidence supporting this element of the classical scheme becomes somewhat ambiguous. To add to the difficulty, several additional stimuli for production of ecdysone have been described.

The relationship between BH and prothoracic glands was initially determined by indirect methods involving ligation, extirpation, and/or implantation (Williams, 1952). Recently Kambysellis and Williams (1972) claim to have shown a more direct interaction using an *in-vitro* system. Inactive, pupal prothoracic glands were stimulated in culture by the addition of active brains. Unfortunately, their assay was based on stimulation of spermatogenesis, an effect not necessarily specific for molting hormones (Takeda, 1972).

Another approach was employed by Oberlander and Schneiderman (1963), who were able to show increased RNA synthesis in the prothoracic-gland cells after stimulation with brains or hormonal extracts. However, Oberlander *et al.* (1965) found that injuries, which would not provoke molting, could also elevate the level of RNA synthesis. The cytological changes in prothoracic-gland cells in response to neurosecretory or traumatic stimulation were somewhat different, but these have not yet been correlated quantitatively with production of ecdysone. It would seem that the ultimate resolution of this question requires direct measurement for production of ecdysone by isolated prothoracic glands in response to pure BH.

Several other agents have been shown or suggested to be involved in the regulation of ecdysone production. Implanted corpora allata stimulated molting in brainless pupae (Williams, 1959; Gilbert and Schneiderman, 1959; Ichikawa and Nishiitsutsuji-Uwo, 1959). That this effect was, in fact, caused by JH was finally demonstrated by Johnson *et al.* (1969). Molting hormone itself was shown to stimulate prothoracic glands (Williams, 1952). Recently, Siew and Gilbert (1971) reported that both JH and ecdysone caused elevated rates of RNA synthesis in prothoracic-gland cells, although ecdysone exerted its effect much more rapidly. It has been speculated that the stimulation of prothoracic glands by ecdysone serves to synchronize the paired glands, whereas stimulation by JH insures that ecdysone is present when peak titers of JH are produced, since JH effects in immature stages are realized only at the time of molting.

It is interesting to note that, although several agents stimulate ecdysone production, no mechanism for turning off its release has yet been described. Since ecdysone itself stimulates quiescent prothoracic glands, control by means of a negative feedback system would seem unlikely. However, Siew and Gilbert (1971) reported that when ecdysone production was initiated normally (by brain hormone), injection of additional ecdysone led to a reduction in RNA synthesis by prothoracic-gland cells.

An additional potential control system is suggested by the observation that the prothoracic glands are innervated in at least some insects (Scharrer, 1964; Srivastava and Singh, 1968). Hintze-Podufal (1970) has even found neurosecretory-type granules in axons extending into the glands. The physiological significance of these observations has yet to be determined.

Finally it was suggested by Karlson and Shaaya (1964) that regulation of titers for ecdysone could be accomplished by adjusting the level of degradative enzymes in the blood rather than the rate of hormonal synthesis, but verification for such a mechanism is still lacking.

JUVENILE HORMONE

While, in terms of the classical scheme, the role of JH in insect development is reasonably well defined, many basic questions remain unanswered. Most prominent among these are questions concerning the possible chemical diversity of JH, its biosynthesis, its mode of action, and the regulation of its production.

The corpora allata have been viewed as the source of JH for a long time, and the recent demonstration of JH synthesis *in vitro* by isolated corpora allata in a defined medium (Judy *et al.*, 1972) seems rather conclusive on this point.

Efforts to identify the chemical structure of JH (Figure 3) culminated in the discovery of two active forms (JH-I, Röller *et al.*, 1967; JH-II, Meyer *et al.*, 1968) from the moth *H. cecropia*. The same two hormones were subsequently found in the closely related moths, *H. gloverii* (Dahm and Röller, 1970) and *S. cynthia* (Röller and Dahm, this volume).

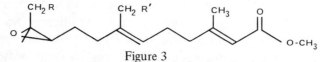

Figure 3

JUVENILE HORMONE

CECROPIA JH I: R = CH_3, R′ = CH_3; MANDUCA JH I: R = H, R′ = H; CECROPIA JH II (MANDUCA JH II): R = CH_3, R′ = H.

The existence of the same two compounds in three different species plus the fact that these hormones produced juvenilizing effects in representatives of a wide range of insect orders, fostered the notion that these may be the juvenile hormones of all insects. However, considering the fact that some insects are relatively insensitive to Cecropia JH and yet respond to minute doses of synthetic analogs that are totally ineffective in Cecropia, the possibility exists that a degree of chemical diversification has occurred among juvenile hormones. This suggestion was reinforced by the discovery of juvabione (Sláma and Williams, 1966), a natural product of certain plants with potent juvenilizing activity specific for certain insects of the family, Pyrrhocoridae.

Very recently we have added more evidence for the possible diversification of JH by describing a new natural hormone from the tobacco hornworm, *Manduca sexta* (Judy *et al.*, 1973). In this species there are also two juvenile hormones, occurring in about equal concentrations, one of which is identical to Cecropia JH-II (Meyer *et al.*, 1968). The second hormone is methyl-10-epoxy-farnesoate, a new natural product but originally identified as an active synthetic compound as early as 1965 (Bowers *et al.*, 1965). Although this new JH is still a closely related homolog of the Cecropia compounds previously described, its discovery does indicate that there is some diversification of the hormonal structure even between the related lepidopteran families of Saturniidae and Sphingidae.

Extensive investigations concerning the nature of JH in other orders have been hampered by the minute quantity of hormone present in most insects at any particular time. Cecropia and its relatives are apparently unique in their ability to sequester high levels of JH in adult abdominal tissue (Williams, 1963). The approach we used to identify the JH of Manduca, however, may greatly facilitate identification of JH from a number of other species. By extirpating active corpora allata from young adult moths and maintaining them for several weeks in a suitable tissue-culture medium, we were able to secure up to a hundred times more hormone from a single pair of glands than could be extracted from a single adult moth. In addition, the procedures for isolating JH from a nearly defined culture medium are far more efficient than those necessary with whole-animal homogenates or even extracts of hemolymph.

Although discovery of new natural juvenile hormones remains for the future, a great deal of effort has already been spent in the synthesis of hundreds of JH analogs. The theoretical feasibility of using JH or JH analogs as third-generation pesticides (Williams, 1967b) has sparked the interest of numerous investigators and led to an ever-increasing accumulation of data on the effects of various compounds on various species of insects under various experimental conditions (see, for example, Sláma, 1971; Jacobson *et al.*, 1972; Staal, 1972; and Pallos and Menn, 1972). Whereas programs of this sort may have a more practical objective, they also serve to extend the basic knowledge of insect endocrinology.

The biosynthesis of JH remains a mystery. Cecropia JH-I and -II, both homosesquiterpenoids, do not appear to follow the biosynthetic pathway of conventional terpenes. Only the derivation of the methyl ester moiety from methionine seems well established (see Metzler *et al.*, this volume; Judy *et al.*,

1973). Degradation of JH, on the other hand, is better understood and initially involves hydrolysis of the ester group and/or hydration of the epoxide (Slade and Zibitt, 1972). Furthermore, Slade and Zibitt (1971) found that JH was decomposed 85 per cent after being incubated *in vitro* only five minutes in hemolymph. The possible significance of these findings in relation to the regulation of JH titers will be discussed below.

The various and sundry effects of JH in insects can be conveniently assembled into three general categories: morphogenetic, gonadotropic, and prothoracotropic. Morphogenetic effects are taken to include behavioral changes, which are probably secondary manifestations of more basic effects on the central nervous system.

The most fundamental morphogenetic effect of JH is the conservation of larval features and the suppression of metamorphosis at each larval molt. Numerous demonstrations of this phenomenon have been reported and reviewed (Wigglesworth, 1970). Typically, removal of the corpora allata from a larval insect causes premature metamorphosis at the next molt. Implantation of additional corpora allata or injection of JH causes supernumery larval molts. Treatment with JH around the time of metamorphosis frequently leads to the formation of inviable larval-pupal or pupal-adult intermediates.

Although JH merely forestalls development to the adult in most instances, it appears to reverse the process by causing adult tissues to reacquire a larval nature in a few controversial cases (Piepho, 1939; Wigglesworth, 1954; Ozeki, 1959; Lawrence, 1966). It is not clear, however, whether differentiated adult cells themselves are reprogrammed or whether they undergo one or more divisions to produce a population of larval-type cells.

Another type of morphogenetic effect for JH is that on embryogenesis. Riddiford and Williams (1967) found that JH applied to young eggs of Pyrrhocoris or Cecropia blocked embryonic development at a specific stage. Additional studies of this sort produced a second unusual finding, namely, that eggs treated after the critical period for blockage of embryonic development hatched into larvae that subsequently developed morphological abnormalities, and, in some cases, were unable to metamorphose. The interpretation of these results was that JH interfered with the genetic programming of tissues, and thus, with their differentiation later during postembryonic development. Willis (1969) suggested as an alternative explanation that JH applied to the embryos affected the programming of the corpora allata to prevent their shutting down in the last larval instar. However, based on data obtained from epidermal transplants, Willis and Lawrence (1970) concluded that JH applied to eggs persists from larval stage to larval stage, possibly in the cuticle, and enough JH remains in the final larval stage to interfere with normal metamorphosis. The more recent work of Riddiford (1971) and Riddiford and Truman (1972) indicates that the deferred action of JH on Pyrrhocoris is not due to persistence but rather, as originally suggested (Willis, 1969), to some type of effect on programming the corpora allata which prevents their being shut off at the time of metamorphosis.

Another interesting example of morphogenetic effect of JH is its role in the degeneration and regeneration of flight muscles. deKort (1969) shows a clear correlation between the reduction of JH titer and the deterioration of flight muscles in the diapausing Colorado beetle. On the other hand, there are the reports of Borden and Slater (1968) using Ips and of Edwards (1970) with Dysdercus which indicate that elevated titers of JH cause deterioration of flight muscles. The mechanism(s) underlying effects of these sorts is not known but may involve the more fundamental action of JH on the central nervous system (deKort, 1969).

The basic gonadotropic functions of JH are the stimulation of protein synthesis in yolk by the fat body and the stimulation of protein uptake in yolk by developing oöcytes. These effects, unlike the morphogenetic effects of JH, are independent of the action of ecdysone. Neurosecretion from the brain may also be involved in stimulating the uptake by oocytes in some species, but the nature of possible interactions with JH is unclear in such cases. The titer of JH is apparently the determining factor in the onset and termination of adult reproductive diapause in females of many species, although other unknown agents may also be involved (see, for example, Bowers and Bickenstaff, 1966).

A clear role has been demonstrated for JH in directing phase polymorphism in Locusta (Staal, 1961). Likewise, JH appears to play significant roles in regulating polymorphism in aphids (White, 1971) and termites (Lüscher, 1963). These effects, as well as effects on secondary sex glands (Willis and Brunet, 1966) and the pheromone production (Borden *et al.*, 1969), are probably related to the gonadotropic functions of JH.

Reference was made earlier to the prothoracotropic effect of JH; again, the physiological significance of this interaction is not known. It is possible that insects have a dual system of control over the prothoracic glands or that JH stimulates production of ecdysone during larval life and brain hormone takes over this function at metamorphosis (Schneiderman and Gilbert, 1964). Indirect evidence for this comes from the findings of Staal (1967, and personal communication) in which early larval Cecropia or Cynthia fail to molt after allatectomy. On the other hand, Akai and Kobayashi (1971) found that a similar effect was brought about by JH injection into last-instar Bombyx larvae. Complex endocrine interactions of this sort, often with contradictory results when different stages or species are tested, continue to defy simple explanations.

Critical to the eventual understanding of the manifold effects of JH is knowledge of its mode of action at the molecular level. Theoretical approaches to this question have been advanced by several investigators. Novák (1967) described a mechanism in which gradient factors bound to DNA condition its capacity for self replication. Loss of these leads to inactivation of DNA molecules, but JH substituting for gradient factor restores activity. Williams and Kafatos (1971) speculatively apply Jacob-Monod principles to the genetic apparatus of insects and see JH as a corepressor of master regulatory genes for pupal and adult syntheses. A third approach (Wigglesworth, 1969) hypothesizes that the basis for JH activity lies in its physio-chemical action on cellular membranes. Accordingly, JH would act indirectly on the genome by causing changes in the ionic composition of the nucleoplasm in a manner similar to that proposed for ecdysone by Kroeger (1963; 1968). Support for this latter view comes from several sources, including Baumann (1968) who detected depolarizing effects on cellular membranes treated with JH-active compounds. Furthermore, Lezzi and Gilbert (1969; 1970) demonstrated the presence of JH-specific puff on the giant chromosomes of Chironomus which would also respond to increases in Na^+ in the nuclear environment. Congote *et al.* (1970) postulate the existence of two different systems; one dependent on sodium and the second directly responsive to hormones.

Whether or not JH interacts directly with the genes, it is well documented that one of its first generalized effects is to bring about increased RNA synthesis. Zalokar (1968) suggests the possibility that the hormone stimulates nucleoside phosphorylases. Congote *et al.* (1970) and Nair and Menon (1972) present evidence that JH increases activity at the transcriptional level, whereas the studies of Ilan *et al.* (1970) point to the translational-level control involving the synthesis or activation of a specific tRNA and its activating enzyme.

A final element in the picture of JH endocrinology is the persistent question of how its production and release are regulated. In larval stages, JH must decrease sharply or lethal anatomical derangements may occur. Yet, during the adult stage, JH is necessary again, at least in some insects, for normal vitellogenesis. Such a regimen would seem to require a rather precise regulatory mechanism.

The corpora allata receive nerves from the brain through the corpora cardiaca as well as from the subesophageal ganglion. In addition, neurosecretory axons from the brain and/or the corpora cardiaca are intimately associated with corpus-allatum cells (Waku and Gilbert, 1964; Tombes and Smith,

1970). Experimental evidence for the participation of both neural and neuro-endocrine stimuli in regulating JH production has been provided by a number of investigators over the past twenty years (Engelmann, 1965; Highnam, 1967). In summary, this evidence suggests that the brain uses certain neural pathways to inhibit the function of the corpora allata, while other neural and/or neuroendocrine stimuli are capable of relieving this inhibition.

Humoral factors also enter into the scheme of JH regulation. In adult female roaches Engelmann (1965) has shown that the activity of corpora allata may depend directly on concentrations of protein in the hemolymph. JH, in turn, stimulates elevated levels of protein in the blood, but the resultant positive feedback cycle is interrupted by absorption of protein into the yolk of maturing oocytes. This system acts in conjunction with, rather than instead of, neural and neuroendocrine stimuli. In addition, Engelmann postulates the existence of an humoral agent from the egg case of a viviparous roach, acting *via* the nervous system to inhibit production of JH. A similar substance, termed the oostatic hormone, has been reported for houseflies (Adams *et al.*, 1968), but its structure and mode of action are not known.

Ecdysone has also been reported to affect the corpora allata by stimulating RNA synthesis and therefore, presumably, the rate of JH production (Siew and Gilbert, 1971). This interaction could insure the simultaneous occurrence of both hormones, a critical factor for normal larval molting. Siew and Gilbert also report that JH itself appears to stimulate the corpora allata, although the need or even the advantage for such an action is difficult to assess.

Other levels of control for JH have been considered and some recent evidence is worth noting. Since JH is a lipid, it may be necessary that it be bound to a water-soluble carrier for transport in the blood. Whitmore and Gilbert (1972) have recently demonstrated binding of JH to a high-density lipoprotein, and it is conceivable that regulation of biosynthesis of the carrier could provide a secondary means of regulating JH titer (see also, Trautmann, 1972). Alternatively, the metabolism of JH by blood-borne (specific ?) esterases (Slade and Zibitt, 1971) could modulate the level of hormone (Whitmore *et al.*, 1972). These latter investigators have found that elevated levels of esterase can be induced in Hyalophora by administration of JH at a time when juvenile hormone should be absent from the blood. Likewise, Weirich (personal communication) has found inverse correlations between esterase and JH levels in Manduca. Although such studies are still very preliminary and it has not been demonstrated that these esterases inactivate endogenous (bound ?) JH, it remains an interesting subject for further investigation.

SUMMARY

It should be apparent, after even so brief a survey, that insect endocrinology has come a long way in a few decades. Perhaps more apparent is the fact that this field has still a long way to go. The classical scheme for the control of insect growth and development represents a milestone in biology, and yet it seems to describe only the top of the iceberg. Concerning only the three major hormones discussed in this chapter, critical questions remain unanswered. The structure of the brain hormone has yet to be determined as well as the active form of ecdysone. Is there a diversity of juvenile hormones among insects and what role, if any, does binding to carrier molecules play in the physiological activity of JH? There are good reasons to reevaluate current opinions on the sources of both BH and ecdysone. Very little is really understood about the mode of action of any of these insect hormones, and the variety of responses elicited by ecdysone and JH suggest that they may have different actions on different target tissues. Finally, the regulation of hormone production for each of the three hormones appears to be far more complex than originally envisioned. Ecdysone and JH levels may not only be controlled by neurosecretions, but both seem to have effects on neurosecretion; each seems capable of stimulating production of the other, and both seem capable of stimulating their own production.

It must be noted, of course, that many of the effects described for these hormones are demonstrated in only one or a few species and should be generalized with caution. Similarly, results obtained with one developmental stage are not necessarily applicable to other stages. Fundamental to any discussion of hormonal titers and interactions is the concept of tissue competence. Is the ability of a target tissue to respond to hormonal stimuli strictly dependent on the presence of the hormone, or are there other subtle and intrinsic requirements which first must be fulfilled in order to render the cells receptive to stimulation?

This brief chapter has been concerned with only those hormones known to play a role in growth and development, but many other hormones and neurohormones also are known in insects (Wyatt, 1972) and the list continues to grow. In the field of insect endocrinology, many years of exciting discovery that will have a beneficial impact on virtually every field of biological research seem inevitable.

References

1. ADAMS, T. S., HINTZ, A. M., and POMONIS, J. G.: Oostatic Hormone Production in Houseflies, *Musca domestica*, with Developing Ovaries. J. Insect Physiol., *14*: 983-993, 1968.
2. AKAI, H. and KOBAYASHI, M.: Induction of Prolonged Larval Instar by the Juvenile Hormone in *Bombyx mori* L. (Lepidoptera: Bombycidae). Appl. Ent. Zool., *6*:138-139, 1971.
3. BAUMANN, G.: Zur Wirkung des Juvenilhormons: Elektrophysiologische Messungen an der Zellmembran der Speicheldrüse von *Galleria mellonella*. J. Insect Physiol., *14*:1459-1476, 1968.
4. BECK. S. D. and ALEXANDER, N.: Proctodone, an Insect Developmental Hormone. Biol. Bull., *126*:185-198, 1964.
5. BODENSTEIN, D.: Contributions to the Problem of Regeneration in Insects. J. Exptl. Zool., *129*:209-224, 1955.
6. BORDEN, J. H., NAIR, K. K., and SLATER, C. E.: Synthetic Juvenile Hormone: Induction of Sex Pheromone Production in *Ips confusus*. Science, *166*:1626-1627, 1969.
7. BORDEN, J. H. and SLATER, C. E.: Induction of Flight Muscle Degeneration by Synthetic Juvenile Hormone in *Ips confusus* (Coleoptera: Scolytidae). Z. Vergl. Physiol., *61*:366-368, 1968.
8. BOWERS, W. S. and BLICKENSTAFF, C. C.: Hormonal Termination of Diapause in the Alfalfa Weevil. Science, *154*:1673-1674, 1966.
9. BOWERS, W. S., THOMPSON, M. J., and UEBEL, E. C.: Juvenile and Gonadotropic Hormone Activity of 10,11-Epoxyfarnesenic Acid Methyl Ester. Life Sci., *4*: 2323-2331, 1965.
10. CHADWICK, L. E.: Molting of Roaches without Prothoracic Glands. Science, *121*: 435, 1955.
11. CHADWICK, L. E.: Removal of Prothoracic Glands from the Nymphal Cockroach. J. Exptl. Zool., *131*:291-305, 1956.
12. CONGOTE, L. F., SEKERIS, C. E., and KARLSON, P.: On the Mechanism of Hormone Action. XVIII. Alterations of the Nature of RNA Synthesized in Isolated Fat Body Cell Nuclei as a Result of Ecdysone and Juvenile Hormone Action. Z. Naturforsch., *25b*:279-284, 1970.
13. DAHM, K. H. and RÖLLER, H.: The Juvenile Hormone of the Giant Silk Moth, *Hyalophora gloveri* (Strecker). Life Sci., Pt. 2, *9*:1397-1400, 1970.
14. deKORT, C. A. D.: Hormones and the Structural and Biochemical Properties of the Flight Muscles in the Colorado Beetle. Meded. Oandboushoges-school Wageningen, Netherlands, *69*:1-63, 1969.
15. DELPHIN, F.: The Histology and Possible Functions of Neurosecretory Cells in the Ventral Ganglia of *Schistocerca gregaria* Forskal (Orthoptera: Acrididae). Trans. Roy. Entom. Soc. Lond., *117*:167-214, 1965.
16. EDWARDS, F. J.: Endocrine Control of Flight Muscle Histolysis in *Dysdercus intermedius*. J. Insect Physiol., *16*:2027-2031, 1970.
17. EDWARDS, J. S.: Neural Control of Metamorphosis in *Galleria mellonella* (Lepidoptera). J. Insect Physiol., *12*:1423-1433, 1966.
18. ENGELMANN, F.: The Mode of Regulation of the Corpus Allatum in Adult Insects. Arch. Anat. Microsc. Morph. Exp., *54*:387-404, 1965.

19. GERSCH, M. and STRÜZEBECHER, J.: Weitere Untersuchungen zur Kennzeichnung des Aktivationshormons der Insektenhaütung. J. Insect Physiol., *14*:87-96, 1968.

20. GERSCH, M.: Über eine Synthese von Ecdyson-^{3}H und Ecdysteron-^{3}H aus Cholesterin-^{3}H in Geschnürten Abdomina von *Mamestra brassicae* Raupen. Experientia, *27*:1475-1476, 1971.

21. GILBERT, L. I.: The Chemistry and Physiology of the Juvenile Hormone of Insects. Ph.D. Thesis. University Microfilms, Inc., Ann Arbor, Mich., 1958.

22. GILBERT, L. I. and KING, D. S. : Physiology of Growth and Development:Endocrine Aspects (II). In: M. Rockstein (ed.), The Physiology of Insecta, 2nd Ed., Vol. 1, New York: Academic Press, 1973 (in press).

23. GILBERT, L. I. and SCHNEIDERMAN, H. A. : Prothoracic Gland Stimulation by Juvenile Hormone Extracts of Insects. Nature, *184:*171-173, 1959.

24. HIGHNAM, K. C. : Insect Hormones. J. Endocr., *39:*123-150, 1967.

25. HINTZE-PODUFAL, C. : The Innervation of the Prothoracic Glands of *Cerura vinula* L. (Lepidoptera). Experientia, *26:*1269-1271, 1970.

26. ICHIKAWA, M. and ISHIZAKI, H. : Protein Nature of the Brain Hormone of Insects. Nature, *198:*308-309, 1963.

27. ICHIKAWA, M. and NISHIITSUTSUJI-UWO, J.:Studies on the Role of the Corpus Allatum in the Eri-silkworm *Philosamia cynthia ricini*. Biol. Bull., *116*:88-94, 1959.

28. ICHIKAWA, M. and NISHIITSUTSUJI-UWO, J. : VII. Effect of the Brain Hormone to the Isolated Abdomen of the Eri-silkworm, *Philosamia cynthia ricini*. Mem. Coll. Sci. Univ. Kyoto, Ser. B, *27:*9-15, 1960.

29. ILAN, J., ILAN, J., and PATEL, N. : Mechanism of Expression in *Tenebrio molitor*. J. Biol. Chem., *245:*1275-1281, 1970.

30. JACOBSON, M., BEROZA, M., BULL, D. L., BULLOCK, H. R., CHAMBERLAIN, W. F., McGOVERN, T. P., REDFERN, R. E., SARMIENTO, R., SCHWARZ, M., SONNET, P. E., WAKABAYASHI, N., WATERS, R. M., and WRIGHT, J. E.: Juvenile Hormone Activity of a Variety of Structural Types Against Several Insect Species. *In*: J. J. Menn and M. Beroza (eds.). Insect Juvenile Hormones: Chemistry and Action, pp. 249-302. New York: Academic Press, 1972.

31. JOHNSON, W. S., CAMPBELL, S. F., KRISHNAKUMARAN, A., and MEYER, A. S. : Total Synthesis of the Racemic Form of the Second Juvenile Hormone (Methyl-12-homojuvenate) from the Cecropia Silk Moth. Proc. Natl. Acad. Sci. USA., *62:*1005-1009, 1969.

32. JUDY, K. J. : Diapause Termination and Metamorphosis in Brainless Tobacco Hornworms (Lepidoptera). Life Sci., pt. 2, *11:*605-611, 1972.

33. JUDY, K. J., SCHOOLEY, D. A., HALL, M. S., BERGOT, B. J., DUNHAM, L. L., and SIDDALL, J. B. : Isolation and Identification of a New Natural Insect Juvenile Hormone from *Manduca sexta* Corpora Allata *in Vitro*. (Manuscript in preparation), 1972.

34. KAMBYSELLIS, M. P. and WILLIAMS, C. M.: *In-vitro* Development of Insect Tissues. I. A Macromolecular Factor Prerequisite for Silkworm Spermatogenesis. Biol. Bull.. *141:*527-540. 1971a.

35. KAMBYSELLIS, M. P. and WILLIAMS, C. M.: *In-vitro* Development of Insect Tissues. II. The Role of Ecdysone in the Spermatogenesis of Silkworms. Biol. Bull., *141:* 541-552, 1971b.

36. KAMBYSELLIS, M. P. and WILLIAMS, C. M. : Spermatogenesis in Cultured Testes of the Cynthia Silkworm: Effects of Ecdysone and of Prothoracic Glands. Science, *175:*769-770, 1972.

37. KARLSON, P. and SHAAYA, E. : Der Ecdysontiter wahrend der Insektenentwicklung. I. Eine Methode zur bestimmung des Ecdysongehalts. J. Insect Physiol., *10:*797-804, 1964.

38. KING, D. S. : Metabolism of α-ecdysone and Possible Immediate Precursors by Insects *in Vivo* and *in Vitro.* Gen. Comp. Endocrinol. (Suppl. Vol.) (in press),1972.

39. KOBAYASHI, M., FUKAYA, M., and MITSUHASHI, J.: Imaginal Differentiation of "Dauer-pupae" in the Silkworm, *Bombyx mori.* J. Sericult. Sci. Jap., *29:*337-340, 1960.

40. KOBAYASHI, M., KIRIMURA, J., and SAITO, M. : Crystallization of the Brain Hormone of an Insect. Nature, *195:*515-516, 1962.

41. KOBAYASHI, M. and YAMAZAKI, M. : The Proteinic Brain Hormone in an Insect, *Bombyx mori* L. Appl. Ent. Zool., *1:*53-60, 1966.

42. KRISHNAKUMARAN, A. : Injury-Induced Molting in *Galleria mellonella* Larvae. Biol. Bull., *142:*281-292, 1972.

43. KROEGER, H.: Cellular Mechanisms Regulating the Activity of Genes in Insect Development. Proc. XVI Intl. Congr. Zool., *4:*251-255, 1963.

44. KROEGER, H. : Gene Activities During Insect Metamorphosis and Their Control by Hormones. *In:* W. Etkin and L. I. Gilbert (eds.). Metamorphosis: A Problem in Developmental Biology, pp. 185-219. New York: Appleton-Century-Crofts, 1968.

45. LAWRENCE, P. A.: The Hormonal Control of the Development of Hairs and Bristles in the Milkweed Bug, *Oncopeltus fasciatus* Dall. J. Exp. Biol., *44:*507-522, 1966.

46. LEZZI, M. and GILBERT, L. I. : Control of Gene Activities in the Polytene Chromosomes of *Chironomus tentans* by Ecdysone and Juvenile Hormone. Proc. Natl. Acad. Sci. USA, *64:*498-503, 1969.

47. LEZZI, M. and GILBERT, L. I.: Differential Effects of K^+ and Na^+ on Specific Bands of Isolated Polytene Chromosomes of *Chironomus tentans.* J. Cell Sci., *6:*615-628, 1970.

48. LOCKE, M. : The Ultrastructure of the Oenocytes in the Molt/Intermolt Cycle of an Insect. Tissue & Cell, *1:*103-154, 1969.

49. LUSCHER, M.: Functions of the Corpora Allata in the Development of Termites. Proc. XVI Intl. Congr. Zool., *4:*244-250, 1963.

50. MARKS, E. P., ITTYCHERIAH, P. I., and LELOUP, A. M.: The Effect of β-Ecdysone on Insect Neurosecretion *in Vitro.* J. Insect Physiol., *18:*847-850, 1972.

51. McDANIEL, C. N. and BERRY, S. J.: Activation of the Prothoracic Glands of *Antheraea polyphemus.* Nature, *214:*1032-1034, 1967.

52. MEYER, A. S., SCHNEIDERMAN, H. A., HANZMANN, E., and Ko, J. H. : The Two Juvenile Hormones from the Cecropia Silk Moth. Proc. Natl. Acad. Sci., USA, *60:*853-860, 1968.

53. MORIYAMA, H., KING, D. S., NAKANISHI, K., OKAUCHI, T., SIDDALL, J. B., and HAFFERL, W.: On the Origin and Metabolic Fate of α-ecdysone in Insects. Gen. Comp. Endocrinol.. *15:*80-87. 1970.

54. NAIR, K. K. and MENON, M.: Detection of Juvenile Hormone-induced Gene Activity in the Colleterial Gland Nuclei of *Periplaneta* by ^{3}H-Actinomycin-D "Staining" Technique. Experientia, *28:*577, 1972.

55. NOVÁK, V. J. A.: The Juvenile Hormone and the Problem of Animal Morphogenesis. *In:* J. W. L. Beament and J. E. Treherne (eds.), Insects and Physiology, pp. 119-132. London: Oliver and Boyd, 1967.

56. OBERLANDER, H.: Effects of Ecdysone, Ecdysterone, and Inokosterone on the *in-vitro* Initiation of Metamorphosis of Wing Disks of *Galleria mellonella*. J. Insect Physiol., *15:*297-304, 1969.

57. OBERLANDER, H., BERRY, S. J., KRISHNAKUMARAN, A., and SCHNEIDERMAN, H. A. : RNA and DNA Synthesis During Activation and Secretion of the Prothoracic Glands of Saturniid Moths. J. Exptl. Zool., *159:*15-32, 1965.

58. OBERLANDER, H. and SCHNEIDERMAN, H. A. : A Study of the Mechanisms of Activation of the Prothoracic Glands. XVI Intl. Congr. Zool., *2:*67, 1963.

59. OZEKI, K. : Secretion of Molting Hormone from the Ventral Glands. Sci. Papers Coll. Gen. Educ. Univ. Tokyo, *9:*256-262, 1959.

60. PALLOS, F. M. and MENN, J. J. : Synthesis and Activity of Juvenile Hormone Analogs. *In*: J. J. Menn and M. Beroza (eds.), Insect Juvenile Hormones: Chemistry and Action, pp. 303-316. New York: Academic Press, 1972.

61. PIEPHO, H.: Raupenhautungen Bereits Verpuppter Hautstücke bei der Wachsmotte *Galleria mellonella* L. Naturwiss., *27:*301-302, 1939.

62. PIEPHO, H. : Zur Frage der Bildungsorgane des Hautungswirkstoffs bei Schmetterlingen. Naturwiss., *35:*94-95, 1948.

63. PIPA, R. L.: Neuroendocrine Involvement in the Delayed Pupation of Space-deprived *Galleria mellonella* (Lepidoptera). J. Insect Physiol., *17:*2441-1450, *1971.*

64. RIDDIFORD, L. M. : Juvenile Hormone and Insect Embryogenesis. Mitteil. Schweizer. Entomol. Gesell., *44:*177-186, 1971.

65. RIDDIFORD, L. M. : Juvenile Hormone in Relation to the Larval-pupal Transformation of the Cecropia Silkworm. Biol. Bull.. *142:*310-325, 1972.

66. RIDDIFORD, L. M. and TRUMAN, J. W. : Delayed Effects of Juvenile Hormone on Insect Metamorphosis are Mediated by the Corpus Allatum. Nature, *237:*458, 1972.

67. RIDDIFORD, L. M. and WILLIAMS, C. M. : The Effects of Juvenile Hormone Analogues on the Embryonic Development of Silkworms. Proc. Natl. Acad. Sci. USA, *57:*595-601, 1967.

68. ROLLER, H., DAHM, K. H., SWEELY, C. C., and TROST, B. M. : The Structure of the Juvenile Hormone. Angew. Chem. Internat. Ed. Engl., *6:*179-180, 1967.

69. ROMER, F. : Hautungshormon in den Oenocyten des Mehlkafers. Naturwiss., *58:* 324-325, 1971.

70. SCHARRER, B.: Histophysiological Studies on the Corpus Allatum of *Leucophaea maderae*. IV. Ultrastructure During Normal Activity Cycle. Z. Zellforsch. Mickros. Anat., *62:*125-148, 1964.

71. SCHNEIDERMAN, H. A. and GILBERT, L. I. : Control of Growth and Development in Insects. Science, *143:*325-333, 1964.

72. SIEW, Y. C. and GILBERT, L. I. : Effects of Moulting Hormone and Juvenile Hormone on Insect Endocrine Gland Activity. J. Insect Physiol., *17:*2095-2104, 1971.

73. SLADE, M. and ZIBITT, C. H.: Metabolism of Cecropia Juvenile Hormone in Lepidopterans. In: A. S. Tahori (ed.), Chemical Releasers in Insects, pp. 45-58. New York: Gordon and Breach, 1971.

74. SLADE, M. and ZIBITT, C. H. : Metabolism of Cecropia Juvenile Hormone in Insects and Mammals. *In*: J. J. Menn and M. Beroza (eds.), Insect Juvenile Hormones: Chemistry and Action, pp. 155-176. New York: Academic Press, 1972.

75. SLÁMA, K. : Insect Juvenile Hormone Analogues. Ann. Rev. Biochem., *40:*1079-1102, 1971.

76. SLÁMA, K. and WILLIAMS, C. M. : "Paper Factor" as an Inhibitor of the Embryonic Development of the European Bug, *Pyrrhocoris apterus.* Nature, *210:*329-330, 1966.

77. SRIVASTAVA, K. P. and SINGH, H. H. : On the Innervation of the Prothoracic Glands in *Papilio demoleus* L. (Lepidoptera). Experientia, *24:*838-839, 1968.

78. STAAL, G. B. : Studies on the Physiology of Phase Induction in *Locusta migratoria migratorioides* R & F. H. Veenman & Zonen N. V. Wageningen, Netherlands, 125 pp., 1961.

79. STAAL, G. B. : Endocrine Aspects of Larval Development in Insects. J. Endocr., *37:*13-14, 1967.

80. STAAL, G. B. : Biological Activity and Bio Assay of Juvenile Hormone Analogs. *In:* J. J. Menn and M. Beroza (eds.), Insect Juvenile Hormones: Chemistry and Action, pp. 69-94. New York: Academic Press, 1972.

81. TAKEDA, N. : Effect of Some Phytoecdysones on the Spermatogenesis of the Slug Moth Prepupa, *Monema flavescens* Walker (Lepidoptera: Heterogeneidae). Appl. Ent. Zool., *7:*37-39, 1972.

82. TOMBES, A. S. and SMITH, D. S. : Ultrastructural Studies on the Corpora Cardiaca-Allata Complex of the Adult Alfalfa Weevil *Hypera postica.* J. Morphol., *132:*137-148, 1970.

83. TRAUTMANN, K. H. : *In-vitro* Studium der Tragerproteine von ^{3}H-markierten Juvenilhormonwirksamen Verbindingen in der Hamolymphe von *Tenebrio molitor* L. Larven. Z. Naturforsch., *27:*263-273, 1972.

84. WAKU, Y. and GILBERT, L. I. : The Corpora Allata of the Silkmoth, *Hyalophora cecropia:* An Ultrastructural Study. J. Morphol., *115:*69-96, 1964.

85. WEIR, S. B. : Control of Moulting in an Insect. Nature, *228:*580-581, 1970.

86. WHITE, D. F. : Corpus Allatum Associated with Development of Wingbuds in Cabbage Aphid Embryos and Larvae. J. Insect Physiol., *17:*761-773, 1971.

87. WHITMORE, D., WHITMORE, E., and GILBERT, L. I. : Juvenile Hormone Induction of Esterases: A Mechanism for the Regulation of Juvenile Hormone Titer. Proc. Natl. Acad. Sci. USA, *69:* 1592-1995, 1972.

88. WHITMORE, E. and GILBERT, L. I. : Haemolymph Lipoprotein Transport of Juvenile Hormone. J. Insect Physiol., (in press), 1972.

89. WIGGLESWORTH, V. B. : Factors Controlling Moulting and "Metamorphosis" in an Insect. Nature, *133:*725-726, 1934.

90. WIGGLESWORTH, V. B. : The Physiology of Insect Metamorphosis. Cambridge University Press, 152 pp., 1954.

91. WIGGLESWORTH, V. B. : Chemical Structure and Juvenile Hormone Activity. Nature, *221:*190-191, 1969.

92. WIGGLESWORTH, V. B. : Insect Hormones. San Francisco: W. H. Freeman & Company, 159 pp., 1970.

93. WILLIAMS, C. M. : Physiology of Insect Diapause. IV. The Brain and Prothoracic Glands as an Endocrine System in the Cecropia Silkworm. Biol. Bull., *103:*120-138, 1952.

94. WILLIAMS, C. M. : The Juvenile Hormone. I. Endocrine Activity of the Corpora Allata of the Adult Cecropia Silkworm. Biol. Bull., *116:*323-338, 1959.

95. WILLIAMS, C. M. : The Juvenile Hormone. III. Its Accumulation and Storage in the Abdomens of Certain Male Moths. Biol. Bull., *124:*355-367, 1963.

96. WILLIAMS, C. M.: Third-generation Pesticides. Scientific American, *217:*13-17, 1967.
97. WILLIAMS, C. M. : The Present Status of the Brain Hormone. *In:* J. W. L. Beament and J. E. Treherne (eds.), Insects and Physiology, pp. 133-139. London: Oliver and Boyd, 1967.
98. WILLIAMS, C. M. : Nervous and Hormonal Communication in Insect Development. Dev. Biol. Suppl., *3:*133-150, 1969.
99. WILLIAMS, C. M. and KAFATOS, F. C. : Theoretical Aspects on the Action of Juvenile Hormone. Mitteil. Schweizer. Entomol. Gesell., *44:*151-162, 1971.
100. WILLIS, J. H. : The Programming of Differentiation and its Control by Juvenile Hormone in Saturniids. J. Embryol. Exp. Morph., *22:*27-44, 1969.
101. WILLIS, J. H. and BRUNET, P. C. J.: The Hormonal Control of Colleterial Gland Secretion. J. Exp. Biol., *44:*363-378, 1966.
102. WILLIS, J. H. and LAWRENCE, P. A. : Deferred Action of Juvenile Hormone Nature, *225:*81-83, 1970.
103. WYATT, G. R. : Insect Hormones. *In:* G. Litwack (ed.), Biochemical Actions of Hormones, pp. 385-490. New York: Academic Press, 1972.
104. YAGI, S., KONDO, E., and FUKAYA, M. : Hormonal Effect on Cultivated Insect Tissues. I. Effect of Ecdysterone on Cultivated Testes of Diapausing Rice Stem Border Larvae (Lepidoptera: Pyralidae). Appl. Ent. Zool., *4:*70-78, 1969.
105. ZALOKAR, M. : Effect of Corpora Allata on Protein and RNA Synthesis in Colleterial Glands of *Blattella germanica.* J. Insect Physiol., *14:*1177-1184, 1968.

BRAIN HORMONE

Masatoshi Kobayashi and Masayoshi Yamazaki

The endocrine function of the insect brain was first suggested by Kopeč (1922). Two decades later, Wigglesworth (1940) demonstrated that the molting of *Rhodnius prolixus* was initiated by a hormonal factor originating from the dorsal region of the protocerebrum containing the neurosecretory cells. Since then, numerous studies on hormonal systems of growth and development have been reported (Wigglesworth, 1953). Many investigations on the system of hormonal action in imaginal differentiation have utilized *Hyalophora cecropia* (Williams, 1946, 1947, 1952), *Bombyx mori* (Kobayashi, 1955, 1957), and other insects.

Williams found that the pupal diapause of the insect is caused by inactivation of the pupal brain. In the classical scheme, brain is activated by exposure to low temperature and secretes brain hormone affecting the prothoracic gland. The latter organ then secretes prothoracic-gland hormone, inducing metamorphosis. Although diapause does not occur in the pupal stage of the silkworm, Kobayashi was able to demonstrate that the brain of the silkworm plays as important a role in the metamorphosis of this moth as it does in other insects.

These experiments have initiated a clearly defined concept for the function of the brain hormone. The hormone stimulates the prothoracic glands to secrete the prothoracic-gland hormone, ecdysone, which acts on the cells of various tissues to provoke growth and differentiation of the insect as a whole. As for the chemical study of brain hormone, the first active extract was prepared by Kobayashi and Kirimura (1958) from brains of the silkworm, *Bombyx mori.* After extensive purification, an active ether-soluble fraction was crystallized and found to show all the physical and chemical properties of cholesterol (Kirimura *et al.,* 1962).

Although the activity of cholesterol was confirmed by Schneiderman and Gilbert (1964), cholesterol is known to be ubiquitous in the tissues of dia-pausing pupae. The ability of the sterol to mimic brain hormone showed a bizarre and often inverse correlation with the amount injected. The nature of the solvent for sterols (9-10 per cent ethanol) proved to be crucial for the activity. Moreover, Karlson and Hoffmeister (1963) studied the biosynthesis of ecdysones in Calliphora larvae and demonstrated that cholesterol is the precursor of ecdysone. From these facts, we are inclined to believe that cholesterol is a substance that mimics the action of brain hormone directly or indirectly.

On the other hand, in 1961 Ichikawa and Ishizaki reported an active extract from the brain that is a water-soluble, heat-stable, and nondialyzable moiety. Subsequently the hormonal extract was found to be resistant to pepsin and trypsin but inactivated by Nagarse and Pronase. On the basis of these latter findings, they concluded that the brain hormone is a protein (Ichikawa and Ishizaki, 1963).

In the course of purification of brain hormone from extract of Bombyx brains, we separated several active fractions by means of counter-current distribution (Kobayashi, 1963), and brain-hormone activity was found in both water-soluble and ether-soluble substances. When water-soluble substances in the extract from Bombyx brains were investigated, the findings of Ichikawa and Ishizaki were confirmed (Kobayashi and Yamazaki, 1966). Then we were able to extract from Bombyx brains a water-soluble, heat-stable material with high activity. Fractionation on Sephadex columns suggested a molecular weight not less than 10,000 and not more than 50,000. The crude extract was purified by chromatography on CM-cellulose. The hormonal activity in the crude extract was found to be resistant to trypsin and chymotrypsin but destroyed by Pronase and Nagarse.

Williams (1967) has also studied the brain hormone and confirmed other investigators' results, but he suspects that the brain hormone is a protein and guesses it may be mucopolysaccharide on the basis of such properties as its heat stability, its lack of specific absorption at 280 mμ., its sensitivity to pepsin, trypsin, and chymotrypsin, and its insensitivity to maneuvers which historically have been used to remove the last traces of protein.

Subsequently, Ishizaki and Ichikawa (1967) have done more work on the purification of brain hormone of the silkworm, *Bombyx mori,* and have reported that the hormone was proved to consist of chromatographically highly heterogeneous molecules, the molecular weight of the major components varying from 9,000 to 31,000. Although they have not investigated properties of the hormone extensively, Ishizaki and Ichikawa (1967) have reported that the brain hormone is bound to DEAE-cellulose but not to CM-cellulose. This result was different from ours (Kobayashi and Yamazaki, 1966), notwithstanding the use of the same material, Bombyx brains. They attributed this difference to the result of methodologies used in the respective laboratories.

When brain hormone was purified from Bombyx-brain extract by Yamazaki and Kobayashi (1969) and the properties of the hormone investigated, the hormone was heat stable, resistant to incubation with chymotrypsin, but inactivated by trypsin, Pronase, or Nagarse. Its molecular weight was estimated by gel filtration on Sephadex G-100 to be 20,000. The isoelectric point of the hormone was pH 8.35-8.65. The most active preparation obtained possibly contains carbohydrate.

Furthermore, these experiments demonstrated that two active fractions were separated by chromatography on CM-cellulose. One of them was fractionated and purified on CM-cellulose, and the properties investigated are recorded in Tables 1 and 2 and Figure 1. Characteristics of the other, unadsorbed on CM-cellulose, could be separated by chromatography on DEAE-cellulose (Figures 2 and 3). These results suggest that the brain hormone of Bombyx consists of several components and that the latter may be the component(s) fractionated by Ishizaki and Ichikawa (1967).

Gersch and Stürzeichung (1968) have reported that the components having brain-hormone activity can be separated from aqueous extract of brains of the cockroach, *Periplaneta americana,* by fractionation on Sephadex G-75. Therefore, with the present evidence, it is reasonable to assume that the brain hormone in insects is proteinic and consists of several kinds of proteins or polypeptides, although their properties are not completely clarified.

In order to reaffirm the endocrine function of brain hormone, the effect of the purified brain hormone from brains of Bombyx pupae on the larval-pupal as well as on the pupal-adult transformation was investigated (Kobayashi, unpublished). As illustrated in Table 3, the result demonstrated that the brain hormone stimulates prothoracic glands to secrete molting hormone.

By means of the procedure previously reported (Ishizaki and Ichikawa, 1967), changes in titer of brain hormone extracted from the brain, head, thorax, and abdomen during the development of *Bombyx mori* from the fourth larval molting up to 6 days after adult emergence were investigated (Ishizaki, 1969). In addition, a few studies on the mode of action of the brain hormone have been done.

The action of the brain hormone on carbohydrate metabolism in the diapausing, brainless pupa of *Samia cynthia* pryeri also was studied (Kobayashi *et al.*, 1967). Injection of the hormone promoted oxygen consumption of the brainless pupa. When ^{14}C-glucose was injected into the brainless pupa, ^{14}C-glucose was incorporated into glycogen in the fat body, whereas ^{14}C-glucose was incorporated into trehalose in blood when ^{14}C-glucose was injected into the hormone-treated, brainless pupa (Tables 4 and 5). These results suggest that the hormone promotes the biosynthesis of trehalose. The same results were obtained in the experiment concerning ecdysone (Kobayashi and Kimura, 1967). These findings may result from indirect function of the brain hormone.

The effect of the brain hormone on nucleic-acid synthesis in the prothoracic gland which is a target organ for the hormone was investigated in the larva of *Bombyx mori* (Kobayashi *et al.*, 1967). It was demonstrated that the hormone does not affect DNA synthesis in the nuclei but promotes RNA synthesis in the nuclei of the prothoracic gland and then newly synthesized RNA transfers into the cytoplasm of the gland. However, the hormone promotes RNA synthesis in the nuclei of other tissues besides the prothoracic gland (Tables 6, 7, 8, and 9).

Burdette and Kobayashi (1968) studied the response of chromosomal puffs to hormones *in vivo*. As can be seen in Table 10, administration of the hormone affected salivary-gland chromosomes of Drosophila. Earlier increase in the size of salivary chromosome puffs chosen as indices to measure response after treatment with the brain hormone was clearly demonstrated by these experiments.

In summary, very active extracts of brain hormone have been obtained and used to elucidate its roles in growth and differentiation. The identification of the chemical nature of the active component(s) now is needed to provide information comparable to that known about juvenile hormones and ecdysones.

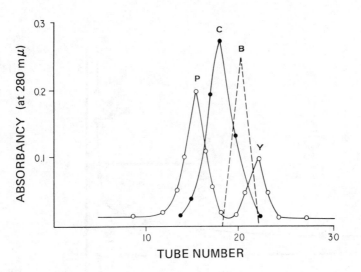

Figure 1

Gel filtration of purified brain hormone and several proteins of known molecular weight on a column of Sephadex G-100. P: Pepsin, C: Chymotrypsin, Y: Yeast cytochrome-C, B: Purified brain hormone.

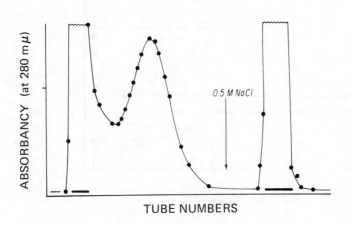

Figure 2

Chromatography of the extract from Bombyx brains on a column of CM-Cellulose. The black band shows the range of brain-hormone activity.

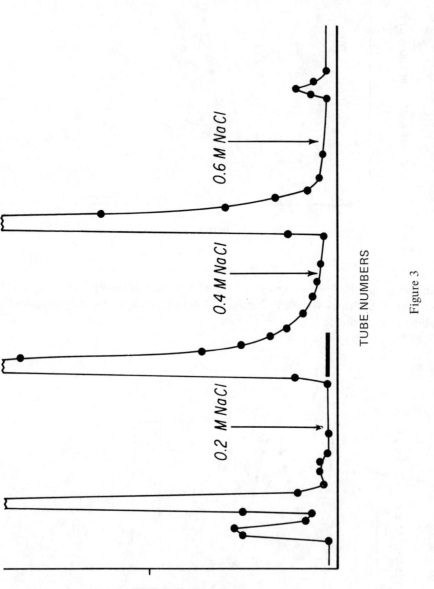

Figure 3

Chromatography of the unabsorbed fraction on CM-cellulose on a column of DEAE-cellulose. The black band shows the range of brain-hormone activity.

TABLE 1

TREATMENTS WITH PURIFIED BRAIN HORMONE

Treatments		No. of Test Objects	No. of Moths Emerged	No. of Pupal Fatalities
Temperature				
	Min.			
100°C.	15	6	5	1
	30	6	6	0
	60	6	3	3
pH	Hr.			
10	24	6	6	0
	48	6	4	1
1.4	24	6	3	1
	48	6	3	1

The results obtained 4 weeks following the injection at 25°C.

TABLE 2

DIGESTION OF PURIFIED BRAIN HORMONE BY PROTEOLYTIC ENZYMES

Digestion	No. of Test Objects	No. of Moths Emerged	No. of Pupal Fatalities
Trypsin			
Hr.			
1	6	2	0
2	6	1	0
Chymotrypsin			
4	6	5	0
24	10	5	2
Pronase			
1	6	2	0
2	6	1	0
Nagarse			
1	6	0	0
2	6	2	0

The results obtained 4 weeks following the injection at 25°C.

TABLE 3

EFFECT OF PROTEINIC BRAIN HORMONE ON THE LARVAL–PUPAL TRANSFORMATION OF DECAPITATED LARVAE

Dose of PBH (Bombyx-unit)	Test Objects	No. of Test Objects	Forms of Result	No. of Larvae, Intermediate Forms, and Pupae Appearing at Hours Indicated after Injection							
				48	72	96	120	144	168	192	218
1/4	DL	7	L	.	.	.	.	.	.	.	.
			I	.	.	1	.	.	.	.	.
			P	.	.	.	.	3	2	.	.
1/2	DL	7	L	1	.	.	.	.	.	.	.
			I	.	.	1	2	.	.	.	.
			P	.	.	.	1	2	.	.	.
1	DL	7	L	1	.	.	.	.	.	.	.
			I	.	.	3	2	.	.	.	.
			P	.	.	.	.	1	.	.	.
0	DL	14	L	.	.	.	.	.	.	.	.
			I	.	.	.	.	.	.	.	.
			P	.	.	.	.	.	.	6	4
1	IA	7	L	.	.	.	.	.	.	.	.
			I	.	.	.	.	.	.	.	.
			P	.	.	.	.	.	.	1	.

The following abbreviations are used: DL, decapitated lavra; IA, isolated abdomen; L, larva; I, intermediate form; P, pupa.

TABLE 4

RELATIONSHIP BETWEEN INSECT HORMONES AND RESPIRATORY RATES
OF BRAINLESS PUPAE OF *SAMIA CYNTHIA*

Injection	Dose (μg.)	O_2 Consumption (1/10 Min./G.)*	CO_2 Output (1/10 Min./G.)*
Proteinic Brain Hormone	60	—	—
Glucose	1	30	37
Glucose	1	13	50
Control (Not Injected)	0	16	46

* Mean value for two pupae

TABLE 5

FATE OF ^{14}C–GLUCOSE IN BRAINLESS PUPAE OF *SAMIA CYNTHIA* PRYERI

Experiments	Radioactivity of Ba ^{14}CO$_3$ (c.p.m./mg. Ba./G.)	Sample	Radioactivity of Trehalose (T) and Glucose (G) (c.p.m./mg./10^3)	T/G	Radioactivity		
					Glyco-gen	Crude Lipid (c.p.m./mg.)	Crude Protein
Proteinic Brain		Blood	2.3	7.2	15	41	49
Hormone (60 μg.)	391	Fat Body	4.0	4.4	129	30	46
Control							
(Not Injected)	94	Blood	4.5	1.2	1	6	23
		Fat Body	2.0	—	2823	3	47

TABLE 6

INCORPORATION OF TRITIATED COMPOUNDS INTO
PROTHORACIC GLAND OF SILKWORM LARVA FOLLOWING INJECTION
OF PROTEINIC BRAIN HORMONE (P B H)

Hours after Injection		1	6	12	18	24
PBH (100 μg.) +	C	+	+	+	+	+
^{3}H-Thymidine (10 μCi.)	N	+ + +	+ + + +	+ + + +	+ + + +	+ + + +
^{3}H-Thymidine (10 μCi.)	C	+	+	+	+	+
	N	+ + +	+ + + +	+ + + +	+ + + +	+ + + +
PBH (100 μg.) + ^{3}H-Uridine (10 μCi.) + Thymidine (6 μg.)	C	+	+ + +	+ + + + +	+ + + +	+ + +
	N	+ + + +	+ + + +	+ + +	+ +	+ +
PBH (100 μg.) + ^{3}H-Uridine (10 μCi.) + Thymidine (6 μg.) + Actinomycin D (3 μg.)	C	+	+ +	+ + +	+ + +	+ + +
	N	+	+ +	+ +	+ +	+ +
^{3}H-Uridine (10 μCi.) + Thymidine (6 μg.)	C	+	+ + +	+ + +	+ + +	+ + +
	N	+	+ +	+ + +	+ +	+

C: Cytoplasm,   N: Nucleus.
Results are based on density in the prothoracic gland incorporating tritiated compounds. Two animals were examined at each hour, and the order of density was scored: $+++++>++++>+++>++>+$.

TABLE 7

INCORPORATION OF TRITIATED COMPOUNDS INTO THE FAT BODY OF SILKWORM
LARVA FOLLOWING INJECTION OF PROTEINIC BRAIN HORMONE (P B H)

Hours after Injection		1	6	12	18	24
PBH (100 μg.) +	C	$\pm$	+	+	+	+
^{3}H-Thymidine (10 μCi.)	N	+	+ + +	+ +	+ +	+ +
^{3}H-Thymidine (10 μCi.)	C	$\pm$	+	+	+	$\pm$
	N	+	+	+	+	+
PBH (100 μg.) + ^{3}H-Uridine (10 μCi.) + Thymidine (6 μg.)	C	+	+ +	+ + +	+ + +	+ +
	N	+ +	+ +	+	+	+
PBH (100 μg.) + ^{3}H-Uridine (10 μCi.) + Thymidine (6 μg.) + Actinomycin D (3 μg.)	C	$\pm$	+	+	+	+
	N	+	+ +	+	+	+
^{3}H-Uridine (10 μCi.) + Thymidine (6 μg.)	C	$\pm$	+ +	+ +	$\pm$	+
	N	+	+ +	+ +	$\pm$	+

TABLE 8

INCORPORATION OF TRITIATED COMPOUNDS INTO THE INTEGUMENT OF SILKWORM
LARVA FOLLOWING INJECTION OF PROTEINIC BRAIN HORMONE (P B H)

Hours after Injection		1	6	12	18	24
PBH (100 μg.) +	C	+	+	+	+	+
^{3}H-Thymidine (10 μCi.)	N	+	+ + +	+ +	+ +	+ + +
^{3}H-Thymidine (10 μCi.)	C	−	+	±	+	±
	N	+	+ +	+ +	+ +	+
PBH (100 μg.) +						
^{3}H-Uridine (10 μCi.) +	C	±	+	+ + +	+ +	+ +
Thymidine (6 μg.)	N	+ +	+	+ + +	+	+
PBH (100 μg.) +						
^{3}H-Uridine (10 μCi.) +	C	±	+	+ +	+ +	+ +
Thymidine (6 μg.) +	N	±	+	+	+	+
Actinomycin D (3 μg.)						
^{3}H-Uridine (10 μCi.) +	C	+	+	+ +	±	+ +
Thymidine (6 μg.)	N	+	+	+ +	±	+

TABLE 9

INCORPORATION OF TRITIATED COMPOUNDS INTO THE MUSCLE OF SILKWORM
LARVA FOLLOWING INJECTION OF PROTEINIC BRAIN HORMONE (P B H)

Hours after Injection		1	6	12	18	24
PBH (100 μg.) +	C	−	+	+	+	+
^{3}H-Thymidine (10 μCi.)	N	+ +	+ + +	+ + +	+ + +	+ + +
^{3}H-Thymidine (10 μCi.)	C	+	+	+	+	±
	N	+	+ + +	+ +	+ +	+
PBH (100 μg.) +						
^{3}H-Uridine (10 μCi.) +	C	+	+ +	+ + +	+	+
Thymidine (6 μg.)	N	+ + + +	+ + +	+ +	±	±
PBH (100 μg.) +						
^{3}H-Uridine (10 μCi.) +	C	±	+	+	+	+
Thymidine (6 μg.) +	N	+	+ +	+ +	+ +	+
Actinomycin D (3 μg.)						
^{3}H-Uridine (10 μCi.) +	C	±	+	+ +	±	+
Thymidine (6 μg.)	N	+	+ +	+ +	±	±

TABLE 10

RESULTS OF TREATING OREGON—R LARVAE WITH PROTEINIC BRAIN HORMONE*†

Puff	Exposure (20 Min.)						Exposure (40 Min.)					
	Control		Brain Hormone (A)		Brain Hormone (B)		Control		Brain Hormone (A)		Brain Hormone (B)	
	Mean	Median	Mean	Median	Mean	Median	Mean	Median	Mean	Median	Mean	Median
2B	1.66	1.65	1.70	1.5	2.03	2.0	1.51	1.50	1.94	2.00	1.84	1.90
71	1.47	1.4	1.6	1.7	1.73	1.7	1.54	1.45	1.78	1.64	1.64	1.45
72	1.23	1.2	1.34	1.3	1.36	1.3	1.28	1.25	1.56	1.60	1.38	1.25
74	1.28	1.3	1.42	1.4	1.62	1.5	1.23	1.20	1.51	1.45	1.61	1.60
75	1.33	1.3	1.47	1.4	1.77	1.7	1.24	1.25	1.60	1.62	1.60	1.60

* Mean and median ratios of diameters of puffs and adjacent bands; 18 observations per puff; (A) Activity of one Bombyx unit/100 μg.; and (B) activity of one Bombyx unit/50 μg.

† Reprinted from Burdette, W. J. and Kobayashi, M. (1969).

References

1. BURDETTE, W. J. and KOBAYASHI, M.: Response of Chromosomal Puffs to Crystalline Hormones *In Vivo*. Proc. Soc. Exptl. Biol. Med., *131*:209, 1969.

2. GERSCH, M. and STÜRZEICHUNG, J.: Weitere Untersuchungen zur Kennzeichung des Aktivationshormons der Insektenhautung. J. Insect Physiol., *14*:87, 1968.

3. ICHIKAWA, M. and ISHIZAKI, H.: Brain Hormone of the Silkworm, *Bombyx mori*. Nature, *191*:933, 1961.

4. ICHIKAWA, M. and ISHIZAKI, H.: Protein Nature of the Brain Hormone of Insects. Nature, *198*:308, 1963.

5. ISHIZAKI, H. and ICHIKAWA, M.: Purification of the Brain Hormone of the Silkworm, *Bombyx mori*. Biol. Bull., *133*:355, 1967.

6. ISHIZAKI, H.: Changes in Titer of the Brain Hormone during Development of the Silkworm, *Bombyx mori*. Develop. Gro. Dif., *11*:1, 1969.

7. KARLSON, P. and HOFFMEISTER, H.: Zur Biogenese des Ecdysones. I. Umwandlung von Cholesterin in Ecdyson. Z. Physiol. Chem., *331*:298, 1963.

8. KIRIMURA, J., SAITO, M., and KOBAYASHI, M.: Steroid Hormone in an Insect, *Bombyx mori*. Nature, *181*:1217, 1962.

9. KOBAYASHI, M.: Relationship Between the Brain Hormone and the Imaginal Differentiation of Silkworm, *Bombyx mori*. J. Sericul. Sci. Jap., *24*:389, 1955.

10. KOBAYASHI, M.: Studies on the Neurosecretion in the Silkworm, *Bombyx mori* L. Bull. Sericul. Exptl. Sta., *15*:181, 1957.

11. KOBAYASHI, M. and YAMAZAKI, M.: Action of Proteinic Brain Hormone to the Prothoracic Gland in an Insect, *Bombyx mori* L. (Lepidoptera: Bombycidae). Appl. Ent. Zool., *1*:53, 1966.

12. KOBAYASHI, M. and KIMURA, S.: Action of Ecdysone on the Conversion of ^{14}C glucose in the Dauer Pupa of the Silkworm, *Bombyx mori*. J. Insect Physiol., *13*:545, 1966.

13. KOBAYASHI, M., KIMURA, S., and YAMAZAKI, M.: Action of Insect Hormones on the Fate of ^{14}C-glucose in the Diapausing Brainless Pupa of *Samia cynthia pryeri* (Lepidoptera: Saturniidae). Appl. Ent. Zool., *2*:79, 1967.

14. KOBAYASHI, M. and KIRIMURA, J.: The Brain Hormone in the Silkworm, *Bombyx mori*. L. Nature, *181*:1217, 1958.

15. KOBAYASHI, M. and YAMAZAKI, M.: The Proteinic Brain Hormone in an Insect, *Bombyx mori* L. Lepidoptera: Bombycidae. Appl. Ent. Zool., *1*:53, 1966.

16. KOPEC, S.: Studies on the Necessity of the Brain for the Inception of Insect Metamorphosis. Biol. Bull., *42*:323, 1922.

17. SCHNEIDERMAN, H. A. and GILBERT, L. I.: Control of Growth and Development in Insect. Science, *143*:325, 1964.

18. WIGGLESWORTH, V. B.: The Determination of Characters at Metamorphosis in *Rhodnius prolixus* (Hemiptera). J. Exptl. Biol., *17*:201, 1940.

19. WIGGLESWORTH, V. B.: The Principle of Insect Physiology. London: Methuen & Co. Ltd., 1953.

20. WILLIAMS, C. M.: Physiology of Insect Diapause: The Role of the Brain in the
     Production and Termination of Pupal Dormancy in the Giant Silkworm,
     Platysamia cecropia. Biol. Bull., *90*:234, 1946.
21. WILLIAMS, C. M.: Physiology of Insect Diapause. II. Interaction Between the Pupal
     Brain and Prothoracic Glands in the Metamorphosis of the Giant Silkworm,
     Platysamia cecropia. Biol. Bull., *93*:89, 1947.
22. WILLIAMS, C. M.: Physiology of Insect Diapause. IV. The Brain and Prothoracic
     Glands as an Endocrine System in the Cecropia Silkworm. Biol. Bull., *103*:120,
     1952.
23. YAMAZAKI, M. and KOBAYASHI, M.: Purification of the Proteinic Brain Hormone
     of the Silkworm, *Bombyx mori*. J. Insect Physiol., *15*:1988, 1969.

MODE of ACTION
of ECDYSONES

Peter Karlson

Ecdysones are substances active as molting hormones in insects. When we coined the term, "ecdysone", we believed that only one substance would exist naturally,the one isolated by us from Bombyx pupae (Butenandt and Karlson, 1954), but soon we discovered that even in Bombyx there are at least two active substances. The second one, described in 1955, was provisionally termed β-ecdysone (Karlson, 1955, 1956a). In re-isolating this compound, Hoffmeister (1966) termed it ecdysterone. Chemically it is 20-hydroxyecdysone and identical with crustecdysone, the crustacean molting hormone, first obtained in extracts from crustaceans in 1955 (Karlson, 1955, 1956a, b) and isolated and identified by Hampshire and Horn (1966).

The chemical structure of a-ecdysone had to be worked out in the days when modern physico-chemical methods were not available. It required much effort to prove that a-ecdysone was a steroid and finally to elucidate the full structure of ecdysone (Figure 1). This was done partly by chemical degradation studies (Karlson *et al.*, 1965), and partly through x-ray analysis of ecdysone crystals (Huber and Hoppe, 1965).

As already mentioned, 20-hydroxyecdysone (Figure 2) occurs in insects and crustaceans. A third compound of this series, 20, 26-dihydroxyecdysone (Figure 3), has recently been isolated from the tobacco hornworm, *Manduca sexta* (Thompson *et al.*, 1967). An excellent review on steroids in insects appeared recently (Robbins *et al.*, 1971).

Many steroids with molting hormone activity, sometimes called "phyto-ecdysones", are found in plants. This field will be summarized below in chapters by Dr. Hikino and Dr. Nakanishi.

Figure 1.   Figure 2.   Figure 3.

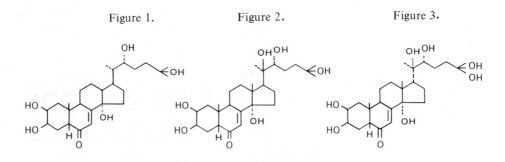

THE ACTION OF ECDYSONES IN VARIOUS INSECTS

In the old literature, many names have been given to the hormone of the prothoracic gland, ecdysone. It has been termed "molting hormone", "pupation hormone", "growth-and-differentiation hormone", etc., according to the type of physiological response under study. In retrospect, this is presumably due to the fact that ecdysone alone, in the absence of juvenile hormone, will lead to progress in development. For a larval molt juvenile hormone must be present as well. It seems appropriate to adhere to the term, "molting hormone", since ecdysone is involved in larval, pupal, and imaginal molts.

Some typical examples of ecdysone-mediated processes are collected in Table 1. It can be seen therefrom that ecdysone is active in all orders of insects studied. It is also effective when ingested by mouth, as borne out by experiments with termites (Karlson and Lüscher, 1958). The dose necessary varies with the species and with the type of response studied. For a more detailed discussion, the reader is referred to earlier reviews (Karlson, 1956a; Gabe *et al.*, 1964; and Novák, 1967).

Table 1.

THE ACTION OF ECDYSONE IN VARIOUS INSECTS*

Order	Species	Experimental Preparation	Type of Response	Dose Necessary[a]
Neuroptera	*Sialis lutaria*	Hibernating larvae	Pupation	50
Isoptera	*Kalotermes flavicollis*	Normal worker larvae	Molting	3
Hemiptera	*Rhodinus prolixus*	Decapitated larvae	Molting	75
Hymenoptera	*Cimbes americana*	Diapause larvae	Initiation of development	660
Lepidoptera	*Ephestia kuehniella*	Ligated larval abdomen	Pupation	50
	Hyalophora cecropia	Brainless dia- pause pupae	Initiation of development	1000
	Samia walkeri	Isolated pupal abdomen	Initiation of development	1330
Diptera	*Calliphora erythrocephala*	Ligated larval abdomen	Puparium formation	1
	Musca domestica	Ligated larval abdomen	Puparium formation	0.3
	Chironomus tentans	Normal late larvae	Puff induction	0.0002

a Expressed in Calliphora units: 1 Call. Unit = 0.01 μg.ecdysone
* For References, see Gabe, Karlson, and Roche, 1964

INDUCTION OF CHROMOSOMAL PUFFS

The most intriguing effect among those listed in Table 1 is, in my opinion, the induction of puffs in salivary-gland chromosomes (Clever and Karlson, 1960). This is a very rapid response, the effect being seen within 30 minutes, and very sensitive, 2×10^{-6} μg. per animal is the threshold dose (Clever, 1961, 1963). For both reasons, we believe that puffing may reflect the primary action of ecdysone at the cellular level.

It was already known at that time that puffs are sites of active RNA synthesis. Therefore, the appearance of a puff should reflect the "activation" of the corresponding gene, i.e., the transcription of this locus into messenger-RNA and eventually the translation into a specific protein (Figure 4). Therefore we drew the conclusion that ecdysone exerts its action by activating certain genes; this might be true for other hormones as well (Karlson, 1961, 1963).

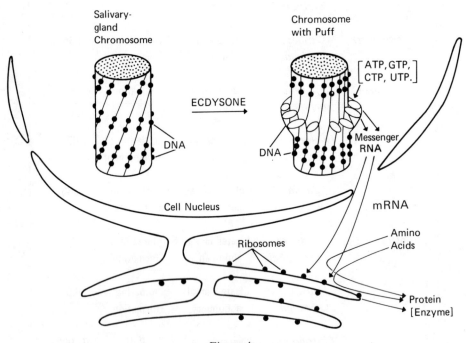

Figure 4.

Mechanism of Action of Ecdysone

The hormone acts first on the DNA producing a puff, which is shown on the left as an unwound region. In the puff, RNA is synthesized from precursors. This RNA is believed to be transferred to the cytoplasm and attached to the ribosomes. As "messenger-RNA," it carries the information about the amino-acid sequence. According to this information, the specific protein is synthesized on the ribosome from activated amino-acids. The whole chain of events explains the formation of specific proteins (e.g., certain enzymes) as the response of the target cell to a hormone. (From Karlson, 1963).

In the scheme given above, the hormone is believed to interact directly with the chromosomal material, whether DNA or a regulatory protein associated with DNA. There is another interpretation of effects of ecdysone on chromosomes; Kroeger and his co-workers (Kroeger, 1963; Lezzi, 1966; and Kroeger and Lezzi, 1966) believe that ecdysone does nothing more than to adjust the intranuclear level of Na^+ and K^+ ions in such a manner that a higher K^+-concentration triggers the induction of puffs, i.e., the activation of genes. This hypothesis is based upon the observation that isolated glands, when explanted and incubated in media of different salinity, developed typical patterns of puffing, and that high K^+-concentration activated the same puff (in *Chironomus thummi*) as ecdysone.

Clever (1968), in a re-investigation, could not reproduce these experiments in *Chironomus tentans*. He found a general and rather irregular stimulation by high concentrations of salt and no difference between K^+ and Na^+ ions as stressed by Kroeger. In *Chironomus thummi*, Kroeger's observations have been confirmed, and the different outcomes of the experiments have been ascribed to differences between the two species. Berendes, working with *Drosophila hydei* also observed salt effects; but they were non-specific, several loci responding to ions but not to ecdysone, others to ecdysone and not to ions, and some both to ecdysone and to high concentrations of salt (see also Ellgaard and Kessel, 1966). It is also known that various other (mis)treatments, i.e., with organic solvents or with thermal shocks, can provoke puffs and alter the puffing pattern in salivary glands. (For review, see Clever, 1968b; Ashburner, 1971). The best estimate, for the time being, is that the salt effects of Kroeger are reproducible artifacts.

In spite of the experimental evidence against the generalized theory of Kroeger, we have taken his arguments quite seriously and have tried to resolve the question with biochemical methods.

BIOCHEMICAL IMPLICATIONS

From the scheme given above, several predictions can be made and tested experimentally: (i) the hormone should be present at its postulated site of action, the nucleus; (ii) as a consequence of gene activation, RNA synthesis should be stimulated; and (iii) biosynthesis of specific proteins (enzymes) directed by the newly formed m-RNA can be anticipated. This is called "enzyme induction".

Some of these predictions (all those arising from induced new-gene activity) also would be consequences of Kroeger's hypothesis. The main difference between his hypothesis and our scheme is the site of action of ecdysone: the cell membrane (or, as Kroeger later modified it, the nuclear membrane) or the nucleus itself, i.e., the chromatin.

Nevertheless, from a more general point of view, as a biochemical proof of our hypothesis, it seemed worthwhile to look also for RNA and protein bio-synthesis. To review this older work briefly, RNA synthesis increased after treatment with ecdysone (Karlson and Peters, 1965 and Sekeris *et al.*, 1965). As for induction of protein synthesis, we were fortunate enough to find a physiologically significant enzyme to investigate: *DOPA* decarboxylase. Earlier work in our laboratory has demonstrated that ecdysone causes changes in tyrosine metabolism, ultimately giving rise to the production of the sclerotizing agent, N-acetyl-dopamin (Karlson and Sekeris, 1969b and 1966b). This whole field has been worked out in detail by Sekeris and co-workers whose work appears elsewhere in this volume.

To solve the crucial question: "Where is the site of action of ecdysone?", we tried to locate labeled ecdysone in homogenates after differential centri-fugation (Karlson *et al.*, 1964). This met with partial success; about 50 per cent of the radioactivity recovered in the epidermis was spun down with the nuclei. More recent experiments of Emmerich (1969) using highly labeled synthetic ecdysone and radioautographic techniques showed indeed more radioactivity at the site of the nuclei than in cytoplasm and membranes. Since these experiments were done with salivary glands (of *Drosophila hydei*), they are a strong argument against Kroeger.

We also found that isolated nuclei are able to respond to ecdysone *in vitro* (Dukes *et al.*, 1966), thus excluding a primary action of ecdysone at the cellular membrane as visualized in Kroeger's first papers. With isolated nuclei from fat-body cells, we have now studied the effect of inorganic ions, ecdysone, and juvenile hormone (Congote *et al.*, 1969).

We found that Na^+, but not K^+, markedly stimulated RNA synthesis in nuclei of isolated fat-body cells. This is at variance with Kroeger's findings. Moreover, the effect of ecdysone (and also juvenile hormone) was seen even in the absence of ions, thus not allowing the action of an "ion pump". This seems to rule out at least the generalized theory of Kroeger. We believe that the experimental results in both types of experiments can best be explained by the assumption that we are dealing here with the well known general effect of higher salt concentration on the binding of protein to DNA. Proteins can be stripped from DNA by salt solutions, and the template activity of chromatin preparations is greatly increased by such treatment. In salivary-gland chromosomes, the critical salt concentration may vary from locus to locus, thus giving a more or less reproducible "artifact pattern".

We have also characterized the RNA produced under treatment with ecdysone and juvenile hormone by hybridization techniques and were able to show that, indeed, new and different species of RNA were synthesized. Details are given by Dr. Sekeris. The observation that juvenile hormone and ecdysone, when applied together, gave less stimulation of RNA synthesis than ecdysone or juvenile hormone alone may be of special biological significance. This may reflect the fact that juvenile hormone preserves the *status quo* or, in other words, inhibits development towards the adult; therefore, those genes determining pupal or imaginal characteristics will not be expressed in the presence of ecdysone plus juvenile hormone, but only by ecdysone alone.

POSSIBLE MECHANISM FOR CONTROL OF TRANSCRIPTION

Having rejected Kroeger's theory on the basis of experimental evidence, it is appropriate to discuss some possible mechanisms for interaction of ecdysone with the chromatin. In the past, we have often interpreted our postulated mechanism of hormonal action (Figure 4) in terms of the Jacob-Monod (1961) model for regulation of genic activity (Karlson, 1966; and Karlson and Sekeris, 1966 b and c). Indeed, the model would fit our experimental findings with ecdysone extremely well; ecdysone acts as an inducer, combining with a postulated repressor and thus triggering induction of puff, RNA synthesis, and synthesis of *DOPA* decarboxylase. It should be stressed, however, that our scheme does not depend on the Jacob-Monod model and was actually proposed before the Jacob and Monod paper was published.

Taking into account the much higher complexity of eucaryonts, especially the organization of the genetic material into a set of chromosomes and the development of nuclear membrane, the indiscriminate application of the Jacob-Monod model actually seems unjustified. It has also been pointed out that higher organisms contain much more DNA than presumably needed for the coding of their proteins, the increase as compared to bacteria being several thousand fold. Moreover, it is known that high organisms contain a fair percentage of redundant DNA and that much of the RNA transcribed never leaves the nucleus but is used and degraded there. One may presume that it serves a regulatory function.

To account for this, several models have been put forward. Mainly two of them will be discussed (Georgiev, 1969; Britten and Davidson, 1969). Both make use of the fact that the first product of transcription in higher organism is a large molecule and that repetitive DNA is scattered throughout the genome.

Georgiev postulates that operons (defined as units of transcription, starting with a promoter region and ending in a terminator region) contain, proximal to the promoter, several other acceptor regions on the DNA used for regulation. The distal part, about half of the operon, represents informational DNA, i.e., structural genes (Figure 5A). In the acceptor part, many sites can be recognized by specific proteins, resulting either in repression (negative control) or derepression (positive control, exerted by removal of histones, for example). On the other hand, the same acceptor DNA might be present in several or many operons, thus forming redundant DNA. This allows a simultaneous control of a whole set of operons and also accounts for a physiological role of redundant DNA sequences that otherwise would be lost during evolution.

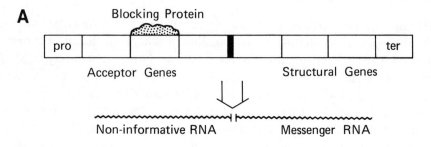

Figure 5a.

The Structure of the Operon in Higher Animals as Proposed by Georgiev (1969)

[pro = promoter region, ter = terminator.] The same acceptor genes may be present in the regulatory part of several operons, thus forming redundant DNA. The non-informative RNA, a by-product of transcription, is confined to the nucleus.

   Britten and Davidson (1969), going one step further, postulate the production of a "second signal" in the form of an activator RNA. This activator RNA is produced by transcription of "integrator genes" linked to a "sensor" (visualized as a protein reacting to metabolites, hormones, etc.). The interaction of the "sensor" with the regulating molecule results in transcription of the integrator genes, producing several activator RNA's (possibly through cleavage of a large RNA). In turn these can combine, in a sequence-specific manner, with receptor genes linked to structural genes. This results in transcription of the structural or "producer" genes yielding m-RNA for translation and possibly also part of the other sequences as non-translatable RNA.
   The salient feature of this model is the postulate that each sensor-integrator unit can contain one or several integrators in common with other units, and that the receptor-structural-gene units also may have some or many receptor regions in common. This is illustrated in Figure 5B for two examples. Thus the integrator genes serve to integrate the activity (transcription) of a variety of receptor-structural-gene units, and each receptor-structural unit can be controlled by several sensor-integrator units. Since the DNA sequences of the same integrator gene in different units are virtually

identical, this accounts for the repetitive sequences of DNA, and the same applies for the identical receptor genes in the different receptor-structural-gene units.

The functional units in this scheme are very similar to Georgiev's "operon". The main difference lies in the postulated production of a second signal (activator RNA) capable of activating, in an integrated or concerted fashion, several other "operons". In Georgiev's scheme, this can only be brought about by putting the same "sensor protein" on all the different

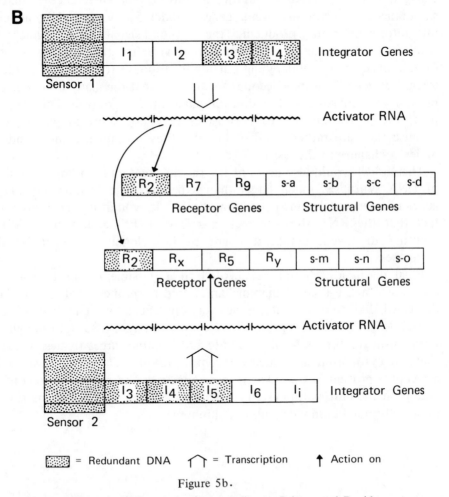

Figure 5b.

Gene Regulation in Higher Animals According to Britten and Davidson

Only two sets of integrator genes and regulatory-structural operons are shown. When sensor 1 is activated, the set of integrator genes is transcribed into activator RNA; this will activate both receptor-structural operons. Sensor 2 will act only on one of those illustrated, but of course on a number of others. The activator RNA involved in regulation makes up for the bulk of RNA confined to the nucleus.

operons. However, the scheme of Britten and Davidson accounts also for the fact that a special RNA of high molecular weight with DNA-like base composition is produced but never translated (D-RNA$_2$ in the terminology of Georgiev); it remains confined to the nucleus and is finally degraded.

Without going into the details, it may be pointed out that the principle of recognition of a piece of DNA and a "signal" in the form of a small molecule (a metabolite, a hormone, or an embryonic inducer) is very much the same in both cases, inherited from the Jacob-Monod model and not principally changed but only modified during evolution. The difference is that, for simultaneous control of several genes, model 5B needs only one sensor-integrator-gene unit, producing the "second-signal RNA" which then regulates many genes. It is tempting to visualize the locus 1-18-C in *Chironomus tentans* undergoing puffing in response to ecdysone as such an integrator gene. This may account for the fact that the many processes set in motion by ecdysone at the time of pupation are controlled through one puff; the activation of producer genes may not show in puffing either because they are rather small or because they are already there and only undergo changes in their size.

This model would also account for the fact that a rather large stimulation of RNA synthesis, much larger than expected from turning on only one gene, is measured by incorporation studies. It would also account for the fact that the RNA shows a high degree of hybridization in our studies, pointing to the fact that it might be homologous to repetitive DNA sequences.

Final discussion should be devoted to a possible receptor protein for ecdysone. In the field of mammalian steroid hormones, proteins have been described that bind these hormones very specifically with a low dissociation constant. These receptor proteins occur only in target tissues; this might be a mechanism for tissues to differentiate and become target tissues. Moreover, there are cytoplasmic and nuclear receptor proteins. There may be a need for a receptor protein in the nucleus to recognize the hormone and to confer its action on the chromatin system. We are now working towards the isolation of an ecdysone-binding protein in Calliphora.

References

1. ASHBURNER, M.: Function and Structure of Polytene Chromosomes During Insect Development. Advances Insect Physiol., 7:1-95, 1970.

2. BRITTEN, R. J. and DAVIDSON, E. H.: Gene Regulation for Higher Cells: a Theory. Science, 165:349-357, 1969.

3. BUTENANDT, A. and KARLSON, P.: Über die Isolierung eines Metamorphose-Hormons der Insekten in Kristallisierter Form. Z. Naturforsch., 9b:389-391, 1954.

4. CLEVER, U.: Gene Activity in the Giant Chromosomes of *Chironomus tentans* and its Relation to Development I. Gene Activation by Ecdysone. Chromosoma, 12:607-675, 1961.

5. CLEVER, U.: Von der Ecdysonkongentration abhängige Genaktivitätsmuster in den Speicheldrüsenchromosomen von *Chironomus tentans.* Dev Biol., 6:73-98,1963.

6. CLEVER, U.: Regulation of Chromosome Function. Ann. Rev. Genet., 2:11, 1968.

7. CLEVER, U. and KARLSON, P.: Induction of Puff Changes in the Salivary Gland Chromosomes of *Chironomus tentans* by Ecdysone. Exptl. Cell Res., 20: 623-626, 1960.

8. CONGOTE, L. F., SEKERIS, C. E., and KARLSON, P.: On the Mechanism of Hormone Action. 13. Stimulating Effects of Ecdysone, Juvenile Hormone and Ions on RNA Synthesis in Fat Body Cell Nuclei from *Calliphora erythrocephala* Isolated by a Filtration Technique. Exptl. Cell Res., 56:338-346, 1969.

9. DUKES,P. P., SEKERIS, C. E., and SCHMID, W.: Wirkung von Ecdyson auf Epidermiszellkerne von *Calliphora*- Larven *in Vitro.* Hoppe-Seyler's Z. Physiol. Chemie, 341: 152-154, 1965.

10. ELLGAARD, E. G. and KESSEL, R. G.: Effects of High Salt Concentration on Salivary Gland Cells of *Drosophila virilis.* Exptl. Cell Res., 42:302-307, 1966.

11. EMMERICH, H.: Anreicherung von Tritiummarkiertem Ecdyson in den Zellkernen der Speicheldrüsen von *Drosophila hydei.* Exptl. Cell Res., 58:261-270, 1969.

12. GABE, M., KARLSON, P., and ROCHES, J.: Hormones in Invertebrates. *In*: M. Florkin and H. Mason (ed.), Comparative Biochemistry, 6:245-298, 1964.

13. GEORGIEV, G. P.: On the Structural Organization of Operon ånd the Regulation of RNA Synthesis in Animal Cells. J. Theor. Biol., 25:473-490, 1969.

14. HAMPSHIRE, F. and HORN, D. H. S.: Structure of Crustecdysone, a Crustacean Molting Hormone. Chem. Commun., pp. 37-38. 1966.

15. HOFFMEISTER, H.: Ecdysteron, ein neues Häutungshormon der Insekten. Angew. Chem. 78:269-270, 1966.

16. HUBER, R. and HOPPE, W.: Zur Chemie des Ecdysons VII. Die Kristall-u. Molekülstrukturanalyse des Insektenverpuppungs-hormons Ecdyson mit der Automatisierten Faltmolekülmethode. Chem. Ber., 98:2403-2424, 1965.

17. JACOB, F. and MONOD, J.: Genetic Regulatory Mechanisms in the Synthesis of Proteins. J. Molec. Biol. , 3:318-356, 1961.

18. KARLSON, P.: Die Prothorakaldrüsenhormone der Insekten: Chemische Eigenschaften und Physiologische Bedeutung. Congres Internat. de Biochemie, Bruxelles, Abstract 12-3, 1955.

19. KARLSON, P.: Biochemical Studies on Insect Hormones. Vitamins and Hormones, 14:227-266, 1956.

20. KARLSON, P.: Chemische Untersuchungen über die Metamorphosehormone der Insekten. Ann. Sci. Nat. Zool., 18:125-137, 1956.

21. KARLSON, P.: Biochemical Mode of Action of Hormones. Dtsch. Med. Wschr., *86*:668-674, 1961.

22. KARLSON, P.: New Concepts of the Mode of Action of Hormones. Persp. Biol.Med., *6*:203-214, 1963.

23. KARLSON, P., HOFFMEISTER, H., HUMMEL, H., HOCKS, P., and SPITTELLER, G.: Zur Chemie des Ecdysons. VI. Reaktionen des Ecdysonmoleküls. Chem. Ber., *98*: 2394-2402, 1965.

24. KARLSON, P. and PETERS, G.: Zum Wirkungsmechanismus der Hormone. IV. Der einfluss des Ecdysons auf den nuclein-saurestoffwechsel von *Calliphora-* Larven. Gen. Compar. Endocr., *5*:252-259, 1965.

25. KARLSON, P. and SEKERIS, C. E.: N-Acetyl-dopamine as Sclerotizing Agent of the Insect Cuticle. Nature, *195*:183-184, 1962.

26. KARLSON, P. and SEKERIS, C. E.: On Tyrosine Metabolism of Insects. IX. Control of Tyrosine Metabolism by Ecdysone. Biochim. Biophys. Acta, *63*:489-495, 1962.

27. KARLSON, P. and SEKERIS, C. E.: Biosynthesis of Catecholamines in Insects. Pharmacol. Rev., *18*:89-94, 1966.

28. KARLSON, P. and SEKERIS, C. E.: Ecdysone, an Insect Steroid Hormone, and Its Mode of Action. Rec. Progr. Hormone Res., *22*:473-502, 1966.

29. KARLSON, P. and SEKERIS, C. E.: Biochemical Mechanisms of Hormone Action. Acta Endocrinologia, *53*:505-518, 1966.

30. KARLSON, P., SEKERIS, C. E., and MAURER, R.:   Zum Wirkungsmechanismus der Hormone. I. Verteilung von Tritium-markiertem Ecdyson in Larven von *Calliphora erythrocephala.* Hoppe-Seyler's Z. Physiol. Chemie, *336*:100-106, 1964.

31. KROEGER, H.: Chemical Nature of the System Controlling Gene Activities in Insect Cells. Nature (London), *200*:1234-1235, 1963.

32. KROEGER, H. and LEZZI, U.: Regulation of Gene Action in Insect Development. Ann. Rev. Entomol., *11*:1-22, 1966.

33. LEZZI, M.: Induktion eines Ecdyson-aktivierbaren Puff in Isolierten Zellkernen von Chironomus durch KCL. Exptl. Cell Res., *43*:571-577, 1966.

34. LUSCHER, M. and KARLSON, P.: Experimentelle Auslösung von Hautungen bei der Termite *Kalotermes flavicollis* (Fabr.). J. Insect Physiol., *1*:341-345, 1958.

35. NOVÁK, V. J. A.: *Insect Hormones,* Second Edition, Methuen, London, 1967.

36. ROBBINS, W. E., KAPLANIS, J. N., SVOBODA, J. A., and THOMPSON, M. J.:   Steroid Metabolism in Insects. Ann. Rev. Entomol., *16*:53, 1971.

37. SEKERIS, C. E., DUKES, P. P., and SCHMID, W.: Wirkung von Ecdyson auf Epidermiszellkerne von *Calliphora*-Larven *in Vitro.* Hoppe-Seyler's Z. Physiol.Chemie, *341*:152-154, 1965.

38. THOMPSON, M. J., KAPLANIS, J. N., ROBBINS, W. E., and YAMAMOTO, R. T.:   20,26-Dihydroxyecdysone, a New Steroid with Molting Hormone Activity from the Tobacco Hornworm, *Manduca sexta* (Johannson). Chem. Commun., *13*:650-653, 1967.

MOLECULAR ACTION
of INSECT HORMONES

Constantin E. Sekeris

S everal mechanisms of action have been proposed recently concerning insect and other hormones, and a tremendous amount of work has been published favoring the one or the other hypothesis. A review of the whole field will not be attempted but will be limited to a discussion of our own work, which was stimulated by the hormone-gene activation hypothesis described by Karlson in this volume (Karlson, 1963; Karlson and Sekeris, 1966a, 1966b:Sekeris, 1971). Salient features of this hypothesis are that hormones act in a way similar to bacterial inducers (Jacob and Monod, 1961), interacting with repressor proteins on the genome, resulting thus in a derepression of the genetic material and transcription of the derepressed genes into messenger RNAs which then will be translated on the ribosomes into specific proteins. The hypothesis predicts the penetration of hormone into the nucleus and its binding to respective nuclear protein(s), differential transcription of gene(s), the appearance of new m-RNA(s) in the cyto-plasm, and the synthesis *de novo* of new proteins.

In order to evaluate critically and to test this hypothesis experimentally, suitable biological systems are needed. Two such systems we have intro-duced in the past years will be described briefly.

SCLEROTIZATION OF INSECT CUTICLE
AND ITS CONTROL BY ECDYSONE

Sclerotization of the insect cuticle during the transformation of a larva to a pupa is brought about by quinone tanning of the cuticular pro-teins (Pryor, 1962). [For more details on the physiology and biochemistry of this process, see Karlson and Sekeris (1964), Sekeris (1965), and Brunet (1965).] In the blowfly, *Calliphora erythrocephala*, N-acetyl dopamine is the precursor of the tanning quinone (Karlson *et al.*, 1962) and is formed in the epidermal cells of the integument from tyrosine by way of 3,4-dihydroxy-phenyalanine (*DOPA*) and dopamine (Sekeris and Karlson, 1962) (Figure 1). [For a review of the biosynthesis of N-acetyl dopamine and the metabolism of tyrosine in late third-instar larvae of *Calliphora erythrocephala*, see Sekeris and Karlson (1966).] A small amount of N-acetyl dopamine is present in early third-instar larvae, and it is increased dramatically just before formation of the puparium. This is the result of the appearance at that time of *DOPA* decarboxylase, one of the principal enzymes involved in the biosynthesis of N-acetyl dopamine. The enzyme is induced by ecdysone (Karlson and Sekeris, 1962). This is suggested by the striking parallelism between enzy-matic activity and titer of ecdysone (Shaaya and Sekeris, 1965) (Figure 2) during the development of the larvae. Further, in blowfly larvae that have been deprived of their ecdysone by ligation, the level of the *DOPA* decar-boxylase remains very low, whereas injection of α- or β-ecdysone induces the rapid appearance of decarboxylase activity (Karlson and Sekeris, 1962) (Figure 3). This increase in enzymatic activity can be prevented by in-jecting the animals with inhibitors of protein synthesis such as puromycin (Figure 4) and inhibitors of RNA synthesis such as actinomycin D (Figure 4), suggesting the synthesis *de novo* of enzymatic protein and the participa-tion of RNA in this process (Sekeris and Karlson, 1964). These inhibitors also affect formation of the puparium (Figure 5). An interesting aspect of these experiments is the importance of exact timing in relation to develop-mental stage when administering the inhibitors, an earlier or later application having very small effects on puparium formation or enzymatic activity. Since actinomycin D acts not only on RNA synthesis but also on RNA degradation and on other processes (Rovera *et al.*, 1970; Stewart and Farber, 1968), we have reinvestigated the relationship of enzymatic induction to RNA syn-

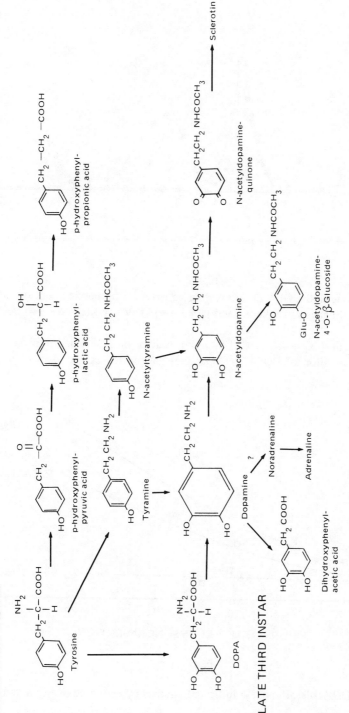

Figure 1

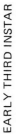

Tyrosine metabolism in third-instar larvae of *Calliphora erythrocephala* (Sekeris and Karlson, 1968).
The main pathway for formation of N-acetyl dopamine is by way of DOPA and dopamine seen in late third-instar larvae.
In early third-instar larvae, some N-acetyl dopamine can be formed by way of tyramine and N-acetyl tyramine.

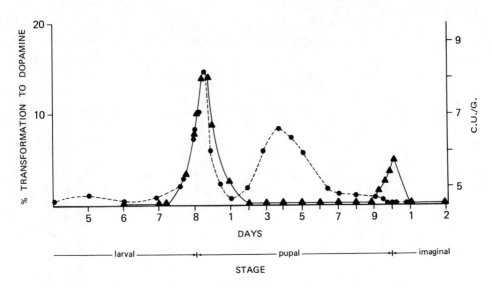

Figure 2

Titer of ecdysone and DOPA decarboxylase activity during development of *Calliphora erythrocephala* (Shaaya and Sekeris, 1965). (●– – –●) Ecdysone titer, (▲——▲) Decarboxylase activity.

Titer of ecdysone (expressed as C.U./G.) and activity of DOPA decarboxylase (as percentage transformation of DOPA to dopamine) are plotted against days of insect life.

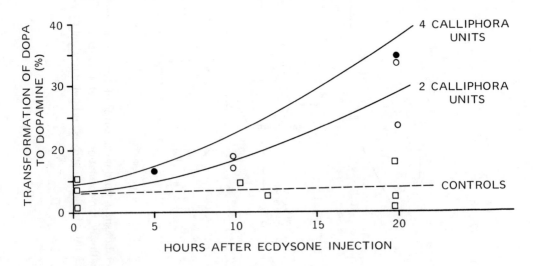

Figure 3

Induction of *DOPA* decarboxylase in ligated animals by ecdysone (Karlson and Sekeris, 1962).

The activity is expressed as percentage transformation of radioactive *DOPA* to dopamine.

thesis using as RNA inhibitor the octapeptide α-amanitin which acts directly on the DNA-dependent RNA polymerase of eucaryotes. [For a review of α-amanitin action, see Fiume and Wieland (1970).]

The effects of the toxin on RNA synthesis of blowfly larvae were studied first. α-Amanitin was tested (a) on RNA synthesis by nuclei isolated from the integument of the larvae, (b) on RNA synthesis by soluble RNA polymerases extracted from the integument of the larvae, and (c) on the incorporation *in vivo* of RNA precursors into RNA.

The results of these experiments appear in Table 1 and in Figures 6 and 7a-c. RNA synthesis in isolated nuclei is inhibited between 40–60 per cent by α-amanitin (Shaaya and Sekeris, 1972), depending on the ionic strength of the incubation medium (Table 1). [See also Seifart and Sekeris (1968).] As in other systems (Fiume and Wieland, 1970) only the RNA polymerase eluting at higher ionic strength from the DEAE-cellulose column corresponding to enzyme II (Blatti *et al.*, 1970) or B (Chambon *et al.*, 1970) is inhibited; whereas the activity of the polymerase corresponding to the nucleolar enzyme I (Blatti *et al.*, 1970) or A (Chambon *et al.*, 1970) is not

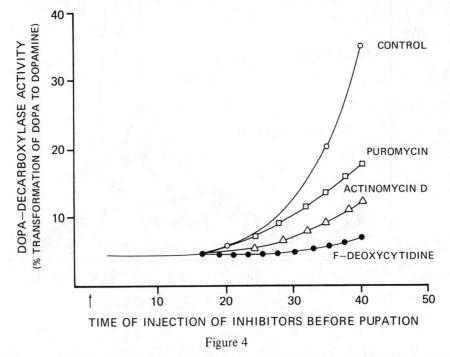

Figure 4

Influence of different inhibitors on the induction of *DOPA* decarboxylase (Sekeris and Karlson, 1962).

The ordinate shows enzymatic activity as percentage transformation of *DOPA* to dopamine; the abscissa, the time of measurement after injection of the substances.

affected at all (Figure 6). However, within 3 to 5 hours after amanitin administration *in vivo*, both DNA-like and ribosomal RNA are inhibited up to 55-
85 per cent. The inhibition of DNA-like RNA can be demonstrated by
pulsing with ^{3}H-orotic acid for 30 minutes *in vivo*, which labels DNA-like
RNA almost exclusively (Shaaya *et al.*, 1971) so that inhibition of RNA
synthesis by α-amanitin under these conditions reflects the inhibition of the

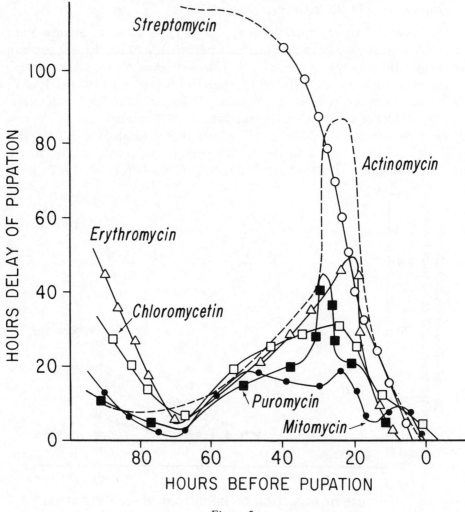

Figure 5

Influence of injection of inhibitors on the pupation of Calliphora larvae (Sekeris and
Karlson, 1964).

The delay of pupation in hours is plotted against the time of injection of the antibiotics
before pupation.

TABLE 1

EFFECT OF α–AMANITIN ON RNA SYNTHESIS
BY ISOLATED NUCLEI FROM EPIDERMIS OF CALLIPHORA LARVAE

Ionic Condition	Total c.p.m. Incorporated into Nuclear RNA		
	Control	α–Amanitin	Per Cent Inhibition
Mn^{2+}	137 122 107	71 68 65	44
$Mn^{2+} + (NH_4)_2 SO_4$	408 410 413	174 177 180	57
Mg^{2+}	103 92 82	45 57 69	40
$Mg^{2+} + (NH_4)_2 SO_4$	279 279 278	98 108 118	61

Nuclei were isolated from the integument by homogenization in 0.25 M. sucrose containing .025 M. KCl, .02 M. $MgCl_2$, and .065 M. tris-HCl at pH 7.55 after filtration through 8 layers of cheese cloth and centrifugation for 5 minutes at 1200 x g., the sediment was taken up in 2 ml. of the same buffer and layered on 20 ml. of 10 per cent (w./v.) Ficoll in the same buffer. The sediment obtained after centrifugation at 1,200 x g. for 20 minutes was taken up in .065 M. tris-HCl at pH 7.9 and used as the nuclear preparation.

The RNA synthesizing mixture consisted of 1 mM. each of ATP, GTP, CTP; 0.1 μCi. ^{14}C-UTP (55 mCi./mM.); 10 μg. creatine phosphokinase, 10 μM. creatine phosphate; 3.0 μM. mercaptoethanol; 0.5 μM. $MnSO_4$ or 3 μM. $MgSO_4$; NH_4SO_4; 0.4 ionic strength; 60 I.U. penicillin G; 20 μM. tris-HCl (pH 7.9). α-Amanitin was added in a dose of 2 μg./ml. Incubation was performed for 10 minutes at 37° C. The measurement of incorporated radioactivity was made by precipitating aliquots on filter paper as described by Lukacs and Sekeris (1967). The values are the average of duplicate experiments (Shaaya and Sekeris, 1972).

DNA-like RNA. By prolonging the duration of the pulse to three hours, ribosomal RNA is also labeled. As illustrated in Figures 7a and 7b, amanitin inhibits the synthesis of ribosomal RNA, almost no labeled ribosomal RNA appearing in the cytoplasm (Figure 7b); whereas the synthesis of t-RNA is affected to a much lesser extent (Figure 7c). Similar effects of α-amanitin *in vivo* have been observed in mammalian systems (Niessing *et al.*, 1970). The discrepancy between findings *in vivo* and *in vitro* have been discussed previously (Niessing *et al.*, 1970).

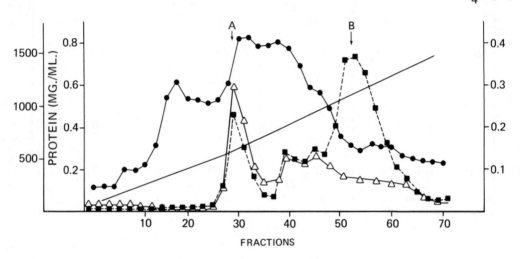

Figure 6

Effect of α-amanitin on the multiple forms of DNA-dependent RNA polymerase from the integument of blowfly larvae. (■----■) Control, (△——△) α-Amanitin-treated, (●——●) Protein, (———) NH$_4$Cl Gradient.

Integument prepared from late third-instar larvae was extracted with .067 M. tris, 1mM. mercaptoethanol, 10 mM. NH$_4$Cl, 10 mM. MgCl$_2$, 0.25 mM. EDTA, and 1 M. (NH$_4$)$_2$SO$_4$ in 20 per cent glycerin at pH 7.9 for one hour and then centrifuged at 45,000 x g. for 15 minutes. Ammonium sulphate was added to the supernatant (final molarity 3.5), and the protein precipitated was collected by centrifugation. Then the sediment was taken up in 0.01 M. tris buffer (pH 7.9) containing NH$_4$Cl, MgCl$_2$, EDTA, and glycerin as above, passed through Sephadex G-25, and chromatographed on DEAE-cellulose.

Elution was performed with an ammonium chloride gradient (0–0.4 M.). The details of the method are published elsewhere. The assay for RNA synthesis is described by Seifart and Sekeris (1969); α-amanitin was added in a concentration of 1 μg./ml.

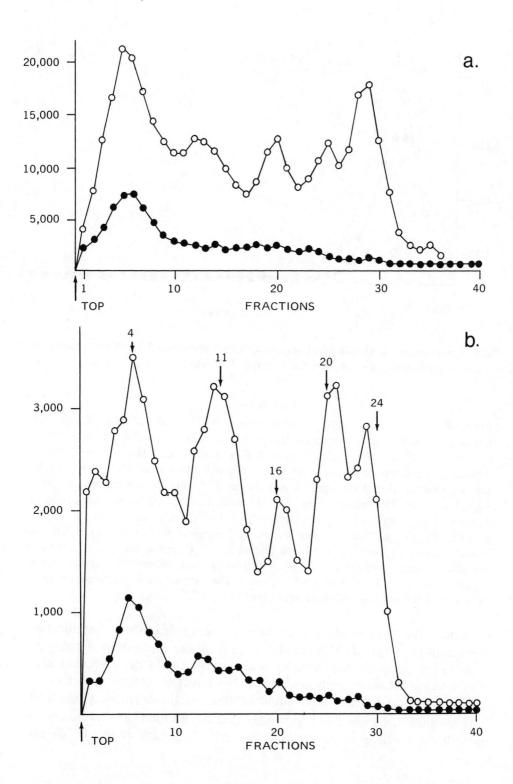

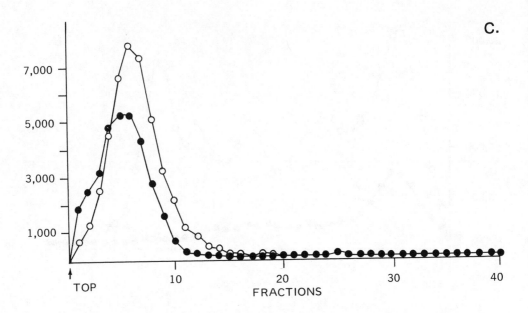

a = Crude nuclear-mitochondrial fraction; b = Crude microsomal fraction; c = Supernatant
(○———○) Controls, (●———●) Amanitin-treated, ▼ S Values.

Figures 7a,b,c

Effect of injection of α-amanitin on incorporation of ^{3}H-orotic acid into RNA of crude
nuclear, microsomal, and supernatant fractions of blowfly larvae. Five μg. amanitin per
animal were injected both 6 and 3 hours before sacrifice and ^{3}H-orotic-acid pulse for
3 hours. The integument of the larvae was homogenized in sucrose-salt buffer, pH 7.55,
the homogenate filtered through 6 layers cheese cloth, and the filtrate centrifuged at
40,000 x g. for 15 minutes to give a crude nuclear-mitochondrial pellet (fraction a).
The supernatant was centrifuged additionally at 250,000 x g. for 60 minutes to give
a crude microsomal fraction (fraction b) and supernatant (fraction c). RNA was
extracted from all three fractions with phenol at 37° C. in the presence of SDS and
bentonite. Sucrose-gradient centrifugation (15-30 per cent sucrose) was carried out at
24,000 r.p.m. for 14 hours in a SW 41 rotor. The method used for measurement of
radioactivity is described by Schutz *et al.* (1968).

Turning then to enzymatic induction, we were able to show that injection
of α-amanitin in ligated Calliphora larvae prior to the application of ecdysone
significantly abolishes the increase in activity of *DOPA* decarboxylase seen
after administration of ecdysone alone. No effect on enzymatic activity is
seen if amanitin is given after administration of the hormone (Figure 8).

It is concluded from this experiment that the hormone affects enzymatic
induction by acting at the transcriptional level (Sekeris *et al.*, 1970) and

that new RNA is needed for the synthesis of the enzyme, very probably among others the m-RNA coding for the *DOPA* decarboxylase. The interpretation of the above data on the basis of a post-transcriptional control, as suggested by Tomkins (Tomkins *et al.*, 1970), is rendered unlikely: no superinduction of *DOPA* decarboxylase can be observed as described for the tyrosine transaminase in hepatoma cells (Tomkins *et al.*, 1970). Early experiments demonstrated that the addition of RNA derived from nuclei in the

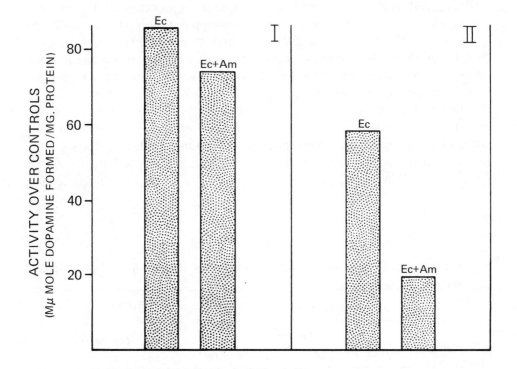

Figure 8

Effects of amanitin on the induction of *DOPA* decarboxylase in ligated Calliphora larvae (Shaaya and Sekeris, Submitted for publication).

Posterior parts of ligated Calliphora larvae were used 24 hours after pupation of the head. a-Amanitin (1 μg./5 μl. insect Ringer's solution) and ecdysone (0.75 μg./5 μl. insect Ringer's solution) were given:
I ecdysone for 5 hours and amanitin for the last 2 hours;
II amanitin for 8 hours and ecdysone for the last 5 hours.
Groups of 15 animals were used for each experiment. Determination of enzyme was performed on the basis of transformation of ^{14}C-*DOPA* to ^{14}C-dopamine which was separated by paper electrophoresis and measured by scintillation counting (Sekeris and Karlson, 1962).

epidermis of ecdysone-induced Calliphora larvae (but not from animals without induction) to a ribosomal system derived from murine liver under conditions of protein synthesis led to the appearance of *DOPA* decarboxylase activity (Sekeris, 1967; Sekeris and Lang, 1964). These experiments suggested the appearance of m-RNA coding for the *DOPA* decarboxylase resulting from the action of ecdysone. Due to the fact that the hepatic ribosomes used have detectable endogenous *DOPA* decarboxylase, it was imperative to show with immunochemical methods that indeed insect *DOPA* decarboxylase is formed *in vitro* under the experimental conditions employed. The rapid progress in the development of systems translating exogenous m-RNA *in vitro* has led us to reconsider and expand our earlier findings additionally, using advanced techniques. Searching for the m-RNA coding of *DOPA* decarboxylase, newly synthesized RNA in the integument of control and hormone-induced animals has been examined by means of double-labeling techniques. As demonstrated previously (Sekeris *et al.*, 1965), both DNA-like and ribosomal RNA synthesis in the nucleus is stimulated by ecdysone within one to two hours (Table 2). Within three hours a significant increase of labeled RNA in microsomal fractions was found. This RNA is mainly of the DNA-like type, so it probably reflects a

TABLE 2

EFFECT OF ECDYSONE ON THE INCORPORATION OF ^{32}P INTO RNA OF EPIDERMIS

Time after Injection of Ecdysone (Hours)	Radioactivity (Counts per Minute per Mg. RNA)					
	Nuclear RNA				Microsomal RNA	
	50° Fraction		65° Fraction			
	Control	Hormone-treated	Control	Hormone-treated	Control	Hormone-treated
1	842	1578	421	1005	550	452
2	2855	3205	2158	2736	2105	1504
3	–	–	–	–	2252	3258

Ligated animals were injected with 5 Calliphora units of ecdysone and 10 μCi. of H_3 $^{32}PO_4$. Controls received only labeled orthophosphate. RNA was prepared at different intervals of time from nuclei and microsomes isolated from the integument of 20 animals (Sekeris *et al.*, 1965).

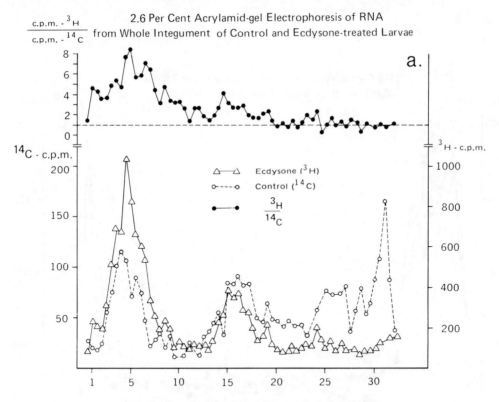

2.6 Per Cent Acrylamid-gel Electrophoresis of RNA
from Whole Integument of Control and Ecdysone-treated Larvae

$$\frac{c.p.m. - {}^{3}H}{c.p.m. - {}^{14}C}$$

a.

${}^{14}C$ - c.p.m.

${}^{3}H$ - c.p.m.

△——△   Ecdysone (^{3}H)

○----○   Control (^{14}C)

●——● $\dfrac{{}^{3}H}{{}^{14}C}$

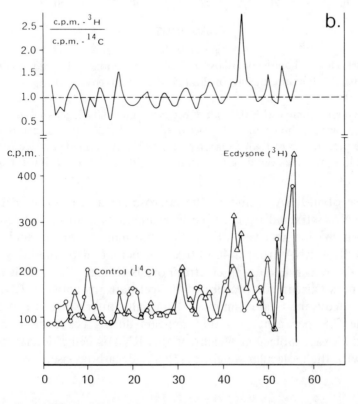

7.5 Per Cent Acrylamid-gel Electrophoresis of RNA
from Whole Integument of Control and Ecdysone-treated Larvae

b.

$$\frac{c.p.m. - {}^{3}H}{c.p.m. - {}^{14}C}$$

c.p.m.

Ecdysone (^{3}H)

Control (^{14}C)

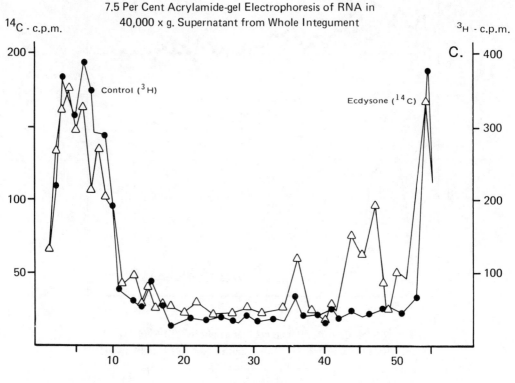

FRACTIONS

Figures 9a,b,c

Acrylamide-gel electrophoresis of RNA derived from whole (a,b) and 40,000 x g. supernatant (c) of the integument of ligated Calliphora larvae (Osang and Sekeris, in preparation).

Ligated larvae were injected with 0.03 μg. β-ecdysone in insect Ringer's solution or with insect Ringer's alone 3 hours prior to sacrifice. ^{3}H- or ^{14}C-orotic acid was injected 1 hour before preparation of RNA (Shaaya et al., 1971). Acrylamide-gel electrophoresis was performed in principle according to Loening (1969). Direction of flow is from right to left.

true increase of m-RNA bound to the microsomes as a result of action by ecdysone. RNA extracted from whole integument of control and ecdysone-treated larvae having received ^{3}H-orotic acid and ^{14}C-orotic acid respectively, as well as RNA from a 40,000 x g. supernatant of the integument, were analyzed by acrylamide-gel electrophoresis (Figures 9a-c). It is evident that differences exist in the profiles of the gel patterns between RNA from control and ecdysone-treated animals. Especially interesting is a peak evident in the 7.5 per cent gels that appears during ecdysone treatment. Currently the exact molecular weight of this RNA is being determined and correlated with the molecular weight of *DOPA* decarboxylase.

THE EFFECTS OF ECDYSONE AND JUVENILE HORMONE ON ISOLATED NUCLEI

As mentioned above, there is no doubt that ecdysone stimulates RNA synthesis in target tissues. Earlier indirect evidence, such as the rapid uptake of ecdysone by the nuclei of the epidermis (Karlson *et al.*, 1964), suggested that the primary reactions leading to increase in RNA synthesis should be sought within the confines of the nucleus as postulated by the hormone-genic activation hypothesis. Therefore, it was thought worthwhile to develop systems utilizing isolated nuclei *in vitro* that would permit a more

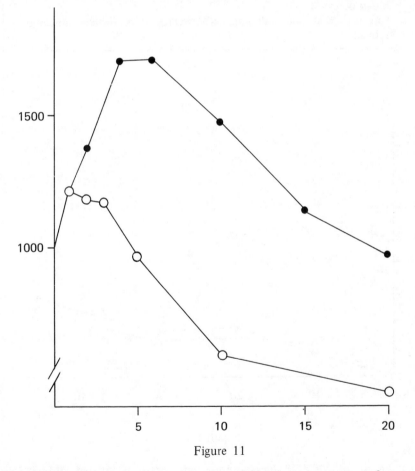

Figure 11

RNA synthesis of fat-body nuclei related to different concentration of magnesium sulfate and manganese (II) sulfate (Congote *et al.*, 1969).

Abscissa: μM. $MgSO_4$ or $MnSO_4$ present in 300 μl. medium; ordinate: ^{14}C-UTP incorporation in c.p.m./A_{260}.

●———● $MgSO_4$, ○———○ $MnSO_4$.

TABLE 3

METHOD FOR ISOLATING FAT–BODY NUCLEI

1. Homogenize fat body in .25 M. sucrose, .025 M. KCl, .02 M. MgCl$_2$, .012 M. ascorbic acid, .05 M. tris, and penicillin G (150 I.U./ml., pH 7.55).
2. Pass through 8 layers of cheese cloth and nylon.
3. Layer filtrate over 10 per cent Ficoll in sucrose-salt buffer and centrifuge at 365 xg. for 20 minutes.
4. Suspend sediment in sucrose-salt medium and filter through nylon (50-μ pores).
5. Pass filtrate through millipore NCW PO12 filters. (Nuclei remain on filters.)

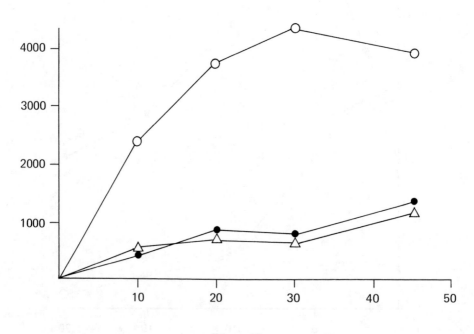

Figure 10

Temporal course of ^{14}C-UTP incorporation into RNA of isolated fat-body nuclei. (○——○) Control Incubation, (△——△) Incubation with Actinomycin D (0.40 μg./ml.), (●——●) Incubation with Ribonuclease (100 μg./ml.).

Fat-body nuclei were incubated in 300 μl. of medium containing: 0.5 mM. each of ATP, GTP, and CTP; 0.2 μCi. ^{14}C-UTP; 3.0 mM. of magnesium sulfate; 60 I.U. penicillin G; and 20 mM. of tris, pH 7.9. [For further details, see Congote *et al.* (1969).]

detailed and thorough examination of the very early effects of hormones on transcription in case they responded to added hormone with increased RNA synthesis. Nuclei were isolated from the integument of late third-instar Calliphora larvae (Sekeris *et al.*, 1965) as well as from the fat body of larvae at different stages of development (Congote *et al.*, 1969). The nuclei of the integument responded to ecdysone with increased RNA synthesis. [For a review of these experiments, see Karlson and Sekeris (1966a).] The system of isolated fat-body nuclei has been developed in collaboration with Dr. L. F. Congote. The nuclei have been isolated by a filtration technique as shown in Table 3. They are able to incorporate radioactive RNA precursors into RNA (Figure 10) in the presence of either Mn or Mg as the bivalent ion (Figure 11). The main features of the system are the following:

a. Both ecdysone and juvenile hormone stimulate the incorporation of labeled precursor into RNA (Table 4). The increase in RNA synthetic capacity of the nuclei as a result of hormonal action is independent of changes in pool size or penetration of precursors into nuclei, since RNA synthesis takes place under conditions of nuclear rupture. There is no difference in ribonuclease activity of the different preparations. Increased transcription very probably reflects a change in the nuclear-chromatin-RNA-polymerase complex (Beato *et al.*, 1970).

b. The hormonal effects are independent of the ionic milieu (See Karlson, this volume, for the significance of this finding).

TABLE 4

RNA–POLYMERASE ACTIVITY OF FAT–BODY NUCLEI TREATED WITH DIFFERENT HORMONES AND IONS (EXPRESSED AS PER CENT ACTIVATION CONTROLS)

Hormonal Treatment	Control	NaCl (50 mM.)	KCl (50 mM.)
Control	0	$40 + 31$ $P < 0.02$	16 ± 33
Ecdysone (1 μG./Ml.)	34 ± 20 $P < 0.01$	$96 + 75$ $P < 0.02$	31 ± 40
Juvenile Hormone (0.1 μG./Ml.)	57 ± 50 $P < 0.05$	41 ± 38 $P < 0.05$	16 ± 39
Juvenile Hormone (0.1 μG./Ml.) and Ecdysone (1 μG./Ml.)	19 ± 33		

All data are expressed as mean $\pm$ confidence interval for $P = 0.05$ and as P level of significance by the t-test (Congote *et al.*, 1969).

c. The effect is dependent on the developmental stage of the larvae from which nuclei were isolated (Congote *et al.*, 1969). Nuclei derived from larvae of an early third-instar respond to juvenile hormone and ecdysone whereas nuclei from late third-instar larvae respond to ecdysone but not to juvenile hormone.

d. Ecdysone and juvenile hormone interact at the nuclear level (Table 4). If both ecdysone and juvenile hormone are added at the same time, no significant difference in RNA synthesis can be seen between nuclei with and without hormonal treatment.

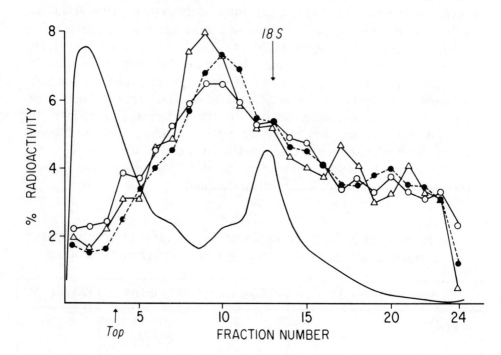

Figure 12

Sucrose density gradient sedimentation profiles of RNA synthesized in isolated fat-body nuclei after hormonal treatment (Congote *et al.*, 1970). (——) A_{254nm}, (●——●) Control, (○——○) Ecdysone-treated Nuclei, (△——△) Juvenile Hormone-treated Nuclei.

The methods for incubation and extraction are described by Schütz *et al.* (1968). Centrifugation continued for 3.5 hours at 60,000 r.p.m. Linear sucrose gradients were 5 to 30 per cent.

TABLE 5

THE EFFECTS OF HORMONES ON HYBRIDIZATION OF RNA SYNTHESIZED *IN VITRO*

Hormonal Treatment	Hybridization Capacity Expressed as Percentage of Controls	P
Controls	100	–
Ecdysone (1 μG./MI.)	143	<0.05
Juvenile Hormone (0.1 μG./MI.)	137	<0.02
Cis, Cis, Trans Isomer of Juvenile Hormone (0.1 μG./MI.)	88	–

The RNA synthesized in isolated nuclei after hormonal treatment was extracted by the hot-phenol method and its hybridization capacity tested as indicated in the section on methods. DNA/RNA = 5:1. The hybridization capacity was calculated and expressed as the percentage over controls. The P values were calculated from 10 experiments (Congote *et al.*, 1970).

TABLE 6

COMPETITIVE DNA–RNA HYBRIDIZATION OF RNA FROM
HORMONE–TREATED NUCLEI

^{3}H-labeled RNA from	RNA Not Radioactive from	Per Cent Inhibition of Hybridization
Ecdysone-treated Nuclei	Nuclei Not Treated	36
	Ecdysone-treated Nuclei	51
Juvenile Hormone-treated Nuclei	Nuclei Not Treated	43
	Juvenile Hormone-treated Nuclei	58

(Congote *et al.*, 1970)

RNA synthesized *in vitro* has been analyzed by different techniques. Sucrose-gradient analysis did not reveal any significant differences in the RNA synthesized in control and in hormone-treated nuclei (Figure 12). However, analysis by DNA-RNA molecular hybridization and hybridization-competition (Tables 5, 6, and 7) revealed:

a. that the hybridization capacity of the hormone-induced RNA is higher than that of the control (Table 5);

b. that labeled RNA derived from ecdysone-treated nuclei is competed to a greater extent with cold RNA derived from ecdysone-treated nuclei than from control preparations; the same is true for preparations treated with juvenile hormone (Table 6);

c. competition of labeled RNA derived from ecdysone-treated nuclei is higher with cold RNA derived from preparations treated with juvenile hormone than from nuclei without treatment (Table 7). The same is true for the competition of labeled "juvenile-hormone" RNA with cold "ecdysone" RNA when compared to cold "control" RNA. It is obvious that under the hybridization conditions applied, most of the RNA has hybridized to repetitive DNA sequences. At the moment a function cannot

TABLE 7

HYBRIDIZATION–COMPETITION STUDIES WITH ECDYSONE AND JUVENILE
HORMONE–EVOKED RNA SPECIES IN FAT–BODY NUCLEI

RNA Labeled with Tritium	Larval Weight (Mg.)	RNA Not Labeled from	Percentage of Initial Hybridization
Nuclei Treated with Ecdysone	51	Nuclei Not Treated	91
		Nuclei Treated with Juvenile Hormone	66
	61	Nuclei Not Treated	64
		Nuclei Treated with Juvenile Hormone	59
Nuclei Treated with Juvenile Hormone	56	Nuclei Not Treated	54
		Nuclei Treated with Ecdysone	42
	56	Nuclei Not Treated	59
		Nuclei Treated with Ecdysone	55

RNA synthesized in nuclei treated with ecdysone was incubated with RNA not labeled from nuclei not treated and with nuclei incubated with juvenile hormone. Labeled RNA: RNA not labeled: DNA = 6:6:1. In the second part of the table, the experimental conditions were the same, but labeled RNA was isolated from nuclei treated with juvenile hormone. The conditions of incubation, extraction of RNA, and hybridization are described by Congote *et al.* (1970).

be ascribed to this RNA. Nevertheless, the results of these experiments speak for the appearance of new species of RNA under the influence of the hormones and suggest further that the transcription of common genes is stimulated by the two hormones. Techniques have now been developed for the hybridization of unique sequences and are being applied currently to analyze further the RNA synthesized *in vitro* under hormonal influence.

In a similar *in-vitro* system that has been developed to test the effects of corticosteroids on RNA synthesis of rat-liver nuclei (Sekeris *et al.*, 1968), the dose of the hormone needed to stimulate RNA synthesis could be reduced from 10^{-5} M. to 10^{-7} -10^{-8} M. when incubation was performed in the presence of cytoplasmic proteins that specifically bind and transport the hormone into the nucleus (Beato *et al.*, 1970; Beato *et al.*, in press). In the experiments described here doses of the insect hormones that probably exceed concentrations *in vivo* have been used. Therefore, it will be of interest to test the effects of possible "receptor" proteins from the respective insect tissues in these *in-vitro* systems.

SUMMARY

Two biological systems are described that offer several advantages for studying molecular mechanisms of action of insect hormones:

a. The effects of ecdysone on RNA synthesis in the integument of larvae and induction of *DOPA* decarboxylase were studied by means of a system in which enzymatic induction was correlated with a specific physiological effect, the tanning of the insect cuticle. The search for m-RNA coding for *DOPA* decarboxylase, which seems to be synthesized in response to ecdysone, is under way with the help of *in-vivo* and *in-vitro* techniques.

b. The action and interaction of ecdysone and juvenile hormone on isolated fat-body nuclei induced quantitative and qualitative changes in RNA synthesis in a system suited for study of the primary steps leading to increased transcription.

Acknowledgement

Thanks are extended to Prof. P. Karlson, Dr. L. F. Congote, Dr. E. Shaaya, and M. Osang for stimulating discussions and fruitful collaborative work and to Mrs. Ch. Pfeiffer, Miss G. Froelich, and Mrs. U. Weiser for capable technical assistance. This work was generously supported by the Deutsche Forschungsgemeinschaft.

References

1. BEATO, M., BRAENDLE, W., BIESEWIG, D., and SEKERIS, C. E.: On the Mechanism of Hormone Action. XVI. Transfer of (1,2-^{3}H) Cortisol from the Cytoplasm to the Nucleus of Rat-Liver Cells. Biochim. Biophys. Acta, *208*: 125-136, 1970.

2. BEATO, M., SCHMID, W., BRAENDLE, W., BIESWIG, D., and SEKERIS, C. E.: Binding of ^{3}H-cortisol to Macromolecular Components of Rat Liver Cells and Its Relation to the Mechanism of Action of Corticosteroids. In: *Advances in the Biosciences,* No. 7. (In press)

3. BEATO, M., SEIFART, K. H., and SEKERIS, C. E.: The Effect of Cortisol on the Binding of Actinomycin D to and on the Template Activity of Isolated Rat Liver Chromatin. Arch. Biochem. Biophys., *138:*272-284, 1970.

4. BLATTI, S. P., INGLES, C.., LINDELL, T. J., MORRIS, P. W., WEAVER, R. F., WEINBERG, F., and RUTTER, W. J.: Structure and Regulatory Properties of Eucaryotic RNA Polymerase. In: Cold Spring Harbor Symposia on Quantitative Biology, Vol. XXXV, p. 649-657, 1970.

5. BRUNET, P. C. J.: The Metabolism of Aromatic Compounds. *In*: Aspects of Insect Biochemistry. Academic Press, 1965.

6. CHAMBON, P., GISSINGER, F., MANDEL. J. L.. KEDINGER, C., GNIAZDOWSKI, M, and MEIHLAC, M.: Purification and Properties of Calf Thymus DNA-Dependent RNA Polymerases A and B. In: Cold Spring Harbor Symposia on Quantitative Biology. 693-707, 1970.

7. CONGOTE, L. F., SEKERIS, C. E. and KARLSON, P.: On the Mechanism of Hormone Action. XIII. Stimulating Effects of Ecdysone, Juvenile Hormone, and Ions on RNA Synthesis in Fat Body Cell Nuclei from *Calliphora erythrocephala* Isolated by a Filtration Technique. Exptl. Cell Res., *56:*338-346, 1969.

8. CONGOTE, L. F., SEKERIS, C. E., and KARLSON, P.: On the Mechanism of Hormone Action SVIII. Alterations of the Nature of RNA Synthesized in Isolated Fat Body Cell Nuclei as a Result of Ecdysone and Juvenile Hormone Action. Z. Naturf., *25b:*279-284, 1970.

9. FIUME, L. and WIELAND, Th.: Amanitins, Chemistry and Action. FEBS Letters, *8:*1-5, 1970.

10. JACOB, F. and MONOD, J.: Genetic Regulatory Mechanisms in the Synthesis of Proteins. J. Mol. Biol., *3:*318, 1961.

11. KARLSON, P. and SEKERIS, C. E.: Zum Tyrosinstoffwechsel der Insekten IX. Kontrolle des Tyrosinstoffwechsels durch Ecdyson. Biochim. Biophys. Acta, *63:*489-495, 1962.

12. KARLSON, P.: New Concepts on the Mode of Action of Hormones. Persp. Biol. Med., *6:*203-214, 1963.

13. KARLSON, P. and SEKERIS, C. E.: Biochemistry of Insect Metamorphosis. Comparative Biochemistry, *6:*221-234, 1964.

14. KARLSON, P. and SEKERIS, C. E.: Biochemical Mechanisms of Hormone Action. Acta Endocrin., *53:*505-518, 1966.

15. KARLSON, P. and SEKERIS, C. E.: Ecdysone, an Insect Steroid Hormone and its Mode of Action. Recent Progr. Horm. Res., *22:*1473-1502, 1966.

16. KARLSON, P., SEKERIS, C. E., and MAURER, H. R.: Zum Tyrosinstoffwechsel der Hormone I. Verteilung von Tritium-markierten Ecdyson in Larven von *Calliphora erythrocephala*. Z. Physiol. Chem., *341:*100-106, 1964.

17. KARLSON, P., SEKERIS, C. E., and SEKERI, K. E.: Zum Tyrosinstoffwechsel der Insekten VI. Identifizierung von N-Acetyl-Dopamin als Tyrosinmetabolit. Z. Physiol. Chem., *327:*86-94, 1962.

18. LOENING, U.: The Determination of the Molecular Weight of Ribonucleic Acid by Polyacrylamide Gel Electrophoresis. The Effect of Changes in Conformation. Biochem. J., *113:*131-138, 1969.

19. LUKACS, I. and SEKERIS, C. E.: On the Mechanism of Hormone Action IX. Stimulation of RNA Polymerase Activity of Rat Liver Nuclei by Cortisol *in Vitro*. Biochim. Biophys. Acta, *134*:85-90, 1967.

20. NIESSING, J., SCHNIEDERS, B., KUNZ, W., SEIFART, K. H. and SEKERIS, C. E.:Inhibition of RNA Synthesis by α-Amanitin *in Vitro*. Z. Naturforsch., *25b*:1119-1125, 1970.

21. PRYOR, M. G. M.: Sclerotization. *In*: Comparative Biochemistry. IV. pp. 371-396, Academic Press, 1962.

22. ROVERA, G., BERMAN, S., and BASERGA, R.: Pulse Labelling of RNA of Mammalian Cells. Proc. Nat. Acad. Sci., *65:*876-883, 1970.

23. SCHÜTZ, G., GALLWITZ, D., and SEKERIS, C. E.: Rapidly Labelled High Molecular RNA from Rat Liver Nuclei. Europ. J. Biochem., *4:*149-156, 1968.

24. SEIFART, K. H. and SEKERIS, C. E.: α-Amanitin, a Specific Inhibitor of Transcription by Mammalian RNA Polymerase. Z. Naturforsch., *24b*:1538-1544, 1969.

25. SEKERIS, C. E.: Action of Ecdysone on RNA and Protein Metabolism in the Blowfly, *Calliphora erythrocephala*. *In:* Mechanism of Hormone Action, pp. 149-164, Thieme, 1965.

26. SEKERIS, C. E.: The Effect of Ecdysone on RNA and Protein Metabolism in Insects. *In*: BBA Library Series, *10:*388-394, 1967.

27. SEKERIS, C. E.: Molecular Action of Ecdysone. *In*: The Action of Hormones, Genes to Population, pp. 7-20, 1971.

28. SEKERIS, C. E., DUKES, P. P., and SCHMID, W.:Wirkung von Ecdyson auf Epidermis-Zellkerne von *Calliphora erythrocephala*. Z. Physiol. Chem., *341:*152-154, 1965.

29. SEKERIS, C. E., HOMOKIN, J., BEATO, M., GALWITZ, D., SEIFART, K. and LUKACS, I.: *"In Vitro"* Action of Cortisol in the Nucleus of the Liver Cell. In: *Advances in the Biosciences, 2*:222-235, 1968.

30. SEKERIS, C. E. and KARLSON, P.: Zum Tyrosinstoffwechsel der Insekten VII. Der Katabolische Abbau des Tyrosins und die Biogenese der Sklerotisierungssubstanz, N-Acetyl-Dopamin. Biochim. Biophys. Acta, *62*:103-113, 1962.

31. SEKERIS, C. E. and KARLSON, P.: On the Mechanism of Hormone Action II. Ecdysone and Protein Biosynthesis. Arch. Biochem. Biophys., *105:*483-487,1964.

32. SEKERIS, C. E. and KARLSON, P.: Biosynthesis of Catecholamines in Insects. Pharmacol. Rev., *18:*89-94, 1966.

33. SEKERIS, C. E. and LANG, N.: Induction of DOPA-Decarboxylase Activity by Insect Messenger RNA in an *in Vitro* Amino-acid Incorporating System from Rat Liver. Life Sciences, *3:*625-633, 1964.

34. SEKERIS, C. E., LANG, N., and KARLSON, P.: Zum Wirkungsmechanismus der Hormone V. Der Einfluss von Ecdyson auf den RNA-Stoffwechsel in der Epidermis der Schmeissfliege *Calliphora erythrocephala*. Z. Physiol. Chem.,*341:*36-43,1965.

35. SEKERIS, C. E., NIESSING, J., and SEIFART, K.H.: Inhibition by α-Amanitin of Induction of Tyrosine Transaminase in Rat Liver by Cortisol. FEBS Letters, *9:*103-104, 1970.

36. SHAAYA, E., SCHNIEDERS, B., KUNG, W., and SEKERIS, C. E.: Characterization of Newly Synthesized RNA in Insects by Chromatography on Columns of Methylated Albumin Kieselguhr and the Study of Its Base Composition. J. Insect Biochem., *1:*113-121, 1971.

37. SHAAYA, E. and SEKERIS, C. E.: Ecdysone During Insect Development III. Activities of Some Enzymes of Tyrosine Metabolism in Comparison with Ecdysone Titer During the Development of the Blowfly, *Calliphora erythrocephala*. Gen. Comp. Endocrin., *5:*35-39, 1965.

38. SHAAYA, E. and SEKERIS, C. E.: FEBS Letters, submitted for publication.

39. STEWART, G. and FARBER, E.: The Rapid Acceleration of Hepatic Nuclear Ribonucleic Breakdown by Actinomycin but Not by Ethionine. J. Biol. Chem., *243:*4479-4485, 1968;

40. TOMKINS, G. M., MARTIN, D. W., JR., STELLWAGEN, R. H., BAXTER, J. D.,MAMONT, P., and LEVINSON, B. B.: Regulation of Specific Protein Synthesis in Eucaryotic Cells. *In*: *Cold Spring Harbor Symposia of Quantitative Biology,* *35*:635-640, 1970.

EFFECTS of
EXOGENOUS MOLTING
HORMONE on PROTEIN
and RNA SYNTHESIS
in INSECT TISSUES

J. A. Thomson

I dentification of the insect molting hormones (MH) and elucidation of the structure of a-ecdysone (Karlson *et al.*, 1965) opened the way for Karlson and his colleagues to make a concerted attack on the problem of the mechanism of action of steroid hormones in general (Karlson, 1963; Karlson and Sekeris, 1966). The abrupt events of metamorphosis in holometabolous insects involve selective cytolysis, differentiation of particular cell types, and morphogenesis; some of these developmental events can be followed *in vitro* as well as *in vivo*. Presumptive target tissues likely to be subject to selective hormonal action are readily identifiable, and in certain Diptera the occurrence of polytene chromosomes permits the correlation of cytological and biochemical analyses, especially of genic activation.

Integration of varied studies of protein and RNA synthesis, especially in the blowfly, Calliphora, has provided evidence of hormonal control of the transcription of specific genetic information in target tissues, and a new overall model of the role of steroid hormones in development has emerged (Karlson, 1963; Karlson, 1967; Karlson and Sekeris, 1966). This model is supported by evidence of rapid effects of exogenous hormone on chromosomal puffing (Clever and Karlson, 1960; later work reviewed by Ashburner,

1970), by the distribution of exogenous hormone in various tissues (Karlson *et al.*, 1964; Thomson *et al.*, 1970), by the effects of the MH on RNA synthesis (Karlson and Peters, 1965; Sekeris, 1965; Lang and Karlson, 1965) and finally by evidence of stimulation of one (or more) specific

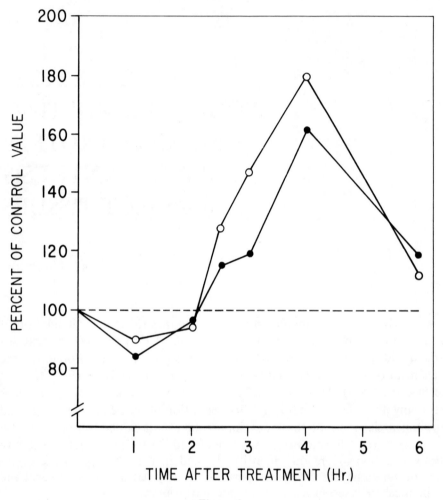

Figure 1.

Temporal course *in vivo* of changes in the incorporation *in vivo* of ^{14}C-leucine into protein of the fat body (●) and body wall (○) in day-8 larvae of *Calliphora stygia*, following injection of 0.2 μg. β-ecdysone per animal. The incorporation time of 1 hour terminated at the time the tissue was collected. The results are based on the ratio of specific activities of purified protein from batches of 5 larvae used as controls and 5 treated with hormone. Each point represents the mean of 2 determinations on separate groups of larvae from the same batch [based on data of Neufeld *et al.* (1968)].

protein species in target tissues treated with the hormone (Karlson and Sekeris, 1962; Sekeris, 1965).

Essentially, the proposed action of MH at the time of puparium formation may be summarized as follows: the hormone stimulates RNA synthesis in certain larval tissues and specifically in the epidermis (Sekeris *et al.*, 1965), leading to the synthesis of *DOPA* decarboxylase (Karlson and Sekeris, 1962), so that cellular metabolism in the epidermis is switched to production of N-acetyl dopamine (Sekeris and Karlson, 1962). Tanning of the puparium then results.

Specificity, and presumably rather direct action, at the genic level is a significant feature of Karlson's (1963, 1967) model of the action of steroid hormones, and this aspect has been widely questioned, particularly by Kroeger (*e.g.* 1967).

GENERAL EFFECTS OF MH ON PROTEIN AND RNA BIOSYNTHESIS

The model of direct and specific hormonal control on read-out at certain genetic loci does not exclude the possibility that MH may be involved in other, perhaps less specific, regulatory processes. Indeed, the broad spectrum of cellular types that show increased protein synthesis (and where examined, increased RNA synthesis) in response to exogenous hormone supports such a view. MH treatment stimulates the synthesis of heterogeneous RNA species in the fat body and integument of Calliphora, nuclear, microsomal, and soluble fractions from these cells show variously enhanced incorporation of precursors with different temporal courses (Neufeld *et al.*, 1968; Feigelson and also Karlson, in discussion, Karlson and Sekeris, 1966). Attention is drawn here to the quite different temporal course for stimulation of RNA synthesis relative to protein synthesis observed in the integument and in fat body (Neufeld *et al.*, 1968).

Enhancement of protein synthesis occurs *in vivo* at certain developmental stages in diverse larval and pupal tissues in insects (Neufeld *et al.*, 1968; Arking and Shaaya, 1969; Sahota and Mansingh, 1970) and in mammalian tissues (Burdette and Coda, 1963; Okui *et al.*, 1968; Chaudhary *et al.*, 1969). The grossly observable stimulation of protein synthesis is of short duration (see below) in insect tissues (Neufeld *et al.*, 1968), and synthesis in treated animals has returned to near control levels before the production of specific proteins such as *DOPA* decarboxylase would be significant (7-10 hours after ecdysone administration; Karlson and Sekeris, 1966). Thus two aspects of this hormonally mediated protein synthesis led us to examine the kinds of proteins involved: first, the wide range of susceptible tissues, and second, the rapid and transitory nature of the response compared with that involved in the synthesis of *DOPA* decarboxylase.

SHORT–TERM EFFECTS OF MH ON PROTEIN BIOSYNTHESIS IN CALLIPHORA

β-Ecdysone is the natural MH of Calliphora (Galbraith *et al.*, 1969a). In mid-third instar larvae, exogenous β-ecdysone produces maximal stimulation of protein synthesis *in vivo* in fat body and body wall (Figure 1.), as well as in salivary gland, approximately 4 hours after injection. The results have been expressed relative to controls injected with water, because handling and injection affect protein and RNA metabolism in some tissues. a-Ecdysone and β-ecdysone are equally effective in stimulating short-term protein synthesis (Neufeld *et al.*, 1968), a result consistent with a rapid conversion of a- to β-ecdysone *in vivo* (King and Siddall, 1969; Galbraith *et al.*, 1969b).

We have consistently seen a brief initial depression of protein synthesis (Figure 1.) preceding stimulation (Neufeld *et al.*, 1968). Other workers (Arking and Shaaya, 1969; Sahota and Mansingh, 1970) have found no evidence of this early reduction in rate of protein synthesis. The experimental systems used differed from ours in both cases, but a convincing explanation for the difference in the immediate response to the hormone cannot be offered at present.

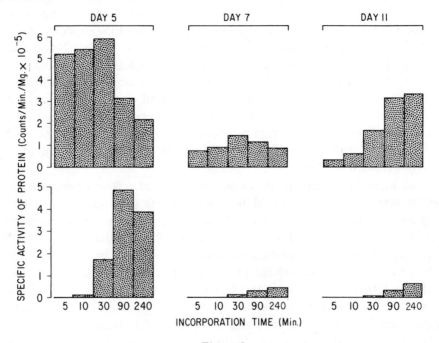

Figure 2.

Temporal course *in vivo* of incorporation of ³H-leucine into fat body (above) and plasma (below) of day-5, day-7 and day-11 (quiescent) larvae of *Calliphora stygia* at specified intervals after injection (based on data of Martin *et al.*, 1969).

The degree of enhancement of protein synthesis following treatment with hormone varies from tissue to tissue and with the stage of development. Fat body shows little response in early third instar (days 3-6) when the normal synthetic activity (Figure 2) of the tissue is very high (Martin *et al.*, 1969). During the wandering stage of mid-third instar (days 7-10) normal protein synthesis in the fat body is much reduced (Figure 2); at this period the effect of injected MH on protein synthesis is most striking. In corresponding wandering stages of development in *C. erythrocephala*, there is a reduction in the number of ribosomes and in the development of the endoplasmic reticulum (Price, 1969), with progressive dimunition in heavy polysome components (Sekeri *et al.*, 1968). The absence of significant short-term hormonal stimulation of protein synthesis in feeding larvae suggests that the synthetic machinery may be saturated in any case at that stage; each of the 11,000 cells of the organ is then synthesizing about 0.4 μg. protein *per diem* based on the data of Martin *et al.* (1969).

At day 11 of development, endogenous MH is present, and the fat body of untreated animals shows increased protein synthesis relative to wandering larvae (Figure 2.). MH injected at this stage again fails to stimulate significant synthetic activity (Neufeld *et al.*, 1968). It is interesting, and perhaps significant, that the intracellular distribution of exogenous ^{3}H-β-ecdysone changes sharply at this developmental stage (Thomson *et al.*, 1970) while alterations in nuclear inclusion ribonucleoprotein can also be detected Thomson and Gunson, 1970).

Does the short-term stimulation of protein synthesis involve new protein species? Does the hormone affect differentially the synthesis of any of the species normally synthesized? We selected the fat body for an examination of these questions because the pattern of protein synthesis during development has been analyzed in detail (Kinnear *et al.*, 1971). This tissue also affords an opportunity to examine the effect of MH on release of protein from the fat-body cells.

Synthesis and release (Figure 2) early in the third instar (days 3-6) (Martin *et al.*, 1969) is followed by a period of uptake (days 7-10) (Martin *et al.*, 1971). The synthesis of each of 22 protein bands was compared by densitometry of radioautographs obtained from electrophoretic separations of isotopically labeled fat-body proteins on acrylamide gels (Thomson *et al.*, 1971). The synthesis of the protein species was not differentially affected by exogenous MH at any developmental stage when examined 4 hours after injection of hormone.

It must therefore be concluded that the short-term effect of exogenous MH on protein synthesis in the fat body of the wandering larva is predominantly (if not entirely) general in nature. There is neither a selective effect on the synthesis of individual proteins nor stimulation of synthesis of new species sufficient to account for the observed over-all increase in protein synthesis.

These non-specific changes in protein synthesis might be related fairly directly to hormonal effects on membrane permeability, electrolyte balance, and transport, the evidence for which has been reviewed by Kroeger (1967). Alternatively, or in addition, the exogenous steroid might act either by changing the pattern of interaction between ribosomes and the endoplasmic reticulum (James *et al.*, 1969), or by affecting the transport of RNA and ribosomal particles from nucleus to cytoplasm (see review by Hamilton, 1971).

The release of proteins from the fat body into the hemolymph (Figure 2) in the normal development of Calliphora has also been examined in detail (Martin *et al.*, 1969; Kinnear *et al.*, 1971) especially for days 3-6 of larval life. The synthesis and release of proteins from the fat body of day-4 larvae was unaffected *in vitro* by the presence of β-ecdysone (5μg./ml.) in the incubation medium, except for the relative suppression (40 per cent of control level) of the appearance in the medium of a lipoprotein designated H4 (Thomson *et al.*, 1971). This lipoprotein is conjugated on release from the fat body and represents quantitatively a major component of the plasma. It is therefore unlikely that synthesis of the apoprotein is suppressed by MH, as this would be readily detectable. Thus β-ecdysone appears to affect either the synthesis in the fat body of the lipid moiety involved, or the conjugation of lipid and apoprotein on release, or both these processes (Thomson *et al.*, 1971).

CONCLUSION

Exogenous MH may have two distinct phases of influence on protein and possibly on RNA synthesis. One effect involves, at certain susceptible stages in development, a general, nonselective, transitory, stimulation of protein synthesis. There is at present no compelling evidence that such over-all enhancement of protein synthesis requires genic participation. The second effect is tissue-specific and also stage-specific; it involves the longer-term synthesis of specific proteins such as *DOPA* decarboxylase in the epidermis of Calliphora. For hormonal effects of this second kind, the work of Karlson and his colleagues provides evidence that the transcription, stabilization, and transport of new mRNA must be involved.

Acknowledgement

Financial support has been received through the Australian Research Grants Committee (Grant D65/15167).

References

1. ARKING, R. and SHAAYA, E.: Effect of Ecdysone on Protein Synthesis in the Larval Fat Body of *Calliphora*. J. Insect Physiol., *15:*287-296, 1969.

2. ASHBURNER, M.: Function and Structure of Polytene Chromosomes During Insect Development. Adv. Insect Physiol., *7:*1-95, 1970.

3. BURDETTE, W. J. and CODA, R. L.: Effect of Ecdysone on Incorporation of ^{14}C-Leucine into Hepatic Protein *in Vitro*. Soc. Exp. Biol. Med., *112*:216-217, 1963.

4. CHAUDHARY, K. D., LUPIEN, P. J., and HINSE, C.: Effect of Ecdysone on Glutamic Decarboxylase in Rat Brain. Experientia, *25*:250-251, 1969.

5. CLEVER, U. and KARLSON, P.: Induktion von Puffveränderungen in dem Speicheldrüsenchromosomen von *Chironomus tentans* durch Ecdyson. Exp. Cell Res., *20*:623-626, 1960.

6. GALBRAITH, M. N., HORN, D. H. S., THOMSON, J. A., NEUFELD, G. J., and HACKNEY, R. J.: Insect Molting Hormones: Crustecdysone in *Calliphora*. J. Insect Physiol., *15*:1225-1233, 1969a.

7. GALBRAITH, M. N., HORN, D. H. S., MIDDLETON, E. J., THOMSON, J. A., SIDDALL, J. B., and HAFFERL, W.: The Catabolism of Crustecdysone in the Blowfly *Calliphora stygia*. J. Chem. Soc. D. Chem. Commun., *1144*:1134-1135, 1969b.

8. HAMILTON, T. H.: Effects of Sexual Steroid Hormones on Genetic Transcription and Translation. *In*: P. O. Hubinont and F. Leroy (ed.), Basic Actions of Sex Steroids on Target Cells, pp. 56-92. Basel: Karger, 1971.

9. JAMES, D. W., RABIN, B. R., and WILLIAMS, D. J.: Role of Steroid Hormones in the Interaction of Polysomes with Endoplasmic Reticulum. Nature, 371-372, 1969.

10. KARLSON, P.: New Concepts on the Mode of Action of Hormones. Perspect. Biol. Med., *6*:203-214, 1963.

11. KARLSON, P.: The Effects of Ecdysone on Giant Chromosomes. RNA Metabolism and Enzyme Induction. *In*: S. G. Spickett (ed.), Endocrine Genetics, pp. 67-76. London: Cambridge University Press, 1967.

12. KARLSON, P. and PETERS, G.: Zum Wirkungsmechanismus der Hormone IV. Der Einfluss der Ecdysons auf den Nucleinsaurstoffwechsel von *Calliphora*-Larven. Gen. Comp. Endocrinol., *5*:252-259, 1965.

13. KARLSON, P. and SEKERIS, C. E.: Zum Tyrosinstoffwechsel der Insekten IX. Kontrolle des Tyrosinstoffwechsels durch Ecdyson. Biochim. Biophys. Acta, *63*:489-495, 1962.

14. KARLSON, P. and SEKERIS, C. E.: Ecdysone, an Insect Steroid Hormone, and Its Mode of Action. Recent Progr. Horm. Res., *22*:473-493, 1966.

15. KARLSON, P., SEKERIS, C. E., and MAURER, R.: Zum Wirkungsmechanismus der Hormone-I. Verteilung von Tritiummarkiertem Ecdyson in Larven von *Calliphora erythrocephala*. Hoppe-Zeyler's Z. Physiol. Chem., *336*:100-106, 1964.

16. KARLSON, P., HOFFMEISTER, H., HUMMEL, H., HOCKS, P., and SPITELLER, G.: Zur Chemie des Ecdysons VI. Reaktionen des Ecdysonmoleküls. Chem. Ber., *98*:2394-2402, 1965.

17. KING, D. S. and SIDDALL, J. B.: Conversion of α-ecdysone to β-ecdysone by Crustaceans and Insects. Nature, *221*:955-956, 1969.

18. KINNEAR, J. F., MARTIN, M-D., and THOMSON, J. A.: Developmental Changes in the Late Larva of *Calliphora stygia*. III. The Occurrence and Synthesis of Specific Tissue Proteins. Austral. J. Biol. Sci., *24*:275-289, 1971.

19. KROEGER, H.: Hormones, Ion Balances and Gene Activity in Dipteran Chromosomes. *In*: S. G. Spickett (ed.), Endocrine Genetics, pp. 55-66. London: Cambridge University Press, 1967.

20. MARTIN, M-D., KINNEAR, J. F., and THOMSON, J. A.: Developmental Changes in the Late Larva of *Calliphora stygia*. II. Protein Synthesis. Austral. J. Biol. Sci., *22*:935-945. 1969.

21. MARTIN, M-D., KINNEAR, J.F., and THOMSON, J.A.: Developmental Changes in the Late Larva of *Calliphora stygia*. IV. Uptake of Plasma Protein by the Fat Body. Austral. J. Biol. Sci., *24*:291-299, 1971.

22. NEUFELD, G. J., THOMSON, J. A., and HORN, D. H. S.: Short-term Effects of Crust-ecdysone (20-Hydroxyecdysone) on Protein and RNA Synthesis in Third-Instar Larvae of *Calliphora*. J. Insect Physiol., *14*:789-804, 1968.

23. OKUI, S., OTAKA, T., UCHIYAMA, M., TAKEMOTO, T., HIKINO, H., OGAWA, S., and NISHIMOTO, N.: Stimulation of Protein Synthesis in Mouse Liver by Insect Molting Steroids. Chem. Pharm. Bull., *16*:384-387, 1968.

24. PRICE, G. M.: Protein Synthesis and Nucleic Acid Metabolism in the Fat Body of the Larva of the Blowfly, *Calliphora erythrocephala*. J. Insect Physiol., *15*:931-944, 1969.

25. SAHOTA, T. S. and MANSINGH, A.: Cellular Response to Ecdysone: RNA and Protein Synthesis in Larval Tissues of Oak Silkworm *Antheraea pernyi*. J. Insect Physiol., *16*:1649-1654, 1970.

26. SEKERI, K. E., SEKERIS, C. E., and KARLSON, P.: Protein Synthesis in Subcellular Fractions of the Blowfly During Different Developmental Stages. J. Insect Physiol., *14*:425-431, 1968.

27. SEKERIS, C. E.: Action of Ecdysone on RNA and Protein Metabolism in the Blowfly, *Calliphora erythrocephala*. *In*: P. Karlson (ed.), Mechanisms of Hormone Action, pp. 149-167. New York: Academic Press, 1965.

28. SEKERIS, C. E. and KARLSON, P.: Zum Tyrosinstoffwechsel der Insekten VII. Der Katabolische Abbau des Tyrosins und die Biogenene der Sclerotisierungsubstanz, N-Acetyldopamin. Biochim. Biophys. Acta, *62*:103-113, 1962.

29. SEKERIS, C. E., LANG, N., and KARLSON, P.: Zum Wirkungsmechanismus der Hormone V. Einfluss von Ecdyson auf den RNA-Stoffwechsel den Epidermis den Schmeissfliege, *Calliphora erythrocephala*. Hoppe-Seyler's Z. Physiol. Chem., *341*:36-43, 1965.

30. THOMSON, J. A. and GUNSON, M. M.: Developmental Changes in the Major Inclusion Bodies of Polytene Nuclei from Larval Tissues of the Blowfly, *Calliphora stygia*. Chromosoma, *30*:193-201, 1970.

31. THOMSON, J. A., KINNEAR, J. F., MARTIN, M-D., and HORN, D. H. S.: Effects of Crustecdysone (20-Hydroxyecdysone) on Synthesis, Release, and Uptake of Proteins by the Larval Fat Body of *Calliphora*. Life Sciences, *10*:203-211, 1971.

32. THOMSON, J. A., ROGERS, D. C., GUNSON, M. M., and HORN, D. H. S.: Developmental Changes in the Pattern of Cellular Distribution of Exogenous Tritium-labelled Crustecdysone in Larval Tissues of *Calliphora*. Cytobios, *6*:79-88, 1970.

EFFECT of INVERTEBRATE HORMONES and ONCOGENIC VIRUSES on POLYTENE CHROMOSOMES

Walter J. Burdette and James E. Carver Jr.

Recognition that the banded pattern observed in some cells represented prophase chromosomes in the larval salivary glands of *Drosophila melanogaster* by Painter (1933) and in the malpighian tubules of *Bibio hortulanus* L. independently by Heitz and Bauer (1933) first provided a means for visualizing the position of genes accurately and later for studying possible causes and effects of genic activation. The polytene nature of these prophase chromosomes proposed by Koltzoff (1934) was incorporated into the interpretation of their morphology; and through fortunate collaboration, Muller, Painter, Patterson, and others correlated the position and type of mutants produced by x-irradiation in Drosophila on crossover maps and salivary-gland chromosomes. Codification of this information into reliable chromosomal maps for different species of Drosophila by Bridges (1935) and later by others then provided means for visual interpretation of location and action of genes that has been invaluable over the years. Polytene chromosomes have been observed both in larval tissues that undergo dissolution with metamorphosis and tissues persisting in the imago. These include salivary glands, fat body, epidermal cells, muscle cells, various parts of the alimentary tract, neural cells, nuclei of trachea, imaginal discs, nurse cells of the ovary, vesiculae seminales, and malpighian tubules. The rediscovery and proper interpretation of the nuclear "cordon cylindrique" seen earlier in the salivary-glands of Chironomids by Balbiani (1881) led to critical observations of puffs and the current interpretation of their relationship to the hormonal control of metamorphosis.

Becker (1959, 1962) tabulated the sequential enlargement of certain regions of the salivary glands in Drosophila and correlated this puffing with the life cycle. After studying these puffed areas in *Chironomus tentans,* Beermann (1952, 1956) became convinced that the increase in size of the puffs which he observed was due to increased activity of genes at the loci of puffs. When morphologic criteria are used, not all puffs relate to molting in Drosophila, although eighty per cent or more are active at specific stages of development; whereas only about ten per cent of the puffing in polytene chromosomes shows developmental specificity in Chironomus. Variations have been found in the puffing pattern between tissues and within salivary glands (Beermann, 1952; Clever, 1962; Berendes, 1966). Puffs have been found to contain RNA in most chromosomes, but both RNA and DNA puffs have been identified in the Sciarinae (Poulson and Metz, 1938; Rudkin and Corlette, 1957; Ficq and Pavan, 1961), and the DNA puffs of *Rynchosciara angelae* observed in one tissue do not appear in another (Breuer and Pavan, 1955).

An increase in size of puffs has been correlated with RNA synthesis as a general rule (Gross, 1957; Pelling, 1964), except for the DNA puffs in the Sciarinae; and, excluding the latter puffs, there has been no consistent correlation between the time of DNA synthesis and puffing (Keyl, 1963; Sebeleva, 1968). Actinomycin D usually inhibits puffing, but the effect varies when results for different loci are compared (Clever, 1967), and induction of puffs can occur when protein synthesis is inhibited by antibiotics (Clever and Beermann, 1963; Ashburner, 1970). After initiation of puffing, the rate of RNA synthesis locally is very rapid, and labeling begins within seconds (Ritossa, 1962).

Proteins stainable with fast or light green at acid pH also have been reported and are identified most easily in puffs recently activated. These proteins may be found both before RNA synthesis is detected and morphologic changes occur (Berendes, 1968) and may not be synthesized at the site of puffs. They seem to be similar to proteins of the ribosomes and are associated with electron-dense granules that have been implicated in the transport process along with tRNA (Swift, 1964; Lezzi, 1967), although the granules are not detected as early as these proteins. Ritossa and Spiegelman (1965) have reported that ribosomal RNA is synthesized under the direction of the DNA in the region of the nucleolar organizer in *Drosophila melanogaster* rather than in the puffs. Steffensen and Whimber (1971) localized tRNA genes in the salivary-gland chromosomes of Drosophila by RNA-DNA hybridization, but a relationship between these sites and *Minute* loci was not established. However, a number of major loci were found to be situated in segments of the chromosomes that puff during larval or prepupal development.

Mutants that are known to prolong the larval stage in Drosophila may or may not be associated with changes in the appearance of polytene chromosomes. In the *l(2)gl* and *giant* mutant stocks, the patterns of puffing vary very little from the normal pattern in *Drosophila melanogaster* (Becker, 1959); but shorter and thicker polytene chromosomes have been observed in the lethal tumor stock, *ltl*, and the *tu^h* stock, and there is some hypertrophy of salivary chromosomes in the *pci* stocks of *Drosophila hydei* (Rodman, 1967a; Kobel and van Breugel, 1968; Ashburner, 1970).

Early studies of Clever and Karlson (1960) and Becker (1959, 1962) identified ecdysones as a major factor in the control of puffing activity. The work of Karlson and colleagues depended on the isolation of the ecdysones, and Becker based his interpretations on separating the posterior part of the salivary gland from the source of hormone by ligation and transplanting glands between animals of different ages. When glands were transplanted, the puffing pattern observed was characteristic of the host, and the stage of puffing was delayed in the posterior portion of the salivary gland isolated by a proximal ligature. We (Burdette, 1962) were able to correlate the titer of ecdysone with the life cycle in Bombyx (Figure 1) and isolated ecdysone from Drosophila (Burdette, 1956), establishing the reality of the hormone in Drosophila and changing titers to which the chromosomal puffs may respond.

Clever and Karlson (1960) have based their interpretations largely on work with the salivary-gland chromosomes of *Chironomus tentans*. For example, it was found that increasing the concentration of ecdysone caused puffs I-18C and IV-2B to persist longer, and a second induction with the hormone was possible after regression (Clever, 1961). On the other hand, puff I-19A regressed when ecdysone was administered in the same series of experiments inducing the puffs just mentioned. The reaction threshold of the various puffs differed, but is has not been clear exactly what factor causes regression of such puffs as IV-2B. Apparently these factors are related to protein synthesis, but the use of inhibitors has not clarified the relationship between the induction of puffs appearing late in relation to those appearing early. The DNA puffs in Sciarinae can be induced with ecdysone (Crouse, 1968), but two Balbiani rings in the prepupae of *Acricotopus lucidos* have been noted to regress after treatment (Panitz, 1964). Panitz also presents evidence

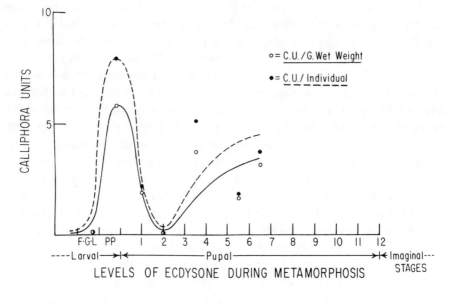

Figure 1

that locus BR-4 in *Acricotopus lucidos* Staeg acts as repressor for the function of H/Q-32, the latter being active in puff formation when BR-4 is inactivated by ecdysone.

An effect of ecdysones on puffing has been established in all the larval tissues that have been studied in Drosophila (Berendes, 1967) and Chironomus (Clever, 1961). Depending on dosage of ecdysone, regions of the chromosomes observed, the time of treatment, and the species used, the puffing pattern in Drosophila may or may not differ from the normal pattern in terms of location and sequence of puffing (Berendes, 1967; Ashburner, 1971). We have found that puffs in Drosophila respond in characteristic fashion to different ecdysones and phytohormones and to proteinic brain hormone and that each compound tested differs from the others in the response it produced (Burdette and Kobayashi, 1969). However, we have found also that not all puffs tested with crude ecdysones responded at a specific time (Burdette and Anderson, 1965), and Ashburner (1970) and others also found that puffs apparently will respond only during sensitive periods. Erratic responses to ecdysones have been obtained *in vitro* (Burdette and Anderson, 1965; Berendes and Boyd, 1969; Ashburner, 1970). Fortunately, improved culture media and techniques have now altered this picture (Ashburner, 1971).

Various treatments in addition to injection of hormones and their analogs are known to affect the puffing pattern in polytene chromosomes, including extremes of heat or cold. Droplets appear in the nuclei of cells with cold treatment, and heat shock results in specific induction of some and regression of other puffs (Ritossa, 1963). Some of the puffs induced by heat shock are not active during normal development, and agents that uncouple oxidative phosphorylation have a similar effect (Ritossa, 1964). Additional puffs may appear after recovery from anoxia (Ashburner, 1970), and we (Burdette and Anderson, 1965) found that CO_2 was effective in causing puffing at specific loci in *Drosophila melanogaster*. Other agents have also been reported to cause changes in puffing pattern, including gibberelin A; acridines; cyclo-heximide; the antibiotics: actinomycin D, oxytetracyclines, and puromycin; thioacetamide; dicyandiamide; tryptophane, ribonuclease; and various saline solutions (Ashburner, 1970; Kroeger and Lezzi, 1966). In addition, cultures of tissues *in vivo* in adult abdomen and cytoplasm of the egg may alter the normal behavior of puffs (Kroeger, 1960).

A number of studies have been carried out on the possible relationship between genic activation, as represented by the pattern of puffing, and secretion of the salivary gland in which polytene chromosomes appear. However, Laufer and Nakase (1965) and others have been able to show that the tissue-specific puffs of the salivary-gland chromosomes are related more to the selective uptake, concentration, and release of secretions than the synthesis of specific constituents in them, and the realization that the gland performs a function as a transport organ as well as one that is primarily secretory has altered the view about an obligate relationship between puffing and cell product in these glands. Berendes (1965) has related activity of puff 47b in *Drosophila hydei* to the presence of secretory granules, and Grossbach (1968) and Beermann (1961) have reported that the location of the gene for secretory granules and puff BR S2 coincide in hybrid Chironomids.

Before crystalline material became available, it was possible to use crude extracts having activity for ecdysones when bioassayed by the Calliphora test. Based on this work and subsequent work with crystalline hormones, Karlson (1965) and Clever (1961) interpreted the prompt response of the salivary-gland chromosomes in Chironomus after exposure to ecdysones as evidence for genic activation and, in general, adopted an interpretation consonant with the Jacob-Monod model for derepression. Recently Karlson (Karlson, this volume) has modified this interpretation, and Kroeger (1967) and Lezzi and Gilbert (1969) and others have pointed out that changes in the ionic concentration and the condition of membranes must be taken into consideration in the interpretation of hormonal effects on chromosomal puffing as well as the direct action of hormone on the process of transcription. The Balbiani rings, I-18C, IV-2B, and BR-1, in *Chironomus tentans* puff when exposed to ecdysone or when isolated nuclei are incubated in a medium rich in K^+. The region I-19A activated by juvenile hormone after 2 to 4 hours (but only after prolonged ecdysone treatment) is also activated by incubating isolated nuclei in a medium rich in Na^+ (Lezzi and Gilbert, 1969). Based on these and other observations, Lezzi and Frigg (1971) have adopted the view that ionic effects on puffing are as specific as hormonal effects and point out that regions of the chromosomes reacting specifically to ecdysone *in vivo* respond to a medium rich in K^+ in isolated nuclei, whereas regions activated by juvenile hormone *in vivo* puff when incubated in media containing Na^+.   They postulate that juvenile hormone increases permeability of the cell membrane permitting sodium ions to gain access to the nucleus of cells, the increasing concentration thus promoting puffing of sodium-sensitive regions. Antagonism between juvenile hormone and ecdysone then would come about because the energy-requiring sodium pump stimulated by ecdysone transports potassium into and sodium out of a cell. By increasing permeability of the cell membrane to sodium, the action of juvenile hormone is opposed to that of ecdysone. Since these mechanisms are not identical, the antagonism would not be a strict one. Lezzi (1970) also has stressed the importance of the ionic environment within the chromosome in interactions between histones and DNA to prevent binding of RNA polymerase at respective chromosomal loci.

The effect of juvenile hormone on puffing has not been as easily determined as the effects of ecdysones and analogs. Laufer and Holt (1970) fed prepupae of *C. thummi* farnesoic-acid derivatives and observed an increase in size of BR IV-B at a time when it is scheduled to regress and inhibition of puffing at nine loci among 91 examined in the treated larvae whose development was arrested after the first three molts. The presence of ecdysone apparently is necessary for normal action of juvenile hormone to occur, and this may explain negative results that have been obtained when animals were tested at a time when levels of ecdysone were low.

Insects have been traditional vectors of many viral diseases in the annals of medicine. The genoid for CO_2 sensitivity has been investigated in Drosophila by L'Heritier (1951), Plus (1954), and others (Burdette, 1958), and virus-like particles infecting Drosophila have been reported by Akai *et al.* (1967). The occurrence of polyhedral virus in *Rynchosciara angelae* causes hypertrophy of the polytene chromosomes, increase in DNA synthesis, chromosomal fragmentation, and the presence of fewer puffs (Pavan and Basile, 1966). The possibility that genetic material may be transferred into the cell by viruses is intriguing, and we have introduced a number of viruses into the alimentary tract or injected them into Drosophila whose puffing pattern was followed subsequently (Burdette, 1959, 1968a, 1968b). So far, we have not found it possible to demonstrate that oncogenic viruses used have been propagated *in vivo,* and studies of salivary-gland chromosomes with fluorescent antibody specific for SV-40 have failed to show any localization either on the cells or at specific sites on the chromosomes. However, there has been a change in the pattern of puffing after administration of viruses and hormones, and studies have been carried out to determine the response of index puffs to crystalline invertebrate hormones and analogs (including phytohormones), to various viruses, and to combinations of them. In order to make sure that there was a reasonable likelihood that the relative size of the puffs is related to content of RNA, puffs were labeled with both tritiated uridine and tritiated thymidine after treatment with oncogenic virus in a pilot study.

METHODS

Larvae of the Oregon R strain of *Drosophila melanogaster* raised on standard culture medium at 25° C. were used for investigating the effects of treatment with hormones and viruses. Salivary glands were removed from the anterior segment of larvae at the times specified in the tables, and then they were compressed and stained with aceto-orcein. The concentrations of hormone administered is expressed as the percentage of weight per volume and 3.0 μl. was injected into each larva. Since it was not possible to exert the same amount of pressure each time chromosomes were compressed in making the preparations, the measurements both of puffs and adjacent bands were made and are given in the tables as the mean ratios of diameters of puffs to adjacent bands. An average of 18 to 36 observations per puff were made in each of the studies on comparison between the action of ecdysterone, inokosterone, ponasterone A, cyasterone, and proteinic brain hormone. Because it was impractical to take measurements of a large number of puffs, index regions were chosen for study. They appear in Table 1 and consist of one

TABLE 1

LOCATION OF INDEX PUFFS

Designation	Location on Map of Salivary-gland Chromosome
B	I:2 B 5–6 + I:2 B 13–17
71	III L:71 C–E
72	III L:72 C–D
74	III L:74 E–F
75	III L:75 B

area on the left end of chromosome I and two areas on chromosome III-L with double puffing. The time at which they puff (Becker, 1959, 1962; Ashburner, 1967) gives reasonable expectation of sensitivity during the time of observation (Figure 2). Measurements for each member of the double puff on the X chromosome at 2 B 5-6; 2 B 13-17 are combined and recorded as a single value. It was not possible to run all types of controls in each experiment, but initially a comparison was made between the puffing pattern without treatment and following injection with 3.0 µl. of modified Ringer solution containing no calcium that was used as vehicle throughout the series of experiments reported.

Figure 2

Pattern of Puffing in *Drosophila melanogaster*

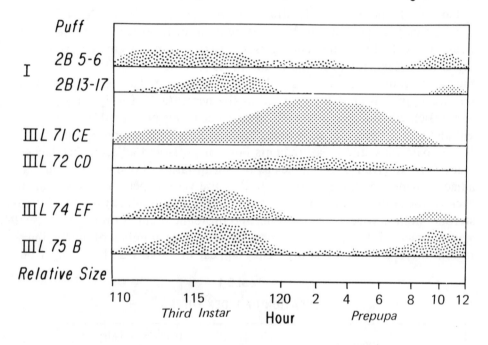

* Modified from Becker (1959), Ashburner (1967, 1969), and Burdette and Anderson (1965)

After hormones were injected into early third-instar larvae in the dilutions indicated in respective tables, observations were made at intervals of 20, 40, 60, and 90 minutes; and results are given respectively for these periods of time. Virus was administered by raising larvae in medium containing virus mixed with yeast in the concentrations indicated in the respective tables. The stock of Rous virus used was stored in concentrations of 1 G. equivalent per milliliter, and the SV 40 contained 4×10^6 plaque-forming units per ml. The Bryan high-titer strain of Rous virus carried Rous-associated virus 2. Potency of each virus was tested by production of fowl sarcomas in the case of the Rous-sarcoma virus and by means of plaque assays in the case of SV 40. After injection of hormone, salivary glands were not removed until the interval specified in the tables had elapsed, since a number of parallel studies *in vitro* did not yield preparations that were equally satisfactory.

In the investigations on labeled puffs, larvae were treated by micro-injection *in vivo* with 0.1 μl. of the Bryan high-titer strain of Rous-sarcoma virus (1:1 dilution) 12 hours before harvesting at the stages indicated in the tables, and modified Drosophila Ringer solution was used for injection of control preparations. Immediately after excision of the glands they were postlabeled *in vitro* by immersing in tritiated uridine. Autoradiographic film was then applied to the preparations, exposed for an appropriate period *in vitro,* developed, and examined. Similar technique was used for labeling the chromosomes with tritiated thymidine.

Measurements of puffed areas in the labeling experiments are expressed in Tables 6-9 as the product of the maximum diameter of the puff times the distance between the nonpuffed adjacent bands. Counts of grains or auto-radiographic-decay spots were made over the areas of the same puffs in the preparations expressed as the ratio of the count over the puff to the count observed over an adjacent standard segment. For the X:2 B ratio listed, the adjacent standard was taken as the segment between the distal end of the puff and the extreme distal end of the chromosome. The nonpuffed area of the chromosome between the proximal limit of puff III L:72 and the distal limit of puff III L:74 was used as a standard for the puffs located on chromosome arm III L.

RESULTS AND DISCUSSION

A comparison of results is recorded in Table 2 for control cultures without treatment and injecting modified Ringer solution. No significant difference in the diameter of puffs was found, suggesting that any differences in the effects of hormones, viruses, and various combinations are not attributable to the saline or used as carrier. Preliminary studies in which the size of puffs after administration of inactivated Rous virus was compared to diameters following injection of saline were inconclusive.

In Table 3, a negative sign before the ratio of diameter of puff to adjacent band following treatment with the hormone at the intervals of time listed indicates that the mean is smaller than the control ratio, a positive sign that it is larger. [The percentage change has been published previously (Burdette, and Kobayashi, 1969).] It is quite apparent that the change in the pattern

TABLE 2

COMPARISON OF RATIOS OF DIAMETERS OF PUFFS TO ADJACENT BANDS WITHOUT
TREATMENT AND 20 MINUTES AFTER INJECTION WITH MODIFIED RINGER SOLUTION

Puff	No Treatment	Modified Ringer Solution
2B	1.47	1.51
71	1.54	1.50
72	1.27	1.28
74	1.24	1.24
75	1.26	1.23

$p > 0.5$

for puffing varies from one puff to the next and also that each hormone
elicits a pattern somewhat different from that of the others tested. Whether
the effect of proteinic brain hormone represents a direct action or is mediated
through the prothoracic gland cannot be stated with certainty, but the latter
may be the mechanism in whole or in part. These studies suggest that the
crystalline hormones tested are each capable of changing the puffing pattern
in the salivary-gland chromosomes of Drosophila in characteristic fashion.

The effect of both DNA and RNA viruses, different strains of the same
virus, and different dilutions of the same virus are given in Tables 4 and 5.
When chromosomes are exposed to 50 per cent concentration of both the
Bryan strain of Rous-sarcoma virus and simian virus 40 respectively, there is
significant reduction in the ratio of puffs to adjacent bands (Tables 4 and 5).
There is only one difference that is significant for the Rous-associated virus 1,
whereas all except one were significantly lowered with the Schmidt-Ruppin
strain of the Rous virus. When SV 40 was administered in various dilutions,
less effect was noted with higher dilutions until there were only two regions
significantly lower than controls when the dilution was 1:15. Information
about these effects are presented graphically in Figures 3a, 3b, and 3c.

Measurements included in Tables 6-9 reveal a reduction in size of puffs
among the preparations treated with Rous virus except for puff III:72 at the
prepupal stage; the largest difference found was at the locus of puff III:71 in
prepupae. Comparison of the corresponding mean ratios for grain counts also
show a consistent reduction among preparations treated with this RNA virus

TABLE 3

MEAN RATIOS OF DIAMETER OF PUFFS TO ADJACENT BANDS

Hormone	Min.	Puff:	2B	71	72	74	75
Ecdysterone	20		+ 1.7[b]	+ 1.6	+ 1.6[b]	+ 1.4	+ 1.5[b]
	40		+ 1.9	+ 1.5	+ 1.4	1.4	+ 1.5
	60		- 1.8	1.6	+ 1.6[b]	- 1.4	- 1.4[b]
	90		1.6	1.7	- 1.5	1.5	- 1.4[c]
Inokosterone	20		+ 1.9[b]	1.5	+ 1.5	+ 1.4	+ 1.5[b]
	40		+ 2.2[b]	+ 1.6[c]	+ 1.5[b]	+ 1.5	+ 1.5
	60		- 1.8	1.6	+ 1.5[c]	- 1.4	- 1.3[b]
	90		+ 1.7	- 1.4[b]	- 1.4[c]	- 1.4	- 1.4[c]
Ponasterone A	20		+ 1.8[b]	1.5	+ 1.5	+ 1.5[b]	+ 1.5[b]
	40		+ 1.9	+ 1.5	+ 1.6[b]	1.4	+ 1.5
	60		1.9	- 1.5	+ 1.5[b]	- 1.4	1.6
	90		1.6	- 1.4[b]	- 1.4[c]	1.5	- 1.5
Proteinic Brain Hormone[a]	20		+ 2.0[b]	+ 1.7[b]	+ 1.4	+ 1.6[b]	+ 1.8[b]
	40		+ 1.8[b]	+ 1.6	+ 1.4	+ 1.6[b]	+ 1.6[b]

a. 1 Bombyx Unit/50 μg.
b. $.0001 \leqslant P < .05$
c. $.05 < P < .10$

TABLE 4

MEAN RATIO[†] OF DIAMETERS OF PUFFS TO ADJACENT BANDS
AFTER EXPOSURE TO ROUS–SARCOMA VIRUS

Puff	Bryan Strain (1:1)		Schmidt–Ruppin Strain (1:1)		Rous-associated Virus I (1:1)	
	Control	Treated	Control	Treated	Control	Treated
2B	1.8	1.5*	1.6	1.4*	2.0	1.7*
71	1.6	1.5*	1.4	1.3*	1.6	1.5
72	1.4	1.2*	1.3	1.2*	1.4	1.3
74	1.4	1.2*	1.3	1.2*	1.4	1.3
75	1.5	1.3*	1.3	1.2	1.4	1.3

* $P < .05$

TABLE 5

MEAN RATIO[†] OF DIAMETERS OF PUFFS
TO ADJACENT BANDS AFTER EXPOSURE TO SV–40

Puff	Control	Dilution			
		1:1	1:5	1:10	1:15
2B	1.9	1.3*	1.4*	1.4*	1.7*
71	1.6	1.2*	1.4*	1.4*	1.5
72	1.4	1.2*	1.2*	1.2*	1.2*
74	1.4	1.1*	1.2*	1.2*	1.3
75	1.4	1.2*	1.2*	1.2*	1.3

†30 Observations Per Puff
* $P < .05$

except for puff III:72. Comparative grain counts for puff III:71 labeled with thymidine show small counts and ratios for both puffed and banded areas, and very little difference in the ratios for puffs in control and treated preparations.

When the ratios between puffs and adjacent bands after administration of inokosterone, ecdysterone, ponasterone, and cyasterone (Tables 10a and 10b) are examined, it is apparent that inokosterone is the most potent of the four. Although a 10 per cent solution of inokosterone shows a significant increase in the ratio for puff 72 only at the end of 90 minutes, there is a prompt response of the other puffs tested. Administration of Rous virus decreased the ratios significantly in 12 of the categories for larvae treated with 10 per cent inokosterone. In no instance was the ratio below that of the value for the control group treated with saline, and in 9 of the groups it was significantly higher. In 12 of the determinations in those treated with 10 per cent inokosterone, the ratios were significantly lower when virus had been administered also. Doubling the amount of inokosterone usually diminished rather than increased the effect, although a significant increase occurred at the end of 90 minutes when puff 74 and 75 were measured. Increasing concentration of inokosterone from 10 to 30 and 50 per cent also failed to increase dramatically the size of the puffs in the group previously treated with Rous virus.

The response of the puffs to ecdysterone was less pronounced than with inokosterone. Ten per cent solution of this hormone induced the 2B puffs later, seemed to inhibit the puff 72, had no significant effect on puff 71, and had a comparable effect only on puff 75. The effect on puff 74 appeared

Figure 3a

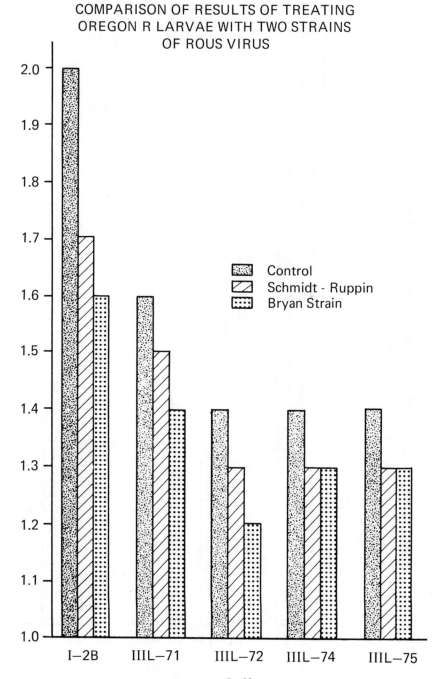

COMPARISON OF RESULTS OF TREATING
OREGON R LARVAE WITH TWO STRAINS
OF ROUS VIRUS

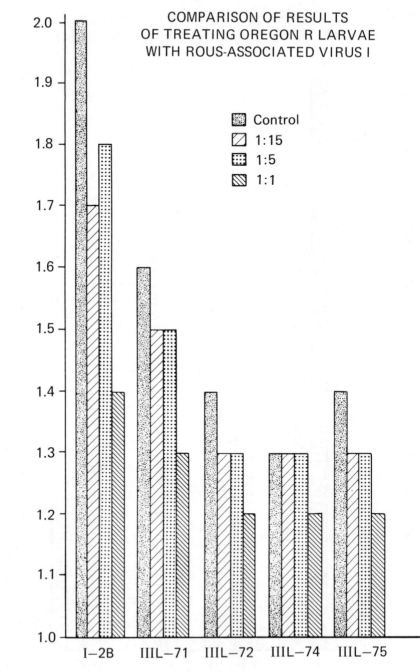

COMPARISON OF RESULTS
OF TREATING OREGON R LARVAE
WITH ROUS-ASSOCIATED VIRUS I

Control
1:15
1:5
1:1

Average Ratio of Breadth of Puffs to Diameter of Adjacent Bands

I−2B   IIIL−71   IIIL−72   IIIL−74   IIIL−75

Puff

Figure 3c

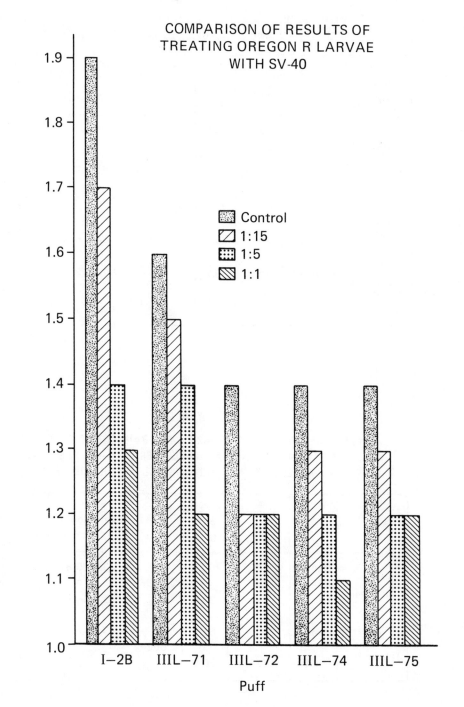

COMPARISON OF RESULTS OF
TREATING OREGON R LARVAE
WITH SV-40

TABLE 6

EFFECT OF ROUS VIRUS ON SIZE AND GRAIN COUNTS OF PUFF X:2B IN
SALIVARY–GLAND CHROMOSOMES LABELED WITH ^{3}H–URIDINE

Larval Age (Hr.)	Class	Number Observed	Mean Area (μ^2)	P	Mean Grain Count Puff/Standard	Ratio	P
110	Control	25	18.9	$<$.002 –	36.0/26.7	1.4	$<$.02 –
	Treated	25	13.4		34.9/31.8	1.1	
115	Control	25	38.0	$<$.002 –	27.8/ 6.3	4.5	$<$.002 –
	Treated	25	28.7		73.8/24.6	3.0	
120	Control	25	30.2	$<$.002 –	51.7/12.3	4.2	$<$.002 –
	Treated	25	27.6		46.4/17.2	2.7	

TABLE 7

EFFECT OF ROUS VIRUS ON SIZE AND GRAIN COUNT OF PUFF III:71
IN SALIVARY–GLAND CHROMOSOMES OF 0–HR. PREPUPAE
LABELED WITH ^{3}H–URIDINE AND ^{3}H–THYMIDINE

Label	Class	Number Observed	Mean Area (μ^2)	P	Mean Grain Count Puff/Standard	Ratio	P
^{3}H Uridine	Control	25	108.6	$<$.002–	73.2/ 9.8	7.5	$<$.002–
	Treated	25	90.5		65.0/14.8	4.4	
^{3}H Thymidine	Control	25	81.5	$<$.002–	3.5/ 9.6	0.4	$<$.05 –
	Treated	25	70.5		5.4/ 6.5	0.3	

TABLE 8

EFFECT OF ROUS VIRUS ON SIZE AND GRAIN COUNT OF PUFF III:72
IN SALIVARY–GLAND CHROMOSOMES LABELED WITH ^{3}H–URIDINE

Larval Age (Hr.)	Class	Number Observed	Mean Area (μ^2)	P	Mean Grain Count Puff/Standard	Ratio	P
120	Control	25	36.4	$<.01-$	11.1/ 8.4	1.3	$<.002-$
	Treated	25	35.8		11.8/11.9	1.0	
0 (Pre–pupae)	Control	25	35.1	$<.002+$	11.2/11.0	1.0	$<.02+$
	Treated	25	36.2		11.5/ 9.6	1.2	

TABLE 9

EFFECT OF ROUS VIRUS ON SIZE AND GRAIN COUNTS OF PUFFS III:74 AND III:75
IN SALIVARY–GLAND CHROMOSOMES LABELED WITH ^{3}H–URIDINE

Puff	Larval Age (Hr.)	Class	Number Observed	Mean Area (μ^2)	P	Mean Grain Count Puff/Standard	Ratio	P
III:74	115	Control	25	34.4	$<.002-$	26.7/6.2	4.3	$<.002-$
		Treated	25	21.3		17.0/6.3	2.7	
III:75	115	Control	25	29.2	$<.002-$	25.7/6.2	4.1	$<.002-$
		Treated	25	20.8		13.8/6.0	2.3	

TABLE 10a

EFFECT OF HORMONES AND ROUS VIRUS ON RATIO OF PUFFS TO ADJACENT BANDS IN SALIVARY–GLAND CHROMOSOMES

| Minutes | Puff | Control | Inokosterone | | | | | | Ecdysterone | | | |
| | | | 10% | | 20% | | 30% | 50% | 10% | | 20% | |
			Alone	+Virus	Alone	+Virus	+Virus	+Virus	Alone	+Virus	Alone	+Virus
20	2B	1.46	2.02*	1.86*	1.56	1.58	1.47	1.83*	1.56	1.49	1.60	1.39†
20	71	1.58	1.79*	1.55†	1.57	1.60	1.65	1.62	1.61	1.61	1.78*	1.54†
20	72	1.38	1.52	1.33†	1.21*	1.33†	1.25	1.36	1.14*	1.15*	1.41	1.39
20	74	1.23	1.44*	1.35*	1.27	1.32	1.26	1.49*	1.26	1.26	1.39*	1.23†
20	75	1.20	1.72*	1.56*†	1.30	1.36*	1.35*	1.71*	1.39*	1.35*	1.47*	1.37*
40	2B	1.65	1.99*	1.94*	1.63	1.54	1.73	1.81	1.75	1.56†	1.58	1.54
40	71	1.64	1.84*	1.66	1.68	1.52	1.69	1.79	1.77	1.62	1.67	1.49†
40	72	1.41	1.49	1.42	1.37	1.33	1.38	1.40	1.38	1.21*†	1.36	1.32
40	74	1.21	1.41*	1.31	1.31	1.34	1.29	1.40*	1.34*	1.20†	1.31	1.22
40	75	1.27	1.68*	1.53*†	1.30	1.33	1.49*	1.59*	1.60*	1.33†	1.41*	1.38
60	2B	1.66	2.01*	1.85*†	1.72	1.44*†	1.82	1.88*	1.88*	1.57†	1.58	1.62
60	71	1.59	1.82*	1.64†	1.74	1.65	1.67	1.69	1.72	1.72	1.63	1.46
60	72	1.37	1.52	1.34†	1.49	1.38	1.34	1.30	1.20*	1.20*	1.43	1.32
60	74	1.30	1.47*	1.41	1.38	1.27	1.30	1.34	1.31	1.22	1.33	1.18*†
60	75	1.39	1.75*	1.51†	1.38	1.33	1.51	1.53	1.68*	1.42†	1.40	1.38
90	2B	1.37	2.05*	1.83*†	1.48	1.55*	1.68*	1.74*	1.70*	1.69*	1.57*	1.80*†
90	71	1.59	1.80*	1.67	1.50	1.60	1.65	1.77	1.59	1.62	1.73	1.76
90	72	1.27	1.47*	1.31†	1.27	1.29	1.30	1.36	1.22	1.22	1.36	1.45*
90	74	1.20	1.58*	1.39*†	1.30*	1.39*	1.46*	1.32*	1.24	1.25	1.33*	1.25
90	75	1.21	1.86*	1.58*†	1.40*	1.41*	1.61*	1.42*	1.46*	1.44*	1.39*	1.43*

* P<.05 Hormone Compared to Modified Ringer Control   † P<.05 Hormone Compared to Hormone & Virus.

TABLE 10b

EFFECT OF HORMONES AND ROUS VIRUS ON RATIO OF PUFFS TO ADJACENT BANDS IN SALIVARY-GLAND CHROMOSOMES

Minutes	Puff	Control	Ponasterone A				Cyasterone			
			10%		20%		10%		20%	
			Alone	+ Virus	Alone	+ Virus	Alone	+ Virus	Alone	+ Virus
20	2B	1.46	1.67*	1.57	1.45	1.76*†	1.58	1.72	1.53	1.66
20	71	1.58	1.81*	1.55†	1.58	1.70	1.70	1.58	1.59	1.69
20	72	1.38	1.43	1.32	1.31	1.32	1.30	1.44	1.33	1.38
20	74	1.23	1.32	1.21	1.23	1.22	1.36*	1.30	1.26	1.39*†
20	75	1.20	1.34*	1.45*†	1.20	1.36*†	1.35*	1.37*	1.26	1.38*
40	2B	1.65	1.68	1.67	1.63	1.53	1.72	1.55	1.50	1.64
40	71	1.64	1.71	1.75	1.63	1.55	1.66	1.64	1.53	1.71†
40	72	1.41	1.38	1.40	1.36	1.22*†	1.40	1.44	1.32	1.38
40	74	1.21	1.29	1.30	1.37*	1.22†	1.22	1.27	1.42*	1.32
40	75	1.27	1.40	1.53*	1.42*	1.38*	1.21	1.25	1.44*	1.38
60	2B	1.66	1.51	1.65	1.53	1.53	1.74	1.54†	1.65	1.44*†
60	71	1.59	1.73	1.73	1.79*	1.56†	1.74	1.68	1.63	1.63
60	72	1.37	1.40	1.34	1.50*	1.16*†	1.49	1.35†	1.38	1.38
60	74	1.30	1.33	1.33	1.37	1.21†	1.37	1.19†	1.37	1.29
60	75	1.39	1.35	1.55*†	1.39	1.44	1.43	1.29	1.38	1.34
90	2B	1.37	1.63*	1.64*	1.65*	1.52†	1.75*	1.60*	1.56*	1.74*
90	71	1.59	1.62	1.50	1.70	1.59	1.68	1.67	1.59	1.68
90	72	1.27	1.37	1.24†	1.48*	1.26†	1.47*	1.38	1.26	1.32
90	74	1.20	1.27	1.24	1.41*	1.16†	1.36*	1.29	1.32	1.38*
90	75	1.21	1.45*	1.39*	1.50*	1.35*†	1.16	1.33*	1.47*	1.46*

* $P < .05$ Hormone Compared to Modified Ringer Control.　† $P < .05$ Hormone Compared to Hormone + Virus.

later and was not sustained. Except for the fact that the hormone in 10 per cent solution seemed to inhibit puff 72 and therefore possibly would not be expected to increase the size of this puff in larvae treated with virus alone, the hormone again increased the size of the puffs significantly beyond the controls or prevented a decrease in the ratio in those animals treated with virus in all but one determination. With 20 per cent solution there was no evidencè of inhibition of puff 72.

Neither ponasterone A nor cyasterone had as great an effect on puffing as inokosterone. Twenty per cent was more effective than 10 per cent ponasterone A only on puff III:74. This was not the case with cyasterone. Again there was evidence that the virus tended to decrease the effect of hormone alone, but the ratios were not significantly lower than those for the control values.

These data as a whole give the impression that the system tested is sufficiently sensitive to make it difficult to standardize, and discrepancies in the general trend are scattered throughout the results; also control values and ranges for the ratios varied from one experiment to the next. In general, however, the hormones increased the size of puffs, and administration of virus alone tended to be assoçiated with puffs smaller than in the controls. The effect of the virus was usually partially or wholly overcome when hormone was administered as well. Hormones tested varied in their effectiveness, and puffs responded in a different manner when results with various hormones were compared. The data obtained from radiolabeling of puffs following treatment with virus along with the published reports on labeling after treatment with ecdysone gives reasonable assurance that the relative size of the puffs reported is related to the content of RNA.

In summary, the inhibition or delay in puffing by the viruses tested, whether the result of slowing development or a direct effect of genic derepression, was often reversed partially or entirely by the hormones tested. Hormones, viruses, and puffs tended to differ one from another in respective effects and responses. Future studies probably will be most informative when newer biochemical methodologies are applied to specific regions of the chromosomes where genes whose action is known are located. Although there is much work to be done in resolving the gross morphological appearance of the chromosome into its ultimate structural components, the polytene state offers many advantages in relating the structure of the metazoan chromosome to biochemical events associated with genic action.

Acknowledgement:

Aided by grants CA 10037 from the U. S. Public Health Service and GF 28889 from the National Science Foundation.

References

1. AKAI, H., GATEFF, E., DAVIS, L. E., and SCHNEIDERMAN, H. : Virus-like Particles in Normal and Tumorous Tissues of Drosophila. Science, *157*:810-813, 1967.
2. ASHBURNER, M. : Patterns of Puffing Activity in the Salivary-gland Chromosomes of Drosophila. I. Autosomal Puffing Patterns in a Laboratory Stock of *Drosophila melanogaster.* Chromosoma, *21*:398-428, 1967.
3. ASHBURNER, M. : Patterns of Puffing Activity in the Salivary-gland Chromosomes of Drosophila. II. The X-Chromosome Puffing Patterns of *D. melanogaster.* Chromosoma, *27*:47-63, 1969.
4. ASHBURNER, M. : Function and Structure of Polytene Chromosomes During Insect Development. Advances in Insect Physiology, *7*:1-95, 1970.
5. ASHBURNER, M. : Induction of Puffs in Polytene Chromosomes of *in-Vitro* Cultured Salivary Glands of *Drosophila melanogaster* by Ecdysone Analogues. Nature New Biology, *230*:222-224, 1971.
6. BALBIANI, E. G. : Sur la Structure du Noyau des Cellules Salivaries chez les Larves de *Chironomus.* Zool. Anz., *4*:637-641; 662-666, 1881.
7. BECKER, H. J. : Die Puffs der Speicheldrusenchromosomen von *Drosophila melanogaster.* I. Beobachtungen zum Zwei Mutanten, *giant* und *lethal-giant-larvae.* Chromosoma, *10*:654-678, 1959.
8. BECKER, H. J. : Die Puffs der Speicheldrusenchromosomen von *Drosophila melanogaster.* II. Die Auslosung der Puffbildung, Ihre Spezifitat und Ihre Beziehung zur Funktion der Ringdruse. Chromosoma, *13*:341-384, 1962.
9. BEERMANN, W. : Chromomerenkonstanz und Spezifische Modifikation der Chromosomenstruktur in der Entwicklung und Organdifferenzierung von *Chironomus tentans.* Chromosoma, *5*:139-198, 1952.
10. BEERMANN. W. : Nuclear Differentiation and Functional Morphology of Chromosomes. Cold Spring Harbor Symposium on Quantitative Biology, *21*:217-232, 1956.
11. BEERMANN, W. : Ein Balbiani-ring als Locus einer Speicheldrusen-mutation. Chromosoma, *12*:1-25, 1961.
12. BERENDES, H. D. : Salivary Gland Function and Chromosomal Puffing Patterns in *Drosophila hydei.* Chromosoma, *17*:35-77, 1965.
13. BERENDES, H. D. : Gene Activities in the Malpighian Tubules of *Drosophila hydei* at Different Stages. J. Exp. Zool., *162*:209-218, 1966.
14. BERENDES, H. D. : The Hormone Ecdysone as Effector of Specific Changes in the Pattern of Gene Activities of *Drosophila hydei.* Chromosoma, *22*:274-293, 1967.
15. BERENDES, H. D. : Factors Involved in the Expression of Gene Activity in Polytene Chromosomes. Chromosoma, *24*:418-437, 1968.
16. BERENDES, H. D. and BOYD, J. B. : Structural and Functional Properties of Polytene Nuclei Isolated from Salivary Glands of *Drosophila hydei.* J. Cell Biol., *41*: 591-599, 1969.
17. BREUER, M. E. and PAVAN, C. : Behaviour of Polytene Chromosomes of *Rhynchosciara angelae* at Different Stages of Development. Chromosoma, *7*:371-386, 1955.
18. BRIDGES, C. B. : Salivary Chromosome Maps. J. Hered., *26*:60-64, 1935.
19. BURDETTE, W. J. : Isolation of Ecdysone from Drosophila. Drosophila Information Service, *20*:107-108, 1956.
20. BURDETTE, W. J. : Cellular Aspects of Tumorigenesis. Ann. N.Y. Acad. Sci., 1068-1071, 1958.

21. BURDETTE, W. J. : Tumors in Drosophila. Biological Contributions, The University
     of Texas, Austin, Pub. No. 5914:57-68, 1959.
22. BURDETTE, W. J.:Changes in Titer of Ecdysone in *Bombyx mori* During Meta-
     morphosis. Science, *135*:432, 1962.
23. BURDETTE, W. J.: Tumors, Hormones, and Viruses in Drosophila. Current Topics
     in Comparative Pathology, Vol. 3, in press, 1973.
24. BURDETTE, W. J.: Visible Alterations in Genic Activation Caused by Hormones and
     Oncogenic Viruses. *In*: Exploitable Molecular Mechanisms and Neoplasia. The
     University of Texas Press, Austin. pp. 507-520, 1968b.
25. BURDETTE, W. J. and ANDERSON, R.: Puffing of Salivary Gland Chromosomes
     after Treatment with Carbon Dixoide. Nature, *208*:409-410, 1965.
26. BURDETTE, W. J. and KOBAYASHI, M.: Response of Chromosomal Puffs to Crys-
     talline Hormones *in Vivo*. Proc. Soc. Exp. Biol. and Med., *131*:209-213, 1969.
27. CLEVER, U.: Genaktivitaten in den Riesenchromosomen von *Chironomus tentans*
     und Ihre Beziehungen zur Entwicklung. I. Genaktivierungen durch Ecdyson.
     Chromosoma, *12*:607-675, 1961.
28. CLEVER, U.: Genaktivitaten in den Riesenchromosomen von *Chironomus tentans*
     und Ihre Beziehungen zur Entwicklung. II. Das Verhalten der Puffs während des
     Letzen Larvenstadiums und der Puppenhautung. Chromosoma, *13*:385-436,
     1962.
29. CLEVER, U.: Control of Chromosome Puffing. *In*: L. Goldstein (ed.), The Control
     of Nuclear Activity. Englewood Cliffs, New Jersey: Prentice Hall, 1967.
30. CLEVER, U. and BEERMANN, W.: Studies of Nucleo-cytoplasmic Interrelations in
     Giant Chromosomes of Diptera. Proc. XVI Internatl. Congress Zoology,
     Washington, D. C., pp. 210-215, 1963.
31. CLEVER, U. and KARLSON, P.: Induktion von Puff-veranderungèn in den Speichel-
     drusenchromosomen von *Chironomus tentans* durch Ecdyson. Exp. Cell Res.,
     20:623-626, 1960.
32. CROUSE, H. V.: The Role of Ecdysone in DNA-puff Formation and DNA Synthesis
     in the Polytene Chromosomes of *Sciara coprophila*. Proc. Natl. Acad. Sci.,U.S.,
     61:971-978, 1968.
33. FICQ, A. and PAVAN, C.: Metabolisme des Acides Nucleiques et des Proteines dans
     les Chromosomes Geants. Path. Biol., Paris, *9*:756-757, 1961.
34. GROSS, J. D.: Incorporation of Phosphorus-32 into Salivary-type Chromosomes
     Which Exhibit Puffs. Nature, London, *180*:440, 1957.
35. GROSSBACH, U.: Cell Differentiation in the Salivary Glands of *Campto-chironomus
     tentans* and *C. pallidufitatus*. Ann. Zool. Fennici, *5*:37-40, 1968.
36. HEITZ, E. and BAUER, H.: Beweise für die Chromosomennatur der Kernschleifen
     in den Knauelkernen von *Bibio hortulanus* L. Z. Zellforsch. Mikrosk. Anat.,
     17:67-82, 1933.
37. KARLSON, P.: Biochemical Studies of Ecdysone Control of Chromosomal Activity.
     J. Cell. Comp. Physiol., *66*:69-76, 1965.
38. KEYL, H.-G.: DNA-Konstanz in Heterochromatin von Glyptotendipes.Exptl. Cell
     Res., *302*:345-347, 1963.
39. KOBEL, H. R. and van BREUGEL, F. M. A.: Observations on *ltl* (*lethal tumorous
     larvae*) of *Drosophila melanogaster*. Genetica, *38*:305-327, 1968.
40. KOLTZOFF, N.: The Structure of the Chromosomes in the Salivary Glands of
     Drosophila. Science, *80*:312-313, 1934.

41. KROEGER, H.: The Induction of New Puffing Patterns by Transplantation of Salivary Gland Nuclei into Egg Cytoplasm of Drosophila. Chromosoma, *11*:129-145, 1960.

42. KROEGER, H.: Hormones, Ion Balances and Gene Activity in Dipteran Chromosomes. Mem. Soc. Endocr., *15*:55-66, 1967.

43. KROEGER, H. and LEZZI, M.: Regulation of Gene Action in Insect Development. A. Rev. Ent., *11*:1-22, 1966.

44. LAUFER, H. and HOLT, Th. K. H.: Juvenile Hormone Effects on Chromosomal Puffing and Development in *Chironomus thummi*. J. Exp. Zool., *173*:341-352, 1970.

45. LAUFER, H. and NAKASE, Y.: Salivary Gland Secretion and Its Relation to Chromosomal Puffing in the Dipteran, *Chironomus thummi*. Proc. Natl. Acad. Sci., U. S., *53*:511-516, 1965.

46. LEZZI, M.: Cytochemische Untersuchungen an Puffs Isolierter Speicheldrusenchromosomen von Chironomus. Chromosoma, *21*:89-108, 1967.

47. LEZZI, M.: Differential Gene Activation in Isolated Chromosomes. International Review of Cytology, *29*:127-168, 1970.

48. LEZZI, M. and FRIGG, M.: Specific Effects of Juvenile Hormone on Chromosome Function. Schweiz. Entomol. Gesellsch., *44*:163-170, 1971.

49. LEZZI, M. and GILBERT, L. I.: Control of Gene Activities in the Polytene Chromosomes of *Chironomus tentans* by Ecdysone and Juvenile Hormone. Natl. Acad. Sci., U. S., *64*:498-503, 1969.

50. L'HERITIER, Ph.: The CO_2 Sensitivity Problem in Drosophila. Cold Spring Harbor Symposium on Quantitative Biology, *16*:99-112, 1951.

51. PAINTER, T. S.: A New Method for the Study of Chromosome Rearrangements and the Plotting of Chromosome Maps. Science, *78*:585-586, 1933.

52. PANITZ, Von R.: Hormonkontrollierte Genaktivitaten in den Riesenchromosomen von *Acricotopus lucidus*. Biol. Abl., *83*:197-230, 1964.

53. PAVAN, C. and BASILE, R.: Chromosome Changes Induced by Infections in Tissues of *Rhynchosciara angelae*. Science, *151*:1556-1558, 1966.

54. PELLING, C.: Ribonucleinsaure-synthese der Riesenchromosomen. Autoradiographische Untersuchungen an *Chironomus tentans*. Chromosoma, *15*:71-122, 1964.

55. POULSON, D. and METZ, C. W.: Studies on the Structure of Nucleolus-forming Regions and Related Structures in the Giant Salivary-gland Chromosomes of Diptera. J. Morph., *63*:363-395, 1938.

56. PLUS, N.: Étude de la Multiplication du Virus de la Sensibilite au Gaz Carbonique chez la Drosophila Bull. Biol. France et Bilg., *88*:248-293, 1954.

57. RITOSSA, F.: Attivita Sintetiche al Livello dei Puffs in *Drosophila busckii*. Atti Ass. Genet. Ital., *7*:147-156, 1962.

58. RITOSSA, F.: New Puffs Induced by Temperature Shock, DNP, and Salicylate in Salivary Chromosomes of *D. melanogaster*. Drosophila Information Service, *37*:122-123, 1963.

59. RITOSSA, F.: Experimental Activation of Specific Loci in Polytene Chromosomes of *Drosophila*. Exp. Cell Res., *35*:601-607, 1964.

60. RITOSSA, F. and SPIEGELMAN, S.: Localization of DNA Complementary to Ribosomal RNA in the Nucleolus Organizer Region of *Drosophila melanogaster*. Proc. Natl. Acad. Sci., U. S., *53*:737-745, 1965.

61. RODMAN, T. C.: Control of Polytenic Replication in Dipteran Larvae. I. Increased Number of Cycles in a Mutant Strain of *Drosophila melanogaster*. J. Cell Physiol., *70*:179-186, 1967.

62. RUDKIN, G. T. and CORLETTE, S. L.: Disproportionate Synthesis of DNA in a Polytene Chromosome Region. Proc. Natl. Acad. Sci., U. S., *43*:964-968,1957.

63. SEBELVA, T. E.: Quantitative Determination of DNA Content during Formation of One of the Puffs and One of the Balbiani Rings in *Chironomus dorsalis*. Cytologia, *10*:765-769, 1968.

64. STEFFENSEN, D. M. and WHIMBER, D. E.: Localization of tRNA Genes in the Salivary Chromosomes of Drosophila by RNA:DNA Hybridization. Genetics, *69*:163-178, 1971.

65. SWIFT, H.: The Histones of Polytene Chromosomes. *In*: J. Bonner and P. Tso (ed.), Nucleohistones. p. 169-183. San Francisco: Holden-Day, 1964.

Assays

BIOASSAY for
BRAIN HORMONE

Masatoshi Kobayashi and Masayoshi Yamazaki

I n Bombyx silkworms diapause does not occur in the pupal stage, and silkworm pupae become moths in about 12 days following pupation at 25° C. However, in an experimental study on the function of the brain during the pupal stage, Kobayashi (1955; 1957; Kobayashi and Kirimura, 1958; Kobayashi and Yamashita, 1959) found that when pupal brains were extirpated immediately after pupation, most did not show any sign of imaginal differentiation and that these brainless pupae proved to be one of the most suitable animals for the assay of brain hormone. Each pupa treated in this way was called a Dauer-pupa, following the nomenclature of Wigglesworth for Dauer-larva.

The F_1-hybrid pupae from crosses between the two Bombyx races, J. 122 and C. 115, were used in the work to be presented and were kept at 25° C. throughout the experiments. The head of each of two controls was incised and not cerebrectomized, whereas the brains of the experimental animals were extirpated. The ordinary pupae of the silkworm became imagines on the eleventh to fourteenth day after pupation; but, when the pupal brain was extirpated immediately after pupation, most pupae did not show any sign of imaginal differentiation for more than 40 days after pupation at 25° C.

As illustrated in Table 1, Dauer-pupa occurred among the pupae operated within 240 minutes after pupation. In both male and female, the earlier the operation was performed, the greater the number of Dauer-pupae obtained.

TABLE 1

RELATIONSHIP BETWEEN THE EXTIRPATION OF BRAIN
AT VARIOUS PERIODS IN EARLY PUPAL STAGE AND
IMAGINAL DIFFERENTIATION IN THE SILKWORM

Series of Experiments	Pupal Age (Minutes)	No. of Pupae	No. of Imagines	No. of Dauer-pupae
Extirpation of Brain	0	654	99	448
	30	86	34	44
	60	49	19	29
	120	44	27	12
	240	45	35	7
Mock Operation	0	83	80	0
No Operation	–	92	90	0

TABLE 2

EFFECT OF IMPLANTATION OF A FRESH BRAIN FROM
BOMBYX MORI INTO EACH DAUER–PUPA AT 25°C

Stage of Donor	No. of Dauer-pupae Recipients	No. of Moths Emerged	Days from Implantation to Emergence	No. of Dead Individuals
Larva	15	14	18 – 25	1
Pupa	33	27	16 – 20	6
Moth	20	10	19 – 25	10
Non-implanted Control	65	0	–	0

Table 2 shows the effect of implantation of a fresh brain from the Bombyx silkworm. When a fresh brain, obtained either from a larva, pupa, or moth was implanted into the head of a Dauer-pupa, the latter became an imago in 16-25 days after implantation, although no imaginal differentiation was observed in the Dauer-pupae that had no implanted brain even though they were kept at 25° C. for 120 days after pupation.

TABLE 3

SEASONAL DIFFERENCES IN THE PERCENTAGE OF DAUER−PUPAE
IN THREE VARIETIES OF THE SILKWORM

Varieties of Silkworm	Rearing Season	No. of Pupae	No. of Imagines (a)	No. of Dauer-pupae * (b)	Percentage of Dauer-pupae (b/a+b)
N122 X C115	Spring	1136 (♀)	155	704	82.0
		1060 (♂)	50	702	93.4
	Summer	255 (♀)	113	91	44.6
		273 (♂)	54	158	74.5
	Late Autumn	242 (♀)	81	121	60.2
		585 (♂)	99	309	75.3
C115	Spring	190 (♀)	65	67	50.8
		116 (♂)	9	63	87.5
	Summer	61 (♀)	35	9	20.5
		49 (♂)	12	17	63.0
	Late Autumn	172 (♀)	70	42	37.5
		149 (♂)	17	29	63.0
N122	Spring	37 (♀)	6	0	0
		53 (♂)	17	0	0
	Summer	107 (♀)	54	0	0
		96 (♂)	37	0	0
	Late Autumn	188 (♀)	84	0	0
		317 (♂)	81	0	0

* Dauer-pupae showed no imaginal differentiation at 25 °C. for 40 days after pupation.

Table 3 gives the seasonal differences in the rates of appearance of Dauer-pupae. The rates of occurrence of Dauer-pupae vary with the varieties and also with the rearing season, even though the operations are made during the same period in the life cycle, *i. e.*, immediately after pupation. After two larval brains were implanted into the fifth abdominal segments of fifth-instar larvae, two different procedures were carried out following pupation of the silkworms on which the operations were performed.

TABLE 4

RELATIONSHIP BETWEEN IMAGINAL DIFFERENTIATION
AND EXTIRPATION OF PUPAL BRAIN

Series of Experiments	No. of Pupae	No. of Imagines (a)	No. of Dauer-pupae (b)	Percentage of Dauer-pupae (b/a+b)
1*	54	12	8	40.0
2**	51	0	18	100.0

* Approximately 24 hours after the fourth molt, two fresh larval brains were implanted into each fifth abdominal segment of fifth-instar larvae; and then, immediately after pupation, the native brain in each pupa was extirpated from the pupae operated on at the larval stage.

** Approximately 24 hours after the fourth molt, the fifth abdominal segment of each larva was wounded without subsequent implantation of a brain; and then, immediately after pupation (as in series 1), the brain was removed from each pupa.

Dauer-pupa showed no imaginal differentiation for 40 days after pupation at 25° C.

In one group of pupae, shown in Table 4, the brain of each host was extirpated immediately after pupation. A positive effect of implanting the brain is evident; all of the nonimplanted controls became Dauer-pupae.

In the other group, included in Table 5, the pupae were ligated at a level between the thorax and abdomen 2 hours after pupation. Then the part anterior to the ligature was removed. With two exceptions, the isolated pupal abdomens in this group showed no imaginal differentiation for 40 days, even though brains had been implanted into each abdomen during the larval stage. Two of the pupae became moths 34-35 days after ligation, but this result could not be repeated when 10 larval brains were implanted into each of 11 abdomens.

It is concluded from these experiments that brain and thoracic segment with prothoracic glands are necessary in Bombyx for the initiation of adult

TABLE 5

EFFECT OF LARVAL BRAIN IMPLANTED INTO ABDOMINAL SEGMENT AT LARVAL
STAGE ON IMAGINAL DIFFERENTIATION OF ISOLATED ABDOMEN OF PUAPE
LIGATED AT LEVEL BETWEEN THORAX AND ABDOMEN

Series of Experiment	No. of Pupae	No. of Imagines (Pupal Time in Days) (a)	No. of Dauer-pupae (b)	Percentage of Dauer-pupae (b/a+b)
3*	61	2 (34 – 35)	10	83.5
4**	53	0	6	100.0
5***	11	0	0	0

* Approximately 24 hours after the fourth molt, two fresh larval brains were implanted into each fifth abdominal segment of the fifth-instar larvae; and then, about 2 hours after pupation, the anterior part of each pupa was cut off after ligating at the level between thorax and abdomen.

** Isolated abdomen from individuals in which approximately 24 hours after the fourth molt, the fifth abdominal segment of each larva was wounded without subsequent implantation of a brain; and then, about 2 hours after pupation (as in series 3) both parts, head and thorax, were cut off.

*** Isolated abdomen from individuals in which approximately 24 hours after the fourth molt, ten fresh brains were implanted into each fifth abdominal segment of the fifth-instar larvae and then, at about 2 hours after pupation, the same fifth-instar operation as in series 3 was carried out.

TABLE 6

IMAGINAL DIFFERENTIATION OF THE DAUER–PUPAE IN THE SILKWORM AT 25°C

Experiments	Series of Experiments (Sex)	Number of Specimens (Pupal Time In Days)*	Days Required for Imaginal Differentiation After Pupation (No. of Imagines)**	Days Survived (No. of Dead Individuals)	No. of Undeveloped Individuals***
Spring Rearing	Females	30 (90)	200 (3) 210 (1) 220 (4) 230 (2) 240 (5) 250 (6) 260 (3) 270 (2)	220 (1) 260 (1) 280 (2)	0
	Males	30 (90)	170 (2) 180 (3) 190 (4) 200 (3) 210 (2) 220 (5) 240 (3) 250 (1)	160 (2) 190 (1) 220 (2) 280 (1) 270 (1)	0

* Pupae deprived of their brains immediately after pupation and kept at 25°C.

** Observation of experimental animals carried out each 10 days beginning at 90 days in the Spring rearing until 300 days after pupation.

*** The results obtained for 300 days at 25°C. after extirpation of pupal brain.

development. The brain first secretes a factor for the activation of the pro-thoracic gland, and the prothoracic gland then releases into the blood a hormone that initiates imaginal differentiation. These interrelationships make the Dauer-pupa a most suitable object for the assay of brain hormone.

The procedure to prepare Dauer-pupae is straightforward. Bombyx pupae consisting of F_1 hybrids between the two races, J. 122 and C. 115, are used as materials immediately after pupation at 25° C. After maintenance at 2.5° C. for several hours to 24 hours to retard circulation of the blood, the brain is extirpated from each pupae. The wounded portion is sealed with melted paraffin, and the resulting brainless pupa (Dauer-pupa) which shows no sign of imaginal differentiation for about 6 weeks may be used at 25° C. in testing for the presence of brain-hormone activity. As indicated in Table 6, most Dauer-pupae are in a diapause-like state for at least 100 days.

Prior to the injection of solution to be tested into Dauer-pupae, sealed paraffin is taken from each pupa and appropriate dilution of test-substance is injected into the pupa through the abdominal intersegmental membrane. The puncture is sealed with melted paraffin, and then the pupae are maintained at 25° C. Usually, the Dauer-pupa injected emerges as a moth in about 3 weeks following the injection of the active substance at 25° C. Extensive experience with the bioassay indicates that it is qualitative for a single concentration, and tests are considered positive when 50 per cent or more of the specimens emerge as moths. Up to the present time, several kinds of insect, such as Antheraea, (Gersch and Sturzeichung, 1968), *Bombyx mori* (Kobayashi and Kirimura, 1958), *Hyalophora cecropia* (Williams, 1967), *Samia cynthia* pryeri, (Kobayashi *et al.*, 1967), and *Samia cynthia* ricini (Ichikawa and Ishizaki, 1961), have been used as test-objects for the brain-hormone assay.

References

1. GERSCH, H. and STÜRZEICHUNG, J.: Weitere Untersuchungen zur Kennzeichung des Aktivationshormones der Insektenhautung. J. Insect Physiol., *14*:87, 1968.
2. ICHIKAWA, M. and ISHIZAKI, H.: Brain Hormone of the Silkworm, *Bombyx mori*. Nature, *191*:333, 1961.
3. KOBAYASHI, M.: Relationship Between the Brain Hormone and the Imaginal Differentiation of the Silkworm, *Bombyx mori*. J. Sericul. Sci. Jap., *24*:389, 1955.
4. KOBAYASHI, M.: Studies on Neurosecretion in the Silkworm, *Bombyx mori* L. Bull. Sericul. Exp. Sta., *15*:181, 1957.
5. KOBAYASHI, M., FUKAYA, S. and MITSUHASHI, J.: Imaginal Differentiation of 'Dauer-pupae' in the Silkworm, *Bombyx mori*. J. Sericul. Sci. Jap., *29*:337, 1960.
6. KOBAYASHI, M. and KIRIMURA, J.: The Brain Hormone in the Silkworm, *Bombyx mori* L. Nature, *181*:1217, 1958.
7. KOBAYASHI, M. and YAMASHITA, Y.: Effect of the Imaginal Differentiation and Activity of the Brain Prothoracic Gland System During the Pupal Stage in the Silkworm, *Bombyx mori*. J. Sericul. Sci. Jap., *28*:67, 1959.
8. KOBAYASHI, M. and YAMASHITA, Y.: Seasonal Differences in the Rates of the Appearance of Dauer-pupa in the Silkworm, *Bombyx mori* L. J. Sericul. Sci. Jap., *27*:93, 1958.
9. WILLIAMS, C. M.: *In*: J.W.L.Beament and J.R.Treharne (ed.), Insect Physiology. p. 133. London: Oliver and Boyd, 1967.

STANDARDIZATION of DIPTERAN BIOASSAY for MOLTING HORMONES

J. A. Thomson

Without a reliable bioassay for molting-hormone (MH) activity, Karlson and his colleagues [see, for example, reviews by Karlson (1956) and Karlson and Sekeris (1966)] would not have been able to extract, purify, and identify ecdysone. The background provided by their work now permits the use of additional chemical, and especially isotopic-tracer, approaches to the identification of MH and related metabolites. Nevertheless, studies of the biosynthesis and of the comparative biological activity of MH and its analogs must still rely on quantitative bioassays.

The best developed bioassay system for MH is based on sclerotization of the dipteran puparium. This test stems from the work of Fraenkel (1935), refined initially by Becker and Plagge (1939). Improvements, or extensions, to the use of other species have been reported by many subsequent authors, including Karlson (1956), Karlson and Shaaya (1964), Kaplanis *et al.* (1966), Ohtaki (1966), Ohtaki *et al.* (1968), Adelung and Karlson (1969), Fraenkel and Zdarek (1970), and Thomson *et al.* (1970). The bioassay depends on the induction of sclerotization in the abdominal cuticle of a dipteran larva when the posterior section of the body is isolated by ligation from the brain/ringgland complex. The posterior section, or test abdomen (Ohtaki *et al.*, 1968) is presumed to be physiologically receptive on the basis of the sclerotization that marks puparium formation (pupariation; Berreur and Fraenkel, 1969) in the anterior portion of the preparation.

It should be emphasized that the need for meticulous control of the physiological state of the test preparations at every stage in the assay arises from the fact that the induced change being measured is not an all-or-nothing response triggered by a dose of hormone above a specific threshold. Rather the hormone is needed over prolonged exposure periods for both the initiation and continuation of metamorphosis (Ohtaki *et al.*, 1968; Zdarek and Fraenkel, 1970). It is thus only to be expected that interruption of the normal developmental sequence at varied times leads to differences in the subsequent response of the preparations to exogenous MH, and that the developmental history of the animals prior to ligation also influences this response.

Failure in the past to use carefully standardized test abdomens has led to considerable discrepancies between laboratories in the magnitude of the "pupariation unit" (Zdarek and Fraenkel, 1970), as for example in Calliphora (Karlson and Sekeris, 1966). Further, conflicting estimates of the relative activity of different MH analogs have appeared in the literature (Thomson *et al.*, 1970). In the sections that follow, the factors known to influence the outcome of the pupariation bioassay are set out in detail.

SELECTION OF SPECIES FOR USE IN THE BIOASSAY

The principal considerations in selection of the species of fly to be used for bioassay are generally:

(a) *Anatomical Suitability*. The pattern of sclerotization of certain species of Diptera would render them quite unsuitable for use in the MH bioassay as normally performed. Larvae of the tsetse fly, Glossina, for example, pupariate posterior to a ligature placed behind the brain before the anterior segment becomes competent to sclerotize (Langley, 1967), indicating exceptionally localized inhibitory influences in the anterior segment. Price (1970) demonstrated very clearly the production of a factor in the midregion of the larva of Calliphora that inhibits sclerotization, and it seems likely that the factor involved is an inhibition of prophenoloxidase activation of low species-specificity produced in the salivary glands of this and other flies, including Drosophila (Thomson and Sin, 1970). Species selected for bioassay work should therefore be suitable for ligation in a consistent position relative to both the brain/ring-gland complex and to sites of inhibitor production. Further, the larvae should withstand handling and ligation satisfactorily; species with a tough integument are most favorable if excessive bleeding, bacterial infection, and tracheal flooding (Thomson *et al.*, 1970) at the site of ligation are to be avoided.

(b) *Yield*. The proportion of suitable test abdomens obtained from each batch of larvae should be sufficient to avoid excessive waste of labor. The predominant related factors are the ability of the animals to withstand ligation without too much damage to tissues, and the degree to which developmental synchrony has been achieved among the larvae of each batch. Wet storage of postfeeding larvae often improves the synchronization of endocrine activation that occurs after transfer of the animals to a dry substrate (Ohtaki, 1966). The time of ligation can thus be reproduced more readily from one batch of larvae to another. Again there are marked differences between species in the response to wet storage: the physiological condition of larvae of *Calliphora stygia*, for example, is more readily standardized by wet storage than is that of *C. erythrocephala* (= *C. vicina* R-D) (Thomson *et al.*, 1970).

(c) *Sensitivity*. The dose-range within which the test-preparations show a linear response to increasing doses of exogenous MH differs from species to species and may vary between batches of the same species. Physiological aspects of this problem are discussed below, but it is clear that sensitivity of the test abdomens is at least partly related to their size. Thus Musca is more sensitive than Calliphora (Kaplanis *et al.*, 1966), and *C. erythrocephala* is more sensitive than *C. stygia* (Thomson *et al.*, 1970).

(d) *Known Identity of Endogenous MH*. Preference should be given to the use of species in which the functional molting hormone (or hormones) of the normal animal at pupariation have been chemically identified. Quantitative calibration of the bioassay can then be based on the natural MH of the species. In both *C. erythrocephala* and *C. stygia*, β-ecdysone (crustecdysone, ecdysterone) is the predominant MH (Galbraith *et al.*, 1969).

CHOICE OF MH STANDARD

Until the identity of the functional MH in Diptera other than Calliphora has been verified chemically, β-ecdysone should be used as a standard for quantitative work (Thomson *et al.*, 1970; Fraenkel and Zdarek, 1970). A-part from its role as the natural MH in Calliphora, β-ecdysone fulfills the criteria of availability and of high solubility with good stability in aqueous solutions.

PREPARATION AND USE OF TEST-ABDOMENS

(a) *Culture Conditions for Larvae.* The production of physiologically uniform batches of larvae for preparation of test abdomens is materially affected both directly and indirectly by culture conditions during larval life. This is especially so in the case of species such as *C. erythrocephala* where synchronization by wet storage (see below) is not particularly effective and the timing of ligation is based on pupariation of a proportion of each batch (Karlson, 1956; Fraenkel and Zdarek, 1970). To achieve uniform development, cultures must be kept relatively uncrowded, (although, if the larvae are too sparse to aggregate in the food, extracorporeal digestion by salivary enzymes is often suboptimal, affecting growth). Karlson (1956) found liver unsuitable for culturing *C. erythrocephala* to be used in bioassay work, and our experience confirms this. Cultures containing liver often become excessively moist in patches and larvae may then be variably inhibited from pupariation. The amount of variation with cultures and success in getting well synchronized test abdomens for bioassay also may vary seasonally (Karlson and Sekeris, 1966), presumably for similar reasons. Disturbance of the animals either through overcrowding or by handling (Mackerras, 1933; Thomson *et al.*, 1970) may have the same effect.

An adequate and reproducible diet during larval development appears particularly necessary in view of the evidence adduced by Fourche (1967) of increased susceptibility of Drosophila larvae to exogenous MH after starvation, (admittedly extreme in these experiments). The fat body in Calliphora is the principal site of breakdown of MH in the larva (Karlson and Bode, 1969). Starvation, with mobilization of lipid and protein reserves, may lead to an increased susceptibility to exogenous MH because of reduced levels of these catabolic enzymes in severely depleted fat body.

Repeated hand sorting of mature, wandering larvae from those in each batch that are still feeding can assist in obtaining reasonably synchronized larvae when wet storage is not appropriate. This is sometimes facilitated by placing the food on aluminum foil (Fraenkel and Zdarek, 1970), so that larvae that have finished feeding move cleanly to a dry substrate. Dry, soft wood sawdust is generally superior to sand as a substrate, because of its absorbent and nonabrasive qualities.

(b) *Synchronization of Development by Wet Storage.* Larval development of certain species (see above) may be synchronized by storage of mature, wandering larvae on wet filter paper covered by a film of free water, which should be changed every 2-3 days. For example, larvae (day 8/9) of *C. stygia* (Thomson *et al.*, 1970) should be wet stored in this way for a minimum of 4-5 days at 20° C., in darkness, before transfer to dry sawdust prior to ligation (Figure 1).

(c) *Ligation.* Anesthesia is readily accomplished by placing the larvae in a deep dish surrounded by melting crushed ice. Silk or synthetic fiber selected for nonslip properties should be used in a single overhand knot. Placement of the ligature requires standardization both to achieve consistency of volume of the test abdomens and a reproducible position relative to the pupariation-inhibiting factors produced posterior to the brain (Price, 1970). The rapid method of ligation used by Staal (1967) for Musca has not proved satisfactory for Calliphora in our hands because of difficulties in controlling placement of the ligature, normally tied just behind the fifth visible segment (compare Fraenkel and Zdarek, 1970), approximately one-third of the length of the body from the anterior end.

(d) *Maintenance after Ligation.* Certain species show a marked tendency for the tracheal trunks to become fluid filled near the site of ligation, and for the adjacent tissues to become necrotic. In *C. stygia*, incubation in an atmosphere of 5 per cent carbon dioxide in oxygen (Thomson *et al.*, 1970) helps to overcome this problem and increases the yield of test abdomens from about 50-60 per cent to 70-80 per cent of the animals ligated. The method may well be effective in other species where local damage from ligation is marked; it does not appear useful in work with *C. vicina*.

Standardization of the time over which pupariation of the anterior portion of the animal is allowed to occur is particularly important. The closer the injection of exogenous hormone to the time of pupariation of the anterior portion of the test preparation, the greater the response to a given dose (Ohtaki *et al.*, 1968; Fraenkel and Zdarek, 1970). Conversely, the greater the delay between ligation and sclerotization of the portion anterior to the ligature (*i. e.*, the earlier relative to normal pupariation that the anterior and posterior portions are separated) the less sensitive will be the resulting test abdomen (Fraenkel and Zdarek, 1970). A 12-hour interval for collection at a standardized time after ligation is generally satisfactory if the larvae are well synchronized.

(e) *Injection of Test Solutions.* Volumes up to 2-3 µl. may be injected into test abdomens with a fine glass micropipette (Thomson *et al.*, 1970), without using a second ligature (Karlson, 1956), but the latter technique becomes desirable to prevent possible leakage when 5-10 µl. or larger volumes

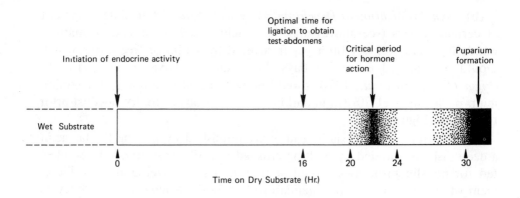

Figure 1

are injected into abdomens of Calliphora. Sensitivity to MH in aqueous solutions increases with injection volume in test abdomens of Calliphora, over the range of 2-10 μl. (Thomson *et al.*, 1970), but the response to a given dose is often reduced when a larger volume is injected.

SCORING THE BIOASSAY

The results of the bioassay are conveniently assessed 24 hours after injection, using the scoring method of Adelung and Karlson (1969). Test abdomens that have only partly sclerotized normally do so progressively from the area around the posterior spiracles towards the ligature, regardless of the position of the injection sites. It is therefore relatively simple to assess the extent of tanning as 0, 25, 50, 75, or 100 per cent of the surface area of the abdomen. Care should be taken to distinguish between tanned, sclerotized abdomens, and those occasional ones that are soft and black or brown as a result of necrosis in bacterially-infected, internal tissues. Such dead preparations are not included in the calculation of the mean percentage response of the injected test abdomens for that sample. Calibration of the assay is achieved when possible by comparison with the response produced by a series of standard MH solutions.

The occurrence of occasional false positive responses among test abdomens has been reported by Ohtaki *et al.* (1968). The program for ligation, injection, and scoring usually can be adjusted to the developmental timetable for each species to avoid this difficulty (*e. g.*, Fraenkel and Zdarek, 1970; Thomson *et al.*, 1970).

The useful range of the bioassay, using volumes of 2 μl. for injection, is 5-50 ng./test abdomen in *C. vicina* and 10-75 ng./test abdomen in *C. stygia*.

PREPARATION OF EXTRACTS FOR TESTING

Certain solvents that have been employed in the preparation of MH extracts are known to cause apparent sclerotization when injected into test abdomens in sufficiently high concentrations (Reay, 1964). Dilute ethanol (5-10 per cent) may safely be used as a solvent when volumes of 2-5 μl. are to be injected into each Calliphora test abdomen. Extensive purification of extracts from animal and plant tissues may be necessary to avoid excess toxicity, and the possibility of concentrating activators or inhibitors of prophenolozidase activity (Thomson and Sin, 1970; Price, 1970) that could affect the bioassay must also be borne in mind until the chemical nature of these components is known.

GENERAL COMMENTS

When careful attention is paid to standardization of the procedure throughout, bioassay methods can provide a reproducible, quantitative evaluation of MH activity. If the identity of the functional MH of the species used for bioassay is known, it seems preferable to express the activity of the unknown sample as the equivalent of a particular dose of purified MH. In the case of *C. stygia* and *C. vicina*, the results of bioassay may be expressed more meaningfully in terms of the amount of β-ecdysone needed per abdomen to produce an equivalent effect. In other species, in which the functional MH has not been identified, results may be expressed more appropriately in pupariation units of MH for that species (Fraenkel and Zdarek, 1970).

It is now clear that the tissues of the isolated abdomen of insects are capable of modifying MH analogs; hydroxylation of α- to β-ecdysone, for example, occurs rapidly in abdominal preparations from Calliphora and Bombyx (King, 1969; Moriyama *et al.*, 1970). As long as the site(s) and route of synthesis of MH remain uncertain, evaluation of the comparative biological activity of MH analogs must proceed in the realization that the observed effects may be due to modification of the analogs by enzymatic systems with specificities and substrate preferences different from those of the normal synthetic pathway.

References

1. ADELUNG, D. and KARLSON, P.: Eine verbesserte, sehr empfindliche Methode zur biologischen Auswertung des Insektenhormones Ecdyson. J. Insect Physiol., *15:*1301-1307, 1969.

2. BECKER, E. and PLAGGE, E.: Über die Puparium-Bildung auslösende Hormon der Fliegen. Biol. Zbl., *59:*326-341, 1939.

3. BERREUR, P. and FRAENKEL, G.: Puparium Formation in Flies: Contraction to Puparium Induced by Ecdysone. Science, *164:*1182-1183, 1969.

4. FOURCHE, J.: Action de l'Ecdysone sur les Larves de *Drosophila melanogaster* soumises au jeûne. Existence d'un Double Conditionnement pour la Formation du Puparium. C. R. Acad. Sci., Paris, D, *264:*2398-2400, 1967.

5. FRAENKEL, G.: A Hormone Causing Pupation in the Blowfly, *Calliphora erythrocephala.* Proc. Roy. Soc., London, Series B, *118:*1-12, 1935.

6. FRAENKEL, G. and ZDAREK, J.: The Evaluation of the *"Calliphora Test"* as an Assay for Ecdysone. Biol. Bull., *139:*138-150, 1970.

7. GALBRAITH, M. N., HORN, D. H. S., THOMSON, J. A., NEUFELD, G. J., and HACKNEY, R. J.: Insect Moulting Hormones. Crustecdysone in *Calliphora.* J. Insect Physiol., *15:*1225-1233, 1969.

8. KAPLANIS, J. N., TABOR, L. A., THOMPSON, M. J.. ROBBINS, W. E., and SHORTLINE, T. I.: Assay for Ecdysone (Moulting Hormone) Activity Using the House Fly, *Musca domestica* L. Steroids, *8:*625-631, 1966.

9. KARLSON, P.: Biochemical Studies on Insect Hormones. Vitam. Horm., *14:* 227-266, 1956.

10. KARLSON, P. and BODE, C.: Die Inaktivierung des Ecdysons bei der Schmeissfliege *Calliphora erythrocephala* Meigen. J. Insect Physiol., *15:*111-118, 1969.

11. KARLSON, P. and SEKERIS, C. E.: Ecdysone, an Insect Steroid Hormone, and its Mode of Action. Recent Progr. Horm. Res., *22:*473-493, 1966.

12. KARLSON, P. and SHAAYA, E.: Der Ecdysontiter während der Insektenentwicklung-I. Eine Methode zur Bestimmung des Ecdysongehalts. J. Insect Physiol., *10:*797-804, 1964.

13. KING, D. S.: Evidence for Peripheral Conversion of α-Ecdysone to β-Ecdysone in Crustaceans and Insects. Gen. Comp. Endocrinol., *13:*512, 1969.

14. LANGLEY, P. A.: Effect of Ligaturing on Puparium Formation in the Larva of the Tsetse Fly, *Glossina morsitans* Westwood. Nature, *214:*389-390, 1967.

15. MACKERRAS, M. J.: Observations on the Life-histories, Nutritional Requirements and Fecundity of Blowflies. Bull. Ent. Res., *24:*353-362, 1933.

16. MORIYAMA, H., NAKANISHI, K., KING, D. S., OKAUCHI, T., SIDDALL, J. B., HAFFERL, W.: On the Origin and Metabolic Fate of α-Ecdysone in Insects. Gen. Comp. Endocrinol., *15:*80-87, 1970.

17. OHTAKI, T.: On the Delayed Pupation of the Fleshfly, *Sarcophaga peregrina* Robineau-Desvoidy. Jap. J. Med. Sci. Biol., *19:*97-104, 1966.

18. OHTAKI, T., MILKMAN, R. D., and WILLIAMS, C. M.: Dynamics of Ecdysone Secretion and Action in the Fleshfly *Sarcophaga peregrina.* Biol. Bull., 135: 322-334, 1968.

19. PRICE, G. M.: Pupation Inhibiting Factor in the Larva of the Blowfly *Calliphora erythrocephala.* Nature, *228:*876-877, 1970.

20. REAY, R. C.: Ability of Various Alcohols to Interfere in the *Calliphora* Bioassay of Ecdysone. Nature, *201:*1329-1330, 1964.

21. STAAL, G. B.: Plants as a Source of Insect Hormones. Proc. K. ned. Akad, Wet. C, *70:*409-418, 1967.

22. THOMSON, J. A. and SIN, Y. T.: The Control of Prophenoloxidase Activation in Larval Haemolymph of *Calliphora.* J. Insect Physiol., *16:*2063-2074, 1970.

23. THOMSON, J. A., IMRAY, F. P., and HORN, D. H. S.: An Improved *Calliphora* Bioassay for Insect Moulting Hormones. Aust. J. Exp. Biol. Med. Sci., *48:*321-328, 1970.

24. ZDAREK, J. and FRAENKEL, G.: Overt and Covert Effects of Endogenous and Exogenous Ecdysone in Puparium Formation of Flies. Proc. Nat. Acad. Sci., U. S., *67:*331-337, 1970.

ASSAYS for
JUVENILE HORMONE

John S. Bjerke and Herbert Röller

Juvenile-hormone activity can be demonstrated by application of a test substance to an insect that is about to undergo a metamorphic molt. As a result of reduced activity of the corpora allata at this stage of development, no surgical procedures are needed to eliminate endogenous juvenile hormone. The various morphogenetic test systems may be divided into two groups, the systemic assays and the so-called cuticle tests.

Systemic tests are those in which the morphogenetic activity of the test substance is evaluated from its effect on the entire body (or whole-body region) of the treated insect. Two useful systems for testing employ Polyphemus and Tenebrio respectively.

    1.   The Polyphemus test. This widely used bioassay which was developed by Williams (1956; Williams and Law, 1965) and Gilbert and Schneiderman (1960; 1961; Schneiderman and Gilbert, 1958; Schneiderman and Gilbert, 1959) utilizes post-diapause pupae (*i. e.,* chilled at 6° C. for several months) of *Antheraea polyphemus.* [Post-diapause pupae of *Hyalophora cecropia* and other saturniids have also been used in similar assays (Gilbert and Schneiderman, 1960; Gilbert and Schneiderman, 1961; Sláma and Williams,

1966; Tsao *et al.*, 1963; Williams, 1956).] The substance to be tested is injected into the dorsal portion of the thorax; retention of pupal characteristics in the forms that emerge from treated animals indicates the presence of juvenile-hormone activity in the material injected.

2.   Tenebrio tests. Yamamoto and Jacobson (1962) and Bowers and Thompson (1963; Bowers *et al.*, 1965) have described systemic bioassays utilizing pupae of *Tenebrio molitor*. The substance to be tested is injected (Yamamoto and Jacobson, 1962; Bowers and Thompson, 1963) or applied topically to the abdominal sternites (Bowers and Thompson, 1963; Bowers *et al.*, 1965); its effect on the development of abdominal structures, specifically urogomphi, genitalia, and gin traps, is evaluated.

The so-called cuticle tests are designed to determine the effect of the test substance on the formation of cuticle in the circumscribed area where the sample is applied. Several test systems have been described:

1.   Wax tests. Post-diapause pupae of *Antheraea polyphemus* (Gilbert and Schneiderman, 1961; Schneiderman, 1961; Schneiderman and Gilbert, 1958; Schneiderman and Gilbert, 1959; Williams and Law, 1965) or *Hyalophora cecropia* (Fisher and Sanborn, 1964) and, more recently, pupae of *Galleria mellonella* (Schneiderman and Gilbert, 1964; Schneiderman *et al.*, 1965; de Wilde *et al.*, 1968) have been used in this sensitive bioassay. The substance to be tested reaches the target tissue, regenerating epidermal cells, by diffusion from wax plugs used to seal small punctures in the prothoracic or mesothoracic tergum of each pupa. The appearance of patches of pupal cuticle over the wounded areas following the adult molt is a positive test for juvenile-hormone activity.

2.   The Rhodnius assay. Various techniques for injection and topical application have been tried in several tests performed on fifth-instar nymphs of *Rhodnius prolixus* (Wigglesworth, 1958; Wigglesworth, 1963). Best results are obtained by spreading the substance to be tested over the fourth abdominal tergite which has previously been abraded by allowing an aqueous suspension of crystalline alumina to dry on its surface. The presence of juvenile-hormone activity in the sample causes the epidermis under the abraded area to produce a patch of nymphal cuticle in the course of the ensuing adult molt.

3.   Tenebrio tests. Three cuticle tests utilizing pupae of *Tenebrio molitor* have been reported. In the micropuncture procedure of Wigglesworth (1958), the cuticle is punctured through droplets of the test-substance which have been applied to the abdominal sternites. In the Tenebrio test of Karlson and Nachtigall (1961), serial dilutions of the test-substance in olive oil are prepared and each concentration is tested in 40 pupae (12-48 hours postpupation). Each animal receives a 0.5 μl. aliquot of the sample injected be-

tween the epidermis and cuticle of an abdominal sternite. Juvenile-hormone activity in the test substance is indicated by the presence in the hatched beetles of spots of pupal cuticle surrounding the punctures, or, respectively, a patch of pupal cuticle over the area where the sample was deposited. The Tenebrio test by Karlson and Nachtigall has been modified by Röller *et al.* (1965; 1969) in several respects.

Pupae 0-27 hours postpupation were used in our assay for some time (Röller *et al.*, 1965; Röller *et al.*, 1969) until it was discovered that the soft, white unsclerotized pupae that are less than approximately 3 hours postpupation had a much lower survival rate than did older pupae. Thereafter, these freshly pupated animals were discarded and pupae 3-27 hours postpupation, which proved to be somewhat more satisfactory, were used (Bjerke, 1970). These animals are much younger and more uniform in age than the pupae in the Tenebrio test of Karlson and Nachtigall [12-48 hours postpupation (1961)].

Furthermore, the animals are punctured intersegmentally between the fourth and fifth abdominal sternites with a 26-gauge needle inserted anteriorly to deposit the standard volume of 1.0 μl. between the epidermis and cuticle of the third abdominal sternite. At least 50 pupae are injected with each concentration of a dilution series. Only beetles on which a patch of typical pupal cuticle can be observed in the third abdominal sternite (over the area where the sample is deposited) are classified as positive. The major difference, however, between our Tenebrio test and that of Karlson and Nachtigall (1961), on which it is based, is in the method of reporting the results. For each assay, we express the numbers of negative, positive, and dead animals as percentages of the total number of pupae used. During routine testing an average mortality of less than 10 per cent of the total pupae injected is observed. The results from assays in which the mortality is more than 20 per cent are disregarded and, if possible, the test is repeated. Karlson and Nachtigall discarded the dead animals and expressed the numbers of negative and positive beetles as percentages of the number of survivors. In so doing, they eliminated a random factor from their results, thus decreasing the variability of their data. When assaying nontoxic substances such as the juvenile hormone, it would have been advantageous to follow the convention of Karlson and Nachtigall in expressing the results. Certain juvenile-hormone mimics and crude oils that we tested, however, produce a mortality in pupae of Tenebrio directly proportional to the dosage. When assaying substances such as these, use of the convention of Karlson and Nachtigall eliminates significant information. A second difference between the two versions is in the definition of the Tenebrio unit. Karlson and Nachtigall defined the Tenebrio-Einheit as "...diejenige Menge wirksamer Substanz, die in 30-50% der Tiere eine positive epidermale Veränderung hervorruft," whereas we established the unit at a single response level of 40 per cent positive of the total pupae injected.

The quantitative aspects of these bioassays are of particular importance in considering their suitability for evaluating the effectiveness of procedures for purification of active extracts of juvenile hormone. Certain methods for applying the sample, *i. e.,* diffusion through abraded cuticle as in the Rhodnius assay, passage through micropunctures as in the Tenebrio test of Bowers and Thompson, and diffusion from wax plugs as in the various wax tests, do not insure that a measured amount is brought quantitatively to the target tissues. Uncontrollable physiological factors such as the variable side effects of wounding in the wax tests and the delay (with concomitant inactivation of the juvenile hormone) that frequently occurs between injection of the sample and resumption of adult development in the Polyphemus test may affect the response significantly. Finally, the methods for quantitating the results must be considered. One approach has been to develop a numerical scoring system similar to those reported for the Polyphemus test [two systems, (Gilbert and Schneiderman, 1960; Williams, 1961)] and the Tenebrio test of Bowers and Thompson by which the animals are rated according to the pupal characteristics that are retained, or the rating scales described for the Tenebrio test of Wigglesworth and the Galleria wax test of Schneiderman *et al.* (1965), that are based on the presence or absence and size of the patches of pupal cuticle produced. The values for the sum or average for each animal or group of animals are then computed to give a score or index indicating the juvenile-hormone activity of the substance tested. When using this approach, it must be assumed that the arbitrary numerical scale based on the magnitude of the response is in fact proportional to the dose as well. The validity of such a proportionality has never been demonstrated. A second approach has been to utilize an experimental design that permits the unit of juvenile-hormone activity to be determined from a standard dose-response curve based on the results of a large number of test animals rated simply on the presence or absence of a given response. With this experimental design, random errors in determining the unit of activity due to biological variability are minimized. It has been adopted in the Tenebrio test of Karlson and Nachtigall (1961), more recently, in the Galleria wax test of de Wilde *et al.* (1968), and in our Tenebrio test (Röller *et al.,* 1965; Röller *et al.,* 1969; Bjerke, 1970), but was not feasible with the Polyphemus test because of the large numbers of animals required (Gilbert and Schneiderman, 1960).

With regard to the accuracy of various bioassays for juvenile hormone, it has been claimed that the Polyphemus test permits comparison of extracts to within a factor of two (Gilbert and Schneiderman, 1961). With a single lot of

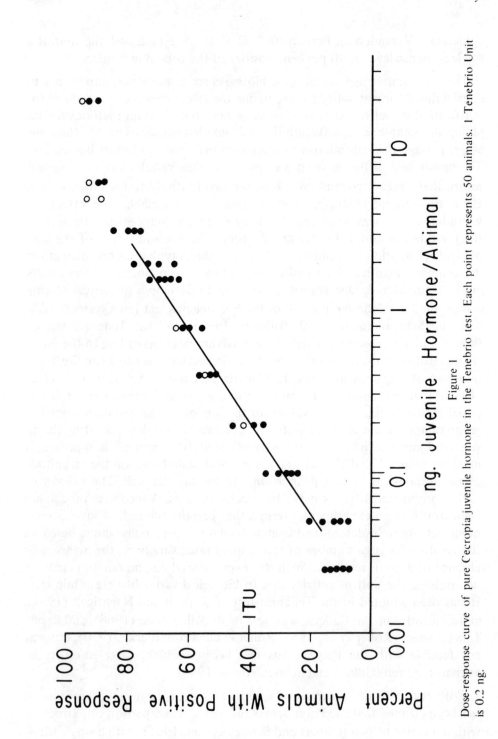

Figure 1

Dose-response curve of pure Cecropia juvenile hormone in the Tenebrio test. Each point represents 50 animals. 1 Tenebrio Unit is 0.2 ng.

twelve pupae, the Galleria wax test also was reported to be "...accurate within a factor of 2" (Schneiderman *et al.*, 1965). Such accuracy cannot be claimed for our Tenebrio test. The range of one confidence interval corresponds roughly to a four-fold difference in concentration of juvenile hormone. This indicates that in at least 90 per cent of the cases, the Tenebrio assay could detect a four-fold difference in the concentration of substance tested. Calculation of the 60 per cent confidence intervals [±4.8 per cent at an injection level of 1 Tenebrio unit (TU); 0.17-0.32 ng. (Figure 1) at a positive response level of 40 per cent] indicates that a two-fold difference in concentration would be detected approximately 60 per cent of the time. In view of the biological variability inherent in the animals tested, the claim of accuracy to within a factor of two would appear to be outstandingly high for an assay of this type. In our version of the Tenebrio test, the variability is indictated by the standard error $^sy.x = 5.51$. Unfortunately, data that would allow us to estimate the variability in the Polyphemus or the Galleria wax test have not been reported. Karlson and Nachtigall (1961) published some replicated data from which the variability of their Tenebrio test can be estimated. The calculated standard errors of 3.6, 5.2, and 12.2 are in the same range as our value of 5.51. While lacking the degree of accuracy claimed for two other juvenile-hormone bioassays, our version of the Tenebrio test does at least compare favorably with the only other test for which an adequate evaluation may be made.

The useful range of the Tenebrio bioassay is between the response levels of 15-70 per cent positive. This corresponds approximately to solutions that contain from 0.05-2.0 ng. of juvenile hormone (0.2-8 TU of juvenile-hormone activity, Figure 1). We did not perform any experiments to determine the least amount of juvenile hormone that could be detected with certainty in this assay.

TABLE 1

SENSITIVITY OF BIOASSAYS FOR JUVENILE HORMONE

Bioassay	Corresponding Animal Unit of *dl* Juvenile Hormone	
Polyphemus test [scored according to Williams (24)]	3+ response:	1×10^{-2} μg.
Tenebrio test (12, 11, 1)	1 Tenebrio Unit:	2×10^{-4} μg.
Polyphemus wax test	1 Polyphemus Unit:	1×10^{-5} μg.
Galleria wax test [performed according to de Wilde (6)]	1 Galleria Unit:	5×10^{-6} μg.

As a basis for comparing the Tenebrio bioassay with two other tests widely used for juvenile hormone from the standpoint of sensitivity, the above figures are pertinent (Table 1). We can consider the Tenebrio test to be approximately 50-fold more sensitive than the Polyphemus test and approximately 20-fold less sensitive than the Polyphemus wax test. The Galleria wax test performed according to de Wilde (de Wilde *et al.*, 1968) was approximately 40 times more sensitive than our Tenebrio test.

Comparing the different known bioassays for juvenile-hormone activity, none is specific for authentic juvenile hormone; it appears on the basis of experiments with various juvenile-hormone analogs that they all have a relatively close range of specificity. Bowers and Thompson (1963) reported that injection of vegetable oils, mineral oil, or oleic acid resulted in the appearance of unpigmented white spots in the hatched beetles of Tenebrio, but it is not clear whether these were pupal cuticle or unsclerotized adult cuticle. When testing certain extracts, we also obtained numerous beetles with unpigmented spots that represented unsclerotized or otherwise abnormal adult cuticle, but did not count these as positive responses. Zlotkin and Levinson, who recently investigated the histological aspects of the Tenebrio test (1968a, 1968b, 1969), reported that such patches of unsclerotized adult cuticle gradually disappeared (1968b). They found that after subcuticular injection of crude oil from *Hyalophora cecropia,* the cuticle produced over the area of sample deposition appeared from the surface to be morphologically identical with pupal cuticle (1969). This agrees with our observation that the two appear identical under the phase contrast microscope (Röller and Finn, unpublished communication). Zlotkin and Levinson demonstrated by biochemical procedures, however, that juvenilized cuticle differs structurally from pupal cuticle in consisting mainly of pupal endocuticle, which represents the last type of cuticle produced by the epidermal cells in the previous molt (1969). Although they emphasize this difference between juvenilized cuticle and pupal cuticle, Zlotkin and Levinson did not study the effects of pure juvenile hormone and implanted corpora allata on the cuticle development and hence overlooked the possibility that a structurally complete pupal cuticle would be formed in the absence of toxic factors which might be present in the oil from *Hyalophora cecropia.* With the help of electron microscopy, Caveney (1970) recently demonstrated that pupal epidermis affected by juvenile-hormone analogs secretes a larvalized exocuticle and a pupal endocuticle. By rigidly defining the criterion for a positive response and by considering all questionable responses as negative, we never were confused by any possible pseudojuvenilizing effects of fatty acids or other components of extracts.

Since culturing *Rhodnius prolixus* is prohibited in some countries (including the United States) and pupae of *Antheraea polyphemus* (and other saturniids) are extremely costly, the Galleria wax test and the Tenebrio test remain as highly sensitive and dependable bioassays for juvenile-hormone activity, advantageous for testing extracts and especially fractions with small yields.

It might be added that several experiments have demonstrated that the biological activity depends largely on the carrier with which it is administered. For example, hormone injected in an aqueous emulsion or in a water-miscible solvent such as dimethyl sulfoxide (DMSO) or 1,2-propanediol, exerts no effect (Wigglesworth, 1963; Röller and Dahm, 1968). These results may be explained by differing degrees of protection and release afforded by the carriers in the presence of degrading enzymes.

Juvenile-hormone activity may also be determined quantitatively on the basis of the much less sensitive gonadotropic response. The response may be measured by the production of protocatechuic-acid glucoside in the colleterial glands (Bodenstein and Shaaya, 1968) or by the growth of terminal oocytes (Bowers *et al.*, 1965) in the allatectomized, ligated, or decapitated adult cockroach, *Periplaneta americana.*

References

1. BJERKE, J. S.: The Purification of Juvenile Hormone from *Hyalophora cecropia* (L.). Doctoral Thesis, University of Wisconsin, Madison, 1970.
2. BODENSTEIN, D. and SHAAYA, E.: The Function of the Accessory Sex Glands in *Periplaneta americana* (L.). I. A Quantitative Bioassay for the Juvenile Hormone. Proc. Nat. Acad. Sci., U. S., *59*:1223, 1968.
3. BOWERS, W. S. and THOMPSON, M. J.: Juvenile Hormone Activity: Effects of Isoprenoid and Straight-chain Alcohols on Insects. Science, *142*:1469, 1963.
4. BOWERS, W. S., THOMPSON, M. J., and UEBEL, E. C.: Juvenile and Gonadotropic Hormone Activity of 10,11-Epoxyfarnesenic Acid Methyl Ester. Life Sci., *4*: 2323, 1965.
5. CAVENEY, S.: Juvenile Hormone and Wound Modelling of Tenebrio Cuticle Architecture. J. Insect Physiol., *16*:1087, 1970.
6. deWILDE, J., STAAL, G. B., deKORT, C. A. D., deLOOF, A., and BAARD, G.: Juvenile Hormone Titer in the Haemolymph and a Function of Photoperiodic Treatment in the Adult Colorado Beetle (*Leptinotarsa decemlineata* Say). Proc. Kon. Ned. Akad. Wetensch. Ser., *C71*:321, 1968.
7. FISHER, F. M. and SANBORN, R. C.: Nosema as a Source of Juvenile Hormone in Parasitized Insects. Biol. Bull., *126*:235, 1964.
8. GILBERT, L. I. and SCHNEIDERMAN, H. A.: The Content of Juvenile Hormone and Lipid in Lepidoptera: Sexual Differences and Developmental Changes. Gen. Comp. Endocr., *1*:453, 1961.
9. GILBERT, L. I. and SCHNEIDERMAN, H. A.: The Development of a Bioassay for the Juvenile Hormone of Insects. Trans. Amer. Microsc. Soc., *79*:38, 1960.
10. KARLSON, P. and NACHTIGALL, M.: Ein Biologischer Test zur Quantitativen Bestimmung der Juvenilhormon-Aktivitat von Insektenextrakten. J. Insect Physiol., *7*:210, 1961.
11. RÖLLER, H., BJERKE, J. S., HOLTHAUS, L. M., NORGARD, D. W., and McSHAN, W. H.: Isolation and Biological Properties of the Juvenile Hormone. J. Insect Physiol., *15*:379, 1969.
12. RÖLLER, H., BJERKE, J. S., and McSHAN, W. H.: The Juvenile Hormone. I. Methods of Purification and Isolation. J. Insect Physiol., *11*:1185, 1965.
13. ROLLER, H. and DAHM, K. H.: The Chemistry and Biology of Juvenile Hormone. Rec. Prog. Horm. Res., *24*:651, 1968.
14. RÖLLER, H. and FINN, W. E.: Unpublished communication.
15. SCHNEIDERMAN, H. A.: The Juvenile Hormone and Other Insect Growth Hormones. Casopis Cesk. Spolecnosti Entomol., *58*:12, 1961.
16. SCHNEIDERMAN, H. A. and GILBERT, L. I.: Control of Growth and Development in Insects. Science, *143*:325, 1964.
17. SCHNEIDERMAN, H. A. and GILBERT, L. I.: The Chemistry and Physiology of Insect Growth Hormone. *In*: D. Rudnick (ed.), Cell, Organism, and Milieu, Symp. Soc. Study Develop. Growth, *17*:157. New York: Ronald Press, 1959.
18. SCHNEIDERMAN, H. A. and GILBERT, L. I.: Substances with Juvenile Hormone Activity in Crustacea and Other Invertebrates. Biol. Bull., *115*:530, 1958.
19. SCHNEIDERMAN, H. A., KRISHNAKUMARAN, A., KULKARNI, V. G., and FREIDMAN, L.: Juvenile Hormone Activity of Structurally Unrelated Compounds. J. Insect Physiol., *11*:1161, 1965.

20. SLÁMA, K. and WILLIAMS, C. M.: The Juvenile Hormone. V. The Sensitivity of the Bug, *Pyrrhocoris apterus*, to a Hormonally Active Factor in American Paper-pulp. Biol. Bull., *130*:235, 1966.
21. TSAO, M.-s., JOU, G.-j., and CHIANG, T.-c.:Studies on the Effects of Juvenile Hormone on the Pupae of Polyvoltine Eri-silkworm *Attacus ricini*. Acta Biol. Exp. Sinica, *8*:538, 1963.
22. WIGGLESWORTH, V. B. : The Juvenile Hormone Effect of Farnesol and Some Related Compounds: Quantitative Experiments. J. Insect Physiol., *9*:105, 1963.
23. WIGGLESWORTH, V. B.: Some Methods for Assaying Extracts of the Juvenile Hormone in Insects. J. Insect Physiol., *2*:73, 1958.
24. WILLIAMS, C. M. : The Juvenile Hormone. II. Its Role in the Endocrine Control of Molting, Pupation, and Adult Development in the Cecropia Silkworm. Biol. Bull., *121*:572, 1961.
25. WILLIAMS, C. M. : The Juvenile Hormone of Insects. Nature (London), *178*:212, 1956.
26. WILLIAMS, C. M. and LAW, J. H. : The Juvenile Hormone. IV. Its Extraction, Assay, and Purification. J. Insect Physiol., *11*:569, 1965.
27. YAMAMOTO, R. T. and JACOBSON, M.: Juvenile Hormone Activity of Isomers of Farnesol. Nature (London), *196*:908, 1962.
28. ZLOTKIN, E. and LEVINSON, H. Z.: Influence of Cecropia Oil on the Cuticle of *Tenebrio molitor*. J. Insect Physiol., *15*:105, 1969.
29. ZLOTKIN, E. and LEVINSON, H. Z.: Influence of Cecropia Oil on Cuticular Phenols in *Tenebrio molitor*. J. Insect Physiol., *14*:1195, 1968a.
30. ZLOTKIN, E. and LEVINSON, H. Z.: Influence of Cecropia Oil on the Epidermis of *Tenebrio molitor*. J. Insect Physiol., *14*:1719, 1968b.

CHROMATOGRAPHIC
DETECTION and IMMUNOASSAY
of INVERTEBRATE HORMONES

Walter J. Burdette

B ioassays of invertebrate hormones continue to serve a very useful purpose, but other approaches to detection that could become more specific and sensitive have been explored and are beginning to yield encouraging results. Principal alternatives that have been used both for isolation and identification of these hormones and analogs are radioimmunoassay and gas-liquid chromatography. A brief description of the current status of these methods is included as a reminder that refinement of assay is not only desirable but also some of these physicochemical methods may well complement traditional bioassays and even supplant them for some purposes.

RADIOIMMUNOASSAY

Radioimmunoassay is carried out by converting hormone to antigen by conjugating with protein and then, after immunizing animals from which antibody is obtained, determining the deficiency in binding labeled hormone to antiserum in the presence of unlabeled hormone from the specimen being tested. Borst and O'Connor (1972) have converted ecdysterone to the oxime acetic acid ether and coupled it to bovine serum albumin *via* the isobutyl-chloroformate mixed anhydride intermediate. After dialysis and hydrolysis, they used the antigen, suspended in Freund's adjuvant, to immunize rabbits with 4.0 mg. initially, followed in six weeks with a booster dose of 1.0 mg. Antiserum collected nine days later was incubated both with ^{3}H-labeled and unlabeled specimens of hormone in borate buffer; the conjugate was precipitated with $(NH_4)_2 SO_4$; and then the pellet was dissolved in Aquasol for scintillation counting. They found that a 10 per cent solution of antiserum would bind virtually 100 per cent of labeled ecdysterone, and the binding was linear with 2 per cent dilution of ecdysterone and amounts of ^{3}H-ecdysterone below 3.0 ng./ml. Both *a*-ecdysone and inokosterone compete with ecdysterone for haptene binding sites, but cholesterol and 3β-hydroxy-5a-cholestan-6-one do not. Although limitations to sensitivity of 200 pg. and competition were encountered, it may be possible to extend the sensitivity to 25 pg. by using labeled ecdysone with higher specific activity that is now available and to resolve the identity of competing analogs by exploiting characteristic binding affinities. The sensitivity of this analysis and the rapidity with which it can be performed when the essential reagents are once prepared are features that encourage continued effort to efface some of the current imperfections of the method and to determine optimum procedures for preparing biological material for its use.

GAS CHROMATOGRAPHY FOR SEPARATION OF ECDYSONES

Another method that has been useful to chemists who have separated and identified invertebrate hormones is gas-liquid chromatography, based on methodologies perfected for separating human steroids. Katz and Lensky (1970) prepared *a*-ecdysone as a derivative of *bis* (trimethylsilyl) acetamide and found that gas chromatographic analysis produced a peak distinct from the solvent and that the peaks of some other steroids, including cholesterol and phytosterols, were embraced by the peak of the solvent and therefore did not interfere with the analysis. Fifty ng. of *a*-ecdysone could be detected by this method at the time of their initial report.

The method of using chromatography to identify and quantify insect molting hormones was extended by Morgan and Woodbridge (1971) who prepared silylated derivatives of *a*-ecdysone and ecdysterone by treating the isomeric *o*-methyloximes with *bis* (trimethylsilyl) acetamide and analyzed them by means of gas-liquid chromatography. They were able to detect ecdysterone in partially purified extracts of *Schistocera-gregaria* nymphs by the procedure they perfected and found that the titer varied from 12 to 240 ng. per individual in nymphs assayed at various ages during the fifth instar.

Miyazaki *et al.* (1972) used both trimethylsilyl ether and heptafluorobutyrate derivatives of phytoecdysones and found that these hormones could be identified in nanogram or picogram quantities by electron-capture techniques. Ponasterone A, ecdysterone, inokosterone, makisterone A and B, cyasterone, and other related steroids were detected by making derivatives and characterizing them by gas chromatography. The heptafluorobutyril derivative of phytoecdysones extracted from Achyranthes could be analyzed at lower temperature than the trimethylsilyl derivative and was detectable at the picogram level in the electron-capture detector and is recommended by these authors for assay of ecdysones in biological systems.

CONCLUSIONS

Considerable progress has been made in identifying invertebrate hormones and ascertaining their concentration in biological systems both by radioimmunoassay and gas chromatography. Although much needs to be done additionally to perfect physicochemical methods and immunoassays for accurate determination of invertebrate hormones in tissues of animals and plants, they represent a promising means to relate accurately the quantity of respective hormones alone or in combination to their biological actions.

References

1. BORST, D. W. and O'CONNOR, J. D.: Arthropod Molting Hormone: Radioimmune Assay. Science, *178:*418-419, 1972.
2. KATZ, M. and LENSKY, Y.: Gas Chromatographic Analysis of Ecdysone. Experientia, *26:*1043, 1970.
3. MIYAZAKI, H., ISHIBASHI, M., and MORI, C.: Gas Chromatographic Separation of Phytoecdysones. J. Chromatographic Sci., *10:*233-242, 1972.
4. MORGAN, E. D. and WOODBRIDGE, A. P.: Insect Molting Hormones (Ecdysones). Identification as Derivatives by Gas Chromatography. Chem. Commun., 475-476, 1971.

Biosynthesis and Degradation of Invertebrate Hormones

BIOSYNTHESIS and
INACTIVATION of ECDYSONE

David Shaw King
and John B. Siddall

Although the fundamental features of the structure and biological function of ecdysone in arthropods have been worked out since its discovery in the early 1930's, knowledge about metabolism of ecdysone is still rather fragmentary (Horn, 1971). Regarding the biosynthetic pathway of ecdysone, it is known only that ecdysone can be derived from cholesterol or 7-dehydrocholesterol and that a-ecdysone is converted into β-ecdysone. The chemical mechanism for inactivation of ecdysone *in vivo* is unknown. Also, the site of production of ecdysone in arthropods remains conjectural. Although it has been widely assumed that the ecdysial gland (insect prothoracic gland, crustacean Y-organ) manufactures and secretes ecdysone in the manner of a normal endocrine gland, none of the surgical extirpation-replacement experiments done to date with ecdysial glands demonstrate unequivocally that ecdysone is actually produced by this gland (Moriyama *et al.*, 1970).

The experiments summarized were designed to extend knowledge about metabolism of ecdysone, namely, to determine whether 22-deoxy-a-ecdysone is a precursor of a-ecdysone in insects, to elucidate the mechanism for inactivation of ecdysone, and to determine the sites in the animal where these various metabolic steps take place. A more detailed account of this work is in press.

METABOLISM OF 22-DEOXY- α -ECDYSONE
A POSSIBLE PRECURSOR OF α-ECDYSONE IN INSECTS

It was found that [22, 23, 24-^{3}H] -22-deoxy-a-ecdysone [specific activity 42 Ci/M.; synthesized by Pd-catalized tritiation of the 22, 23-allene (Siddall, 1969)] was rapidly metabolized (about 70 percent after 4 hours) by *Manduca sexta* prepupae *in vivo* to a-ecdysone, β-ecdysone, 26-hydroxy-β-ecdysone, and a very polar metabolite designated compound A. As only microgram quantities of the radiolabeled metabolites were available for analysis, elucidations of structure were achieved by utilizing radio-thin-layer chromatographic and microchemical techniques.

It was also found that 22-deoxy-a-ecdysone is the major tetrol intermediate in the metabolism of 22, 25-dideoxy-a-ecdysone to a-ecdysone.

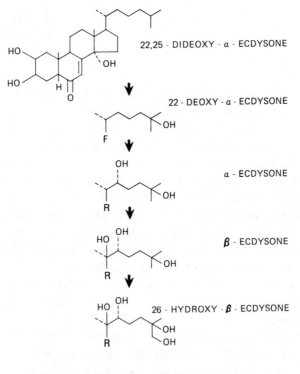

Figure 1.

Sequential metabolism of 22, 25-dideoxy-a-ecdysone in Manduca prepupae *(in vivo* and *in vitro).*

Since 25-deoxy-*a*-ecdysone, 25-deoxy-*β*-ecdysone (ponasterone-A), and 22-deoxy-*β*-ecdysone were not detected in these experiments, it appears that sidechain hydroxylation of 22, 25-dideoxy-*a*-ecdysone in Manduca takes place in a definite sequence, first at C-25, then at C-22β_F, C-20a_F, and C-26 (stereo-chemistry unknown)(Figure 1). In contrast, metabolism of 22, 25-dideoxy-*a*-ecdysone in *Gastrimargus africanus* (grasshopper) nymphs, *Sarcophaga bullata* (blowfly) prepupae, and *Dermestes maculatus* (hide beetle) prepupae [as well as Musca adults (Robbins *et al.*, 1971)] leads to complex mixtures of polar steroids containing little or no *a*- or *β*-ecdysone, thus indicating that 22, 25-dideoxy-*a*-ecdysone is not a normal ecdysone precursor in these insects. The possibility remains, however, that this compound could be a natural precursor of ecdysones in Manduca, as suggested by Kaplanis *et al.*, (1969). Experiments attempting to demonstrate its biosynthesis from radiolabeled cholesterol have not as yet been successful; hence the question of whether this compound as well as 22-deoxy-*a*-ecdysone are indeed natural intermediates in the biosynthesis of ecdysone requires further investigation.

MECHANISM FOR INACTIVATION OF EXOGENOUS ECDYSONES

Although the results of Heinrich and Hoffmeister (1970) showing production of ecdysone glucosides by the Calliphora fat body *in vitro* have been confirmed in Manduca, inactivation of exogenous ecdysone *in vivo* is brought about by the formation of sulfate esters. Experiments involving solvolysis *in vivo* of the highly polar metabolites of *a*-ecdysone (compound A) with anhydrous dioxane containing 1 per cent acetic acid, as well as enzymatic hydrolysis with crude sulfatase preparations, indicate that compound A is a complex mixture of sulfated ecdysones (*a*, *β*, and 26-hydroxy-*β*) and other unidentified polar steroids. The pyridinium salt of compound A has the same mobility on silica chromatoplates as the pyridinium salt of the synthetic monosulfate of *a*-ecdysone.

Preliminary experiments done in collaboration with H. Hikino and Y. Ohizumi indicate that compound A in Bombyx is a steroid sulfate and not a sidechain-cleavage fragment as previously suspected (Moriyama *et al.*, 1970). Whether ecdysone glucosides are obligatory intermediates in formation of sulfate ester, which hydroxyl group is sulfated, and where the sulfotransferase is located in the insect are important questions that are presently being investigated.

Figure 2. summarized the current picture for biosynthesis of ecdysones and the excretion of ecdysones into the gut in both free (Hoffmeister *et al.*, 1965) and conjugated forms.

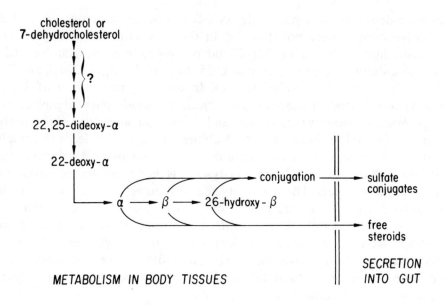

Figure 2.

Summary diagram for biosynthesis, metabolism, and excretion of ecdysone in Manduca.

THE SITES OF METABOLISM OF a-ECDYSONE AND DEOXYECDYSONES

Since the site for biosynthesis of ecdysone is not yet known, it seemed desirable to determine which tissues in the body of insects are responsible for the various metabolic steps mentioned above. These experiments were done by incubating tissues isolated from Manduca prepupa in saline along with the radiolabeled precursors *in vitro* for 2-4 hours. The results obtained to date are presented in Table 1. Efficient conversion of 22,25-dideoxy-a-ecdysone, a-ecdysone, β-ecdysone, and 26-hydroxy-β-ecdysone, as well as the production of ecdysone conjugates, was found to take place in isolated fat body and malpighian tubules. None of the indicated conversions was found to take place in blood, muscle, salivary gland, or oenocytes, although the gut and body wall were capable of metabolizing a- to β-ecdysone, but no farther. Isolated prothoracic gland is unable to metabolize a- to β-ecdysone, and a single preliminary experiment has demonstrated that metabolism of 22,25-dideoxy-a-ecdysone by this tissue, although very efficient (50 per cent conversion after 3.5 hours), stops at a-ecdysone. The latter result is particularly enigmatic in view of the fact that experiments attempting to demon-

ABILITY OF ISOLATED MANDUCA PREPUPAL TISSUES
TO METABOLIZE DEOXYECDYSONES *IN VITRO* [a]

Tissue	Conversion of α-to β- ecdysone	Ecdysone conjugation	Metabolism of 22– deoxy – α - ecdysone	Metabolism of 22 , 25 – dideoxy - α -
Fat body	+	+	+	+
Malpighiam tubules	+	+b	+	+
Body wall	+	−		
Gut	+	−		
Blood	−	−	−	−
Muscle	−	−		
Salivary gland	−	−		
Oenocytes	−	−		
Prothoracic gland	−	−		+c

[a] Metabolism of deoxyecdysones was not tested for all tissues.
[b] Nature of conjugates not determined.
[c] Metabolism stops at α-ecdysone.

strate the production of ecdysone from radiolabeled cholesterol by isolated ecdysial glands have not been successful. It seems clear that the ecdysial gland does not produce β-ecdysone (King, 1969); the role of the gland in the production of α-ecdysone remains conjectural, and is presently under investigation.

Acknowledgement

We wish to thank B. J. Bergot for excellent technical assistance in many phases of this work, and Drs. D. H. S. Horn and H. Hikino for the gift of various ecdysones.

References

1. HEINRICH, G.and HOFFMEISTER, H.: Bildung von Hormonglykosiden als Inaktivie-rungsmechanismus bei *Calliphora erythrocephala*. Z. Naturforsch, *25b*:358-361, 1970.

2. HOFFMEISTER, H., RUFER, C., and AMMON, H.: Ausscheidung von Ecdyson bei Insekten. Z. Naturforsch, *20b*:130-133, 1965.

3. HORN, D. H. S.: The Ecdysones. *In:* Jacobson and D. G. Crosby.(ed.).Naturally Occurring Insecticides, pp. 333-459. New York: Marcel Dekker Inc., 1971.

4. KAPLANIS, J. N., ROBBINS, W. E., THOMPSON, M. J., and BAUMHOVER, A. H.: Ecdysone Analog: Conversion to α-Ecdysone and 20-Hydroxyecdysone by an Insect. Science, *166*:1540-1541, 1969.

5. KING, D. S.: Evidence for Peripheral Conversion of α-Ecdysone to β-Ecdysone in Crustaceans and Insects. Gen. Comp. Endocrinol., *13*:512, 1969.

6. KING, D. S.: Metabolism of α-Ecdysone and Possible Immediate Precursors by Insects *in Vivo* and *in Vitro*. Gen. Comp. Endocrinol., in press.

7. MORIYAMA, H., NAKANISHI, K., KING, D. S., OKAUCHI, T., SIDDALL, J. B., and HAFFERL, W.: On the Origin and Metabolic Fate of α-Ecdysone in Insects. Gen. Comp. Endocrinol., *15*:80-87, 1970.

8. ROBBINS, W. E., KAPLANIS, J. N., THOMPSON, M. J., and SVOBODA, J. A.: Chemistry and Biological Activity of the Ecdysones and Ecdysone Analogues. Reported at the Second International Congress of Pesticide Chemistry, Tel Aviv., 1970.

9. SIDDALL, J. B.: Synthetic Studies on Insect Hormones. *In:* Insect-Plant Interactions. Natl. Acad. Sci., U. S., Work Conference Report, pp. 70-72, 1969.

SOME ASPECTS of the BIOSYNTHESIS of the MOLTING HORMONES in CALLIPHORA

J. A. Thomson, D. H. S. Horn,
M. N. Galbraith, and E. J. Middleton

The early finding by Karlson and Hoffmeister (1963) that exogenous cholesterol can be utilized *in vivo* for the synthesis of molting hormone (MH) in *Calliphora erythrocephala* appeared to pave the way for the analysis of the biosynthetic pathway involved, but relatively little progress in establishing the early steps seems to have been made so far. We are concerned here to review briefly the following questions relating to MH synthesis:

(1) Which hormonally active compounds are produced in Calliphora, and when?
(2) Is the synthesis of intermediate storage precursors indicated?
(3) Where does the synthesis of MH occur?

Developmental changes in the total endogenous MH of the brown blowfly, *Calliphora stygia,* follow a pattern (Galbraith *et al.,* 1969a; and more extensive unpublished data) comparable, (after adjustment for a small difference in the length of life-cycle) with that described for *C. erythrocephala* by Shaaya and Karlson (1965). A transitory peak appears just after puparium formation. A second, lower but more sustained, peak follows 1-2 days later and extends over the next 3-4 days of imaginal development. The only MH contributing to the activity of extracts prepared at each of these peak stages is β-ecdysone (Galbraith *et al.,* 1969a). There are thus two temporally separated phases of β-ecdysone activity during development in Calliphora for which different precursors or intermediates might conceivably be available *in vivo.* Our work so far has concentrated on the synthesis of MH at the first of these periods.

Time of Synthesis

An indirect approach to the question of the time of synthesis of MH can be made from the pattern of incorporation of $(1-^3H)$-cholesterol into β-ecdysone. If the final steps of the synthesis utilized inactive intermediates previously sequestered and stored, perhaps in a specific type of cell, it would be expected that the efficiency for utilization of ^3H-cholesterol might change according to the time of its administration. Injection of ^3H-cholester-

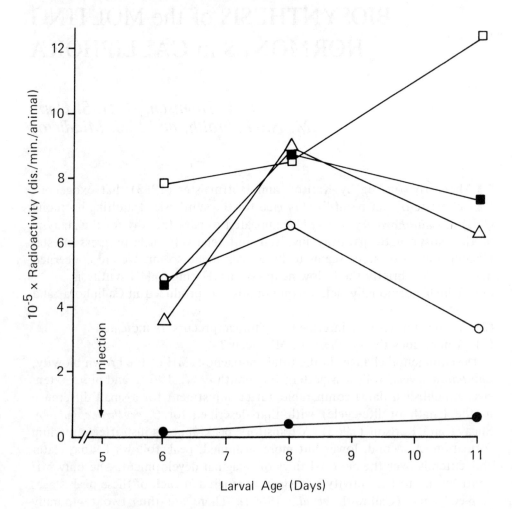

Figure 1.
Distribution of radioactivity in larval tissues of *C. stygia* at intervals after injection of ^3H-cholesterol (2.0 μCi.) into day-5 larvae. Day-11 samples comprised animals at the white puparial stage. Plasma □, body wall ■, fat body △, gut ○, brain/ring gland complex ●.

ol into feeding and wandering larvae of Calliphora does not significantly improve the efficiency of incorporation of the label into β-ecdysone (measured 6 hours after puparium formation) relative to experiments in which the cholesterol is given either just before (Galbraith et al., 1970), or at, puparation. Thus rapid incorporation of ^{3}H-cholesterol at, and just after, puparium formation provides evidence that synthesis occurs from initial precursors derived directly from the pool of plasma cholesterol.

The total plasma cholesterol in *C. stygia* increases rapidly over the last 3 days of larval life (mid- to late-wandering period), although the volume of hemolymph drops over this time (Kinnear et al., 1968). If ^{3}H-cholesterol is injected into the hemocoele of mid-feeding larvae (Figure 1), the radio-activity is rapidly taken up by the gut, body-wall tissues, and fat body. In the last three days of larval life, labeled material is mobilized into plasma, especially from the gut and fat body. Virtually all the plasma label at puparium formation is due to unchanged free cholesterol or to cholesterol associated with lipid. Levinson and Shaaya (1966) reported the occurrence of an unique steroidal metabolite just prior to puparium formation in *C. erythrocephala*, but we have been unable to identify a similar component in *C. stygia.*

Sites of Synthetic Activity

Moriyama et al. (1970) have drawn attention very cogently to the lack of compelling evidence that MH itself is synthesized in the ecdysial glands. As these authors point out, the gland may produce an enzyme or enzymes involved in the biosynthetic transformation of the steroid nucleus elsewhere, or it may produce one or more tropic factors controlling MH biosynthesis.

We have attempted, without success, to obtain evidence of production of MH in the brain-ring gland complex of Calliphora by incubation of this tissue *in vitro* in a medium containing plasma from larvae previously injected with ^{3}H-cholesterol of high specific activity (Figure 1). It was hoped by this means to insure that the cholesterol would be available to the incubated tissues in a normal form, biologically available. No evidence of MH synthesis was found in this instance, but the approach seems worth extending to other tissues.

It should, of course, be kept in mind that the tissues of the abdomen in Calliphora are certainly not competent to synthesize MH from cholesterol if isolated by ligation before the critical period for secretory activity of the ring gland. Moriyama et al. (1970) and King (1969) have reported unequivocal evidence for the conversion of a- to β-ecdysone in the isolated abdomen of Calliphora, an hydroxylation well established as occurring rapidly in the intact animal (King and Siddall, 1969; Galbraith et al., 1969b).

A study of the tissue distribution of MH activity in *C. erythrocephala* over the period from 30 hours before puparium formation to 5 hours after this event (Shaaya, 1969) revealed significant MH activity in hemolymph and fat body 15-20 hours prior to pupariation. Shaaya observed MH activity in integumental tissue 10 hours later, and by 5 hours after formation of puparium the MH content of the integument accounted for 27.5 per cent of the total hormone in the insect. These data show relatively little rise in the hormonal content of hemolymph from 20 hours before to 5 hours after pupariation, consistent with a transport rather than reservoir role of the hemolymph as emphasized by Ohtaki, Milkman, and Williams (1968). Gradually increasing MH levels in the fat body, and the sharper rise in integument, follow patterns similar to those observed after administration of exogenous a-ecdysone (Karlson *et al.*, 1964) and do not suggest the location of hormonal biosynthesis.

The Biosynthetic Pathway

In spite of the relatively large pool (40 μg./animal) of cholesterol present in *C. stygia* at the time of puparium formation, the conversion of exogenous ^{3}H-cholesterol to β-ecdysone is sufficiently high (0.015 per cent) to permit the testing of intermediates, which might be farther along the pathway towards β-ecdysone, for their ability to replace cholesterol in the biosynthesis of MH. (1-^{3}H)-7-Dehydrocholesterol is converted to β-ecdysone almost twice as efficiently as cholesterol during the first few hours after formation of puparium (Galbraith *et al.*, 1970). 7-Dehydrocholesterol may not, however, be a preferred substrate in this case, because the pool size (2 μg./animal) is much lower than that of cholesterol. More convincingly, 7-dehydrocholesterol administered with ^{3}H-cholesterol does not suppress the utilization of the cholesterol in the hormonal biosynthesis (Galbraith *et al.*, 1970). In these experiments, the steroids to be tested have been injected into late third-instar larvae shortly before formation of puparium as colloidal suspensions, often in solutions of oleate, and utilization may reflect, in part, availability in a form biologically usable.

In earlier work on Calliphora (Thomson *et al.*, 1969), it was suggested that side-chain hydroxylation might precede modification of the steroid nucleus of cholesterol during the course of the biosynthesis of MH. This sequence now seems unlikely, since neither 22- nor 25-hydroxycholesterol is significantly incorporated into β-ecdysone in *C. stygia* (Galbraith, Horn, Middleton, and Thomson, unpublished), and it appears more probable that the 5-ene system of cholesterol must be altered before side-chain hydroxylation can proceed.

Among the MH analogues that have been examined as possible close precursors of β-ecdysone are 22-deoxy-α-ecdysone and 22, 25-di-deoxy-α-ecdysone. At the time the puparium is formed both are converted to α-ecdysone, β-ecdysone, and more polar metabolites (unpublished data) in *C. stygia.* No significant amount of α-ecdysone can be obtained from bulk extractions of Calliphora (Galbraith *et al.,* 1969a), so that neither 22-deoxy- nor 22-25-di-deoxy-α-ecdysone are likely to be normal precursors of β-ecdysone. It is similarly possible to exclude 25-deoxy-α-ecdysone as a normal intermediate.

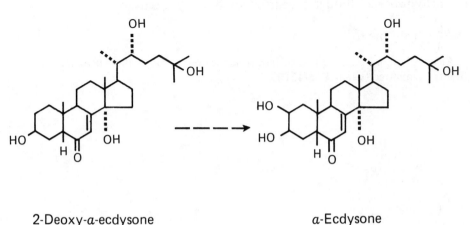

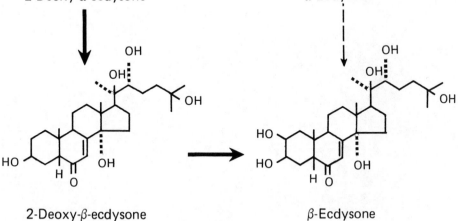

Figure 2.

Probable immediate precursors of β-ecdysone in Calliphora.

In pupariating Calliphora, this compound yields both inokosterone and ponasterone A (Thomson *et al.*, 1969), neither of which is a usual endogenous component. Preferential hydroxylation of 25-deoxy-*a*-ecdysone at the C-20 position, to give ponasterone A rather than *a*-ecdysone, apparently occurs in this case. The ponasterone A is then hydroxylated at about equal rates at C-25 and C-26 to yield *β*-ecdysone and inokosterone respectively. 2-Deoxy-*a*-ecdysone (Chong *et al.*, 1970) and 2-deoxy-*β*-ecdysone (Galbraith *et al.*, 1968) are both highly active in the Calliphora test, suggesting very efficient conversion to *β*-ecdysone as shown in Figure 2. Thus, at the present time, it appears most plausible that the biosynthesis of *β*-ecdysone may normally proceed through precursors of 2-deoxy-*a*-ecdysone.

Acknowledgement

Financial support for this work has been received through the Australian Research Grants Committee (Grant D65/15167).

References

1. CHONG, Y. K., GALBRAITH, M. N., and HORN, D. H. S.: Isolation of Deoxycrustecdysone, Deoxyecdysone, and a-Ecdysone from the Fern *Blechnum minus*. J. Chem. Soc. D., Chem. Commun., *1278*:1217-1218, 1970.

2. GALBRAITH, M. N., HORN, D. H. S., MIDDLETON, E. J., and HACKNEY, R. J.: Structure of Deoxycrustecdysone, a Second Crustacean Molting Hormone. J. Chem. Soc. D. Chem. Comm., *1274*:83-85, 1968.

3. GALBRAITH, M. N., HORN, D. H. S., MIDDLETON, E. J., and THOMSON, J. A.:The Biosynthesis of Crustecdysone in the Blowfly *Calliphora stygia*. J. Chem. Soc. D. Chem. Commun., *1824*:179-180, 1970.

4. GALBRAITH, M. N., HORN, D. H. S., MIDDLETON, E. J., THOMSON, J. A., SIDDALL, J. B., and HAFFERL, W.:The Catabolism of Crustecdysone in the Blowfly *Calliphora stygia*. J. Chem. Soc. D. Chem. Commun., *1144*:1134-1135, 1969b.

5. GALBRAITH, M. N., HORN, D. H. S., THOMSON, J. A., NEUFELD, G. J.,and HACKNEY, R. J.:Insect Molting Hormones: Crustecdysone in *Calliphora*. J. Insect Physiol., *15*:1225-1233, 1969a.

6. KARLSON, P. and HOFFMEISTER,H.:Zur Biogenese des Ecdysons I. Umwandlung von Cholesterin in Ecdyson. Hoppe-Seyler's Z. Physiol. Chem., *331*:298-300, 1963.

7. KARLSON, P., SEKERIS, C. E., and MAURER, R.: Zum Wirkungsmechanismus der Hormone-I. Verteilung von Tritiummarkiertem Ecdyson in Larven von *Calliphora erythrocephala*. Hoppe-Seyler's Z. Physiol. Chem., *336*:100-106, 1964.

8. KING, D. S.: Evidence for Peripheral Conversion of a-Ecdysone to β-Ecdysone in Crustaceans and Insects. Gen. Comp. Endocrinol., *13*:512, 1969.

9. KING, D. S. and SIDDALL, J. B.: Conversion of a-Ecdysone to β-Ecdysone by Crustaceans and Insects. Nature, *221*:955-956, 1969.

10. KINNEAR, J. F., MARTIN, M. D., THOMSON, J. A., and NEUFELD, G. J.: Developmental Changes in the Late Larva of *Calliphora stygia* I. Hemolymph. Aust. J. Biol. Sci., *21*:1033-1045, 1968.

11. LEVINSON, H. and SHAAYA, E.: Occurrence of a Metabolite Related to Pupation of the Blowfly *Calliphora erythrocephala* Meig. Rivista. Parassit., *27*:203-209, 1966.

12. MORIYAMA, H., NAKANISHI, K., KING, D. S., OKAUCHI, T., SIDDALL, J. B.,and HAFFERL, W.: On the Origin and Metabolic Fate of a-Ecdysone in Insects. Gen. Comp. Endocrinol., *15*:80-85, 1970.

13. OHTAKI, T., MILKMAN, R. D., and WILLIAMS, C. M.: Dynamics of Ecdysone Secretion and Action in the Fleshfly *Sarcophaga peregrina*. Biol. Bull., *135*:322-334, 1968.

14. SHAAYA, E.: Der Ecdysontiter während der Insektenentwicklung, VI. Untersuchungen über die Verteilung des Ecdysons in verschiedenen Geweben von *Calliphora erythrocephala* und über seine biologische Halbwertzeit. Z. Naturforsch., *24b*:718-721, 1969.

15. SHAAYA, E. and KARLSON, P.: Der Ecdysontiter während der Insektenentwicklung-II. Die postembryonale Entwicklung der Schmeissfliege *Calliphora erythrocephala* Meig. J. Insect Physiol., *11*:65-69, 1965.

16. THOMSON, J. A., SIDDALL, J. B., GALBRAITH, M. N., HORN, D. H. S., and MIDDLETON, E. J.: The Biosynthesis of Ecdysones in the Blowfly *Calliphora stygia*. J. Chem. Soc. D. Chem. Commun., *641*:669-670, 1969.

The METABOLISM
of the SYNTHETIC
ECDYSONE ANALOG, 1α- ³H-22,25-
BISDEOXYECDYSONE in RELATION
to CERTAIN of ITS BIOLOGICAL
EFFECTS in INSECTS

J. N. Kaplanis, S. R. Dutky,
W. E. Robbins, and M. J. Thompson

Certain naturally occurring ecdysones and synthetic ecdysone analogs exhibit a variety of biological activities in insects (Robbins *et al.*, 1968, 1970; Williams and Robbins, 1968). Particularly interesting among the synthetic analogs is the steroid 22,25-bisdeoxyecdysone (2β,3β,14α-trihydroxy-5β-cholest-7-ene-6-one, Figure 1) that was synthesized and first shown to have molting-hormone activity by Hocks and coworkers (Hocks *et al.*, 1966). In addition to possessing molting-hormone activity in insects (Hocks *et al.*, 1966; Robbins *et al.*, 1970) and a crustacean (Krishnakumaran *et al.*, 1970), this analog also terminates diapause (Kaplanis *et al.*, 1969; Wright, 1969), disrupts larval growth and development (Earle *et al.*, 1970; Robbins *et al.*, 1968, 1970), and inhibits ovarian maturation and reproduction in adult insects (Earle *et al.*, 1970; Kaplanis *et al.*, 1972; Robbins *et al.*, 1968,

161

1970). In order to obtain information on the action of this steroid, the metabolism of radiolabeled 22,25-bisdeoxyecdysone is being studied in relation to its biological effects in insects. This communication is concerned with the metabolism of the analog in relation to two of these biological activities: termination of pupal diapause in the tobacco hornworm, *Manduca sexta* (L.), and the inhibition of ovarian development in the adult house fly, *Musca domestica* (L.)

Figure 1

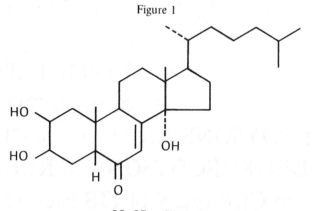

22, 25 – Bisdeoxyecdysone

MATERIALS AND METHODS

Labeled Compound

The 1α-^{3}H-22,25-bisdeoxyecdysone was synthesized from 1α-^{3}H-cholesterol according to procedures used for the preparation of the unlabeled compound (Thompson *et al.*, 1970). During the ten-step synthesis of the 1α-^{3}H-22,25-bisdeoxyecdysone from 1α-^{3}H-cholesterol, there was no change in specific activity based on that calculated from the starting material. The observable specific activity of the tritium-labeled analog was 1720 d.p.m./μg. Column and thin-layer chromatography showed the labeled compound to have a radiochemical purity of greater than 98 per cent.

Assay for Molting Hormones (MH)

The house-fly assay (Kaplanis *et al.*, 1966) was used to detect MH activity during fractionation and to assess the activity of purified or crystalline ecdysones and/or analogs following their isolation. The compounds or fractions were injected into the insect either as aqueous solutions, or if insoluble in water, as 5 per cent hydroxy lecithin emulsions (Louloudes *et al.*, 1962). [1]

[1]   Mention of a proprietary product in this paper does not constitute an endorsement of this product by the United States Department of Agriculture.

Termination of Pupal Diapause

The $1a-{}^{3}H$-22.25-bisdeoxyecdysone (specific activity, 1720 d.p.m./μg.) was administered at 10 μg. per gram of body weight (1 μg./1 μl., in 60 per cent acetone solution) by injection with a microsyringe into the abdomen of diapausing male tobacco hornworm pupae collected in the field (Kaplanis et al., 1969). The externally visible character of eye pigmentation (Williams, 1968) served as a valid and reliable indicator for ascertaining termination of diapause or spontaneous development, or both, in the intact organism. With pigmentation of the eye as the criterion, 621 insects were harvested 7.5 to 8.5 days after injection and kept frozen until they were processed.

Inhibition of Ovarian Development

For this study the $1a-{}^{3}H$-22,25-bisdeoxyecdysone was diluted with unlabeled 22,25-bisdeoxyecdysone to give a final specific activity of 5100 d.p.m./mg. In each of 28 one-gallon glass containers, 300 newly-emerged adult house flies (250 females, 50 males) were held for 4 days on a diet (LeBreque et al., 1960) containing an inhibitory concentration (0.1 per cent) of the ${}^{3}H$-analog (Robbins et al., 1970). At the end of 4 days the sex of the flies was determined, they were frozen, and their excreta were collected from the glass containers by rinsing alternately with aliquots of water and methanol. The solvent mixture was reduced under vacuum, and the extractives were stored in methanol until they were processed.

Extraction, Fractionation, and Isolation of Metabolites from Biological Material

Detailed procedures for extracting and fractionating small to large quantities of biological material have been described elsewhere (Kaplanis et al., 1966). Essentially the same procedures were used in these metabolic studies, however, for the sake of continuity a general treatment of this facet, including certain modifications and supplementary procedures, is presented. Insects were homogenized in a blender with methanol. After the homogenate was transferred to centrifuge cups and centrifuged at 2200–3000 r.p.m. for 10 minutes, the supernatant was removed and the residue was rehomogenized and/or extracted two additional times with 75 per cent methanol. After centrifugation, the supernatants were collected, pooled, and reduced nearly to dryness in vacuum. The residue was partitioned between water and butanol, and the water phase was re-extracted with ¼ to ½ volumes of butanol. When necessary, the phases were separated by centrifugation. The aqueous phase was extracted two additional times with butanol, and the combined butanol extracts (base treatments were omitted in these studies) were taken to dryness. The residue was then partitioned between equal volumes of 70 per cent methanol and n-hexane, the 70 per cent methanol phase was reduced to dryness, and the crude extractive was stored in methanol. The crude extractives in these studies were first chromatographed on silicic acid $\underline{2/}$ (Kaplanis *et al.*, 1969) and eluted with increasing concentrations of methanol in benzene (Table 1). Fractions containing 5, 10, and 25 per cent methanol in benzene eluted 22,25-bisdeoxyecdysone, *a*-ecdysone plus 20-hydroxyecdysone and 20,26-dihydroxyecdysone, respectively. The 25 per cent methanol-in-benzene fraction also eluted other polar compounds. Finally, elution with methanol removed the extremely polar compounds. The counter-current-distribution (CCD) system of cyclohexane, butanol, and water (5:5:10) was used to separate and purify *a*-ecdysone and 20-hydroxyecdysone. Counter-current-distribution systems of cyclohexane, butanol, and water (2:8:10 and 1:9:10) were also used to detect and purify the 20,26-dihydroxyecdysone.

Chromatography on either Woelm alumina (neutral grade I + 20 per cent water) or on silicic acid (Kaplanis *et al.*, 1966) was used to purify the ecdysones following counter-current distribution. It should be pointed out that chromatography on alumina, however, was not necessarily used in the sequence given above but on occasion was also used earlier in the fractionation scheme. When sufficient quantities of the ecdysones were available, the compounds were crystallized from ethyl acetate.

Thin-layer Chromatography

Preparative silica gel G plates (20 x 20 cm. and 10 x 20 cm.) were used for separation, purification, or for tentative identification of metabolites by co-chromatography with authentic standards. The developing solvent system used was chloroform-ethanol (95 per cent) 8:2 or variations of this system. The compounds were visualized directly under ultraviolet light or sprayed with vanillin-sulfuric acid reagent (Stahl, 1965). For identification, the areas of silica gel G containing the metabolites were scraped into centrifuge tubes and extracted several times with methanol. The methanol extracts were held for further analysis.

$\underline{2/}$ Unisil, 100 to 200 mesh, Clarkson Chemical Co., Williamsport, Pennsylvania.

TABLE 1

COLUMN–CHROMATOGRAPHIC ANALYSES* OF TOTAL ³H–COMPOUNDS ISOLATED FROM TOBACCO HORNWORMS FOLLOWING INJECTION WITH ³H–22,25–BISDEOXYECDYSONE

Fraction	Volume (ml.)	Total d.p.m ($\times 10^5$)	Per Cent of Total	House-fly Units (Per Cent of Total)
Benzene-Methanol (95:5)				
1	3550	15.0	10.7	0.6
2	1775	1.6	1.1	0.1
3	1775	0.7	0.5	0.1
Benzene-Methanol (90:10)				
4	940	7.5	5.3	12.0
5	940	23.0	16.4	50.0
6	940	15.0	10.7	25.0
7	940	4.5	3.2	5.0
8	940	4.4	3.1	1.5
9	940	4.5	3.2	0.5
10	940	3.3	2.4	0.2
Benzene-Methanol (75:25)				
11	940	28.0	19.9	2.0
Methanol				
12	940	30.0	21.4	2.0
Water				
13	940	3.0	2.1	1.0

*   Column 9.5 cm. (I.D.) × 2.3 cm. high. 80.0 G. of silicic acid.

Enzymic Hydrolysis of Polar Fractions

The polar fractions from the column were incubated with either a β-gluco-sidase or sulfatase preparation [3] in a 0.2 M. sodium acetate-acetic acid buffer system (pH 6.3) for 24 hours (Colowick and Kaplan, 1955). The buffer solution was then extracted three times with equal volumes of butanol. The extracts were pooled, radioassayed, and fractionated on silicic-acid columns, as described above, to determine the percentage hydrolysis and the nature of the radioactive compounds.

Instrumentation

An International model PR-2 portable refrigerated centrifuge was used to centrifuge extracts. Counter-current distribution was made with a manually operated Craig-Post 60-tube train with 10 ml. volumes for upper and lower phase or a 50-tube, Craig-Post automatic counter-current-distribution instrument 100 ml. for upper and lower phase. Ultraviolet spectra were taken in methanol with a Bausch and Lomb Spectronic 505 spectrophotometer. Mass spectra were measured by using the LKB Model 9000 gas-chromatograph mass spectrometer; samples were introduced directly into the ionization chamber, and the ionization energy was 70 ev. Nuclear magnetic resonance (NMR) spectra were recorded at 60 Mc. with a Varian-A-60A NMR spectrometer by using deuterated chloroform or pyridine as the solvent and tetramethylsilane as the internal NMR standard.

RESULTS

Metabolism of 1α-^{3}H-22,25-Bisdeoxyecdysone During Termination of Diapause in Pupae of the Tobacco Hornworm

The crude extractive from 621 (1.99 kg.) tobacco hornworms contained 1.9×10^7 d.p.m. of the injected radioactivity. Most of the remaining radio-activity could be accounted for in the aqueous phase, and solids to give a total recovery of approximately 80 per cent of the administered dose. When chromatographed on silicic acid about 10 per cent of the radioactivity and less than 1 per cent of the biological activity was eluted in the fraction for 22,25-bisdeoxyecdysone (fraction 1, Table 1). Thin-layer chromatography (TLC) of this fraction, however, yielded several radioactive zones, and the

[3]   β-Glucosidase: One mg. liberates approximately 2.5–7.0 μmoles of glucose per minute from saticin at pH 5.25 and 37° C.

Sulfatase Type H-2: One unit will hydrolyze 1 μmole of nitrocatechol sulfate per hour at pH 5.0 and 37° C.

Sulfatase Type III: One mg. will hydrolyze 8.5 μ moles of nitrocatechol sulfate per hour at pH 5.0 and 37° C.

zone for 22,25-bisdeoxyecdysone contained about half of the total radio-activity. NMR and mass spectra established this compound to be 22,25-bisdeoxyecdysone.

About 36 per cent (5.0×10^6 d.p.m.) of the recovered radioactivity and 92 per cent of the total biological activity were eluted in column fractions 4 through 7 (Table 1) that contain a-ecdysone and 20-hydroxyecdysone (Kaplanis et al., 1969). Additional purification by chromatography of the pooled fractions of a-ecdysone and 20-hydroxyecdysone over alumina resulted in about 65 per cent reduction in mass without any loss either in biological activity or radioactivity. The methanol eluate from the alumina column (5.15×10^6 d.p.m.), when subjected to 60 counter-current trans-fers, gave two major peaks when analyzed with ultraviolet light and radio-assay. The relative distribution of the radioactive peaks was about 72 per cent in tubes 9 through 31 and 28 per cent in tubes 32 through 50, coinci-ding with the tubes expected to contain 20-hydroxyecdysone and a-ecdy-sone, respectively. Radioactive peaks were found to parallel closely the peaks obtained by ultraviolet spectroscopy. The radioactive compounds in tubes 13 through 26 purified by silicic-acid chromatography and recrystallization from ethyl acetate, yielded 2.82 mg. of 20-hydroxyecdysone [specific ac-tivity, 760 d.p.m./μg. (theoretical, 1581 d.p.m./μg.)]. After fractionation and crystallization from ethyl acetate, the apolar compound (tubes 36 through 48) yielded 0.54 mg. of a-ecdysone [specific activity, 802 d.p.m./ μg. (theoretical, 1636 d.p.m./μg.)]. The physical properties, including NMR and mass spectra of the crystalline 20-hydroxyecdysone and a-ecdysone from the hornworm, were identical to those of authentic standards; and the compounds were found to be radiochemically pure by column chroma-tography and thin-layer chromatography. When fractions 8 through 11 (4.02×10^6 d.p.m., Table 1) were pooled and fractionated by CCD, several radioactive peaks were detected, including a peak associated with 20,26-dihydroxyecdysone (tubes 0–8, 2.3×10^6 d.p.m.). Exhaustive purification by CCD in a solvent system of cyclohexane, butanol, and water (2:8:10 and 1:9:10), column chromatography on silicic acid, and thin-layer chroma-tography indicated that only about 10 per cent (3.0×10^5 d.p.m.) of the total radioactivity present in fractions 8 through 11 is 20,26-dihydroxy-ecdysone.

The final major column fraction (fraction 12, Table 1) contained a sub-stantial amount of radioactivity (21 per cent) but only a small amount of MH activity. Preliminary to enzymatic hydrolysis, aliquots of fraction 12 were refractionated on silicic acid and about 95 to 98 per cent of the radio-activity was again eluted in the polar fractions (benzene-methanol, 75:25) and methanol. To determine if the ^{3}H-polar compounds were steroidal conjugates, aliquots of fraction 12 were hydrolyzed with either β-glucosidase or sulfatase preparations following which the extracts were examined by column chromatography. About 15 to 25 per cent was hydrolyzed with the β-glucosidase whereas 75 to 85 per cent was hydrolyzed with the preparation of sulfatase.

The remaining portion of fraction 12 (2.34 x 10^6 d.p.m.) was hydrolyzed with the sulfatase and then chromatographed on silicic acid (Table 2). Analyses of fraction 1 from this column by thin-layer chromatography gave several radioactive zones. A zone that accounted for about 60 per cent of the total radioactivity from the plate appeared to be 22,25-bisdeoxyecdysone. Comparative analyses by thin-layer chromatography, nuclear magnetic resonance, and mass spectroscopy confirmed the identity of this compound to be 22, 25-bisdeoxyecdysone.

Column fractions 4 through 6 (8.4 x 10^5 d.p.m., Table 2), which elute a-ecdysone and 20-hydroxyecdysone, were fractionated by counter-current distribution (60 tubes). About 6.0 per cent (3.3 x 10^4 d.p.m.) of the total radioactivity from the counter-current was associated with the tubes (12 through 27) that contain 20-hydroxyecdysone and 94.0 per cent (6.0 x 10^5 d.p.m.) with the tubes (34 through 50) that contain a-ecdysone. The minor component from the counter-current distribution was purified additionally by column chromatography, and analyses by co-chromatography on thin-layer chromatography and mass spectrometry showed it to be 20-hydroxyecdysone. The tubes (34 through 50) from counter-current distribution containing the a-ecdysone fraction were bioassayed and then purified by column chromatography on silicic acid. Analyses of this major component by mass spectrometry and nuclear magnetic resonance showed it to be a-ecdysone.

Metabolism of 1a-^{3}H-22,25-Bisdeoxyecdysone in the Adult House Fly

The crude extractives from 6,700 adult female flies (125 G.) and their excreta contained a total of 2.0 and 9.2 mg.-equivalents of ^{3}H-compounds, respectively. A high percentage of the recovered radioactive material from the flies (73.0 per cent) and excreta (56.0 per cent) behaved chromatographically in a manner similar to 22,25-bisdeoxyecdysone (fraction 1, Table 3). Additional purification by preparative TLC and subsequent analyses by NMR and mass spectrometry confirmed that this ^{3}H-compound was 22,25-bisdeoxyecdysone. When column fractions 3 through 6 were fractionated by counter-current distribution, about 9 and 21 per cent of the radioactivity was associated with 20-hydroxyecdysone from the flies and excreta, respectively. However, refractionation of this radioactive material by counter-current and thin-layer chromatography indicated that only trace amounts behaved similarly to 20-hydroxyecdysone (1.5 μg.-³H-equivalents). When bioassayed, this material was found to be inactive in the MH assay. Analyses of fractions 4 through 6 (Table 3) by CCD showed that 80–90 per cent of the radioactivity partitioned like *a*-ecdysone. When this material was fractionated by thin-layer chromatography, 66 and 58 per cent of the radioactivity from the flies and excreta, respectively, behaved like *a*-ecdysone. The biological activity in both cases was also associated with this zone. Mass spectral analyses showed this compound to be a pentahydroxy steroid, how-

TABLE 2

COLUMN–CHROMATOGRAPHIC ANALYSES* OF THE POLAR FRACTION[†] FROM
TOBACCO HORNWORMS FOLLOWING HYDROLYSIS OF THE FRACTION
WITH A SULFATASE PREPARATION

Fraction	Volume (ml.)	Total d.p.m. $(\times 10^5)$	Per Cent of Total
Benzene-Methanol (95:5)			
1	3550	8.20	34.5
2	1775	1.14	4.8
3	1775	0.18	0.8
Benzene-Methanol (90:10)			
4	940	4.80	20.2
5	940	2.80	11.8
6	940	0.77	3.2
Benzene-Methanol (75:25)			
7	940	2.88	12.1
Methanol			
8	940	3.00	12.6

* 9.5 cm. (I.D.) × 2.3 cm., 80 G. silicic acid.
† Fraction 12, Table 1.

ever, with fragmentation pattern distinct and different from that of a-ecdysone. Two refractionations on silicic acid of fraction 7 (Table 3) in search of 20,26-dihydroxyecdysone resulted in most of the radioactivity being eluted in fraction 8. Approximately 2.4 μg.-^{3}H-equivalents was accounted for in the fraction and this was inactive in the MH assay.

A substantial amount of radioactivity, particularly from the excreta, was eluted in the polar fractions (fraction 8). When these fractions were first incubated with β-glucosidase, about 35 per cent of the radioactivity from the adults and 66 per cent from the excreta was hydrolyzed to ^{3}H-steroidal moieties that eluted in the earlier column fractions on silicic acid (fractions 1 through 6). When ^{3}H-polar metabolites from the flies and excreta that remained unchanged following hydrolysis with β-glucosidase were incubated with the sulfatase preparation, an additional 45 and 15 per cent, respectively, of the radioactive compounds were hydrolyzed. When the ^{3}H-steroid moieties of the conjugates from the feces were examined by thin-layer chromatography and mass spectrometry, only a small amount of 22,25-bisdeoxyecdysone was found. Three tetrahydroxy steroids were present as indicated by thin-layer chromatography and mass spectrometry. One of the tetrahydroxy steroids was inseparable from 22,25-bisdeoxyecdysone by thin-layer chromatography. The two other tetrahydroxy steroids, both of which showed the typical ultra-violet spectrum for an a,β-unsaturated ketone, were more polar than the parent compound by thin-layer chromatography. In addition, a pentahydroxy steroid similar or identical to the one described above was present in the conjugates also.

DISCUSSION

The results from these studies with labeled 22,25-bisdeoxyecdysone during termination of diapause in the tobacco hornworm and inhibition of ovarian development in the female fly point to some interesting similarities and differences in the metabolism of this steroid in the two insects. The high percentage of the 22,25-bisdeoxyecdysone found in the house fly and excreta may in part be due to its limited absorption from the intestinal tract; adult flies injected with the ^{3}H-analog show an efficient metabolism of the analog, with only about 5 per cent of the radioactive compounds in the flies and excreta behaving as unmetabolized [3]H-22,25-bisdeoxyecdysone. [4/] These latter results are similar to those observed with diapausing tobacco-hornworm pupae in which the unchanged analog accounted for less than 5 per cent of the total radioactivity.

[4/]   Kaplanis, J. N., Dutky, S. R., Robbins, W. E., and Thompson, M. J. (Unpublished data).

TABLE 3

COLUMN–CHROMATOGRAPHIC ANALYSES* OF THE ^{3}H–COMPOUNDS ISOLATED FROM THE HOUSE FLIES AND THE EXCRETA. FLIES WERE FED ON A DIET CONTAINING 0.1 PER CENT ^{3}H–22,25–BISDEOXYECDYSONE

Fraction	Total d.p.m. (x 10^3)		Per Cent of Total	
	Adult	Excreta	Adult	Excreta
Benzene-Methanol (95:5)				
1	80.0	260.0	72.7	56.3
2	1.3	2.0	1.2	0.4
3	0.5	0.9	0.5	0.2
Benzene-Methanol (90:10)				
4	2.0	4.5	1.8	1.0
5	2.8	7.2	2.5	1.6
6	3.9	4.9	3.5	1.1
Benzene-Methanol (75:25)				
7	2.6	47.3	2.4	10.2
Methanol				
8	17.0	135.0	15.4	29.2

* 2.2 cm. (I.D.) x 2.35 cm., 4.5 G. silicic acid for extracts from excreta; 3.3 cm. (I.D.) x 2.4 cm., 10.13 G. silicic acid for extracts from adult flies.

Although hydroxylation is the major metabolic modification in both the hornworm and the adult house fly, the metabolic pathways do differ in the two insects. In the house fly, the ^{3}H-ecdysone analog is not converted in significant detectable amounts to any of the insect ecdysones but is metabolized into unidentified tetrahydroxy and pentahydroxy steroids. In the hornworm, however, conversion of the synthetic ecdysone analog to the insect ecdysones—*a*-ecdysone, 20-hydroxyecdysone, and 20,26-dihydroxyecdysone—represents a major metabolic pathway. An explanation for the difference in metabolism in the hornworm and the house fly is that the mechanism for biosynthesis of ecdysone would be expected in pupae during metamorphosis, but the mechanism may well be absent in adult insects.

Formation of *a*-glucosides has been reported previously as a means for inactivation of ecdysones in immature *Calliphora erythrocephala* (Meigen)

(Heinrich and Hoffmeister, 1970); and the sulfates of neutral sterols such as cholesterol, campesterol, and β-sitosterol have been isolated from the meconium of the tobacco hornworm (Hutchins and Kaplanis, 1969). Conjugation is also a major metabolic pathway for the labeled 22,25-bisdeoxyecdysone and/or its metabolites in the tobacco hornworm and the house fly. Sulfates were the predominant conjugates in the more polar fraction from the hornworm and the adult house fly, whereas β-glucosides were the predominant conjugates in the excreta of the house fly. However, when 22, 25-bisdeoxyecdysone was injected into the adult house fly, [4] the polar fraction from the flies and excreta were found to be principally sulfate conjugates. The predominance of the β-glucosides found in the excreta following oral administration of the analog could be related either to the intestinal route of absorption or to the activity of intestinal microorganisms or both. From these studies it appears that both glucosides and sulfates play a role in inactivation of insect ecdysones and related steroids.

In the adult house fly the steroidal moieties of the conjugates were unidentified tetrahydroxy and pentahydroxy steroids plus very small amounts of 22,25-bisdeoxyecdysone. The composition of the steroid moieties of the conjugates from the tobacco hornworm was qualitatively similar to that found for the unconjugated or free forms: 22,25-bisdeoxyecdysone, α-ecdysone, and 20-hydroxyecdysone. Quantitatively, however, there was a difference; α-ecdysone was present as conjugates in much greater amounts than was the 20-hydroxyecdysone, whereas 20-hydroxyecdysone was the major component in the free form. The observed efficient inactivation of α-ecdysone by conjugation may explain why this compound is tolerated in high doses by diapausing hornworm pupae [5] without causing abnormal development, whereas equivalent doses of 20-hydroxyecdysone disrupt development, an effect previously reported for diapausing *Samia cynthia* (Drury) silkworm pupae (Williams, 1968). In addition to serving as a means for inactivating ecdysones, conjugation may also be a mechanism for regulating the biosynthesis and titer of 20-hydroxyecdysone in certain insects.

The results of these studies indicate that the synthetic analog or its metabolites trigger the biochemical mechanism for the biosynthesis of the ecdysones from endogenous steroid precursors in the diapausing pupa of the tobacco hornworm and that the synthetic analog also serves as a precursor for this insect's molting hormones. The specific activity of the crystalline ecdysones from the hornworm is about 50 per cent of theoretical, indicating that approximately one-half of both the α-ecdysone and the 20-

[5]   Kaplanis, J. N., Robbins, W. E., and Thompson, M. J. (Unpublished data).

hydroxyecdysone was derived from the ^{3}H-22,25-bisdeoxyecdysone and the other half was derived from endogenous steroid precursors. The reports that ^{3}H-a-ecdysone is converted to 20-hydroxyecdysone (Cherbas and Cherbas, 1970; Galbraith et al., 1969; King and Siddall, 1969; Moriyama et al., 1970), taken together with these findings that the three insect ecdysones are biosynthesized from a common precursor, confirms our premise (Thompson et al., 1967) that these three steroids are metabolites in the biosynthetic scheme of the ecdysones.

The relationship between metabolism of 22,25-bisdeoxyecdysone and its activity in the female house fly is unresolved at this point. The compound could exert its effect through hydroxylation to more active metabolites, such as the unidentified tetrahydroxy and pentahydroxy steroid metabolites that are inactivated in turn by conjugation to form glucosides and sulfates. Alternately, the synthetic analog could be active *per se,* and its inactivation may proceed through the observed combination of hydroxylation and conjugation. A final decision on the relationship between metabolism and activity of the synthetic ecdysone analog in the fly, however, must await the characterization and biological evaluation of the hydroxylated metabolites.

SUMMARY

The metabolism of labeled $1a$-^{3}H-22,25-bisdeoxyecdysone was studied in relation to the termination of pupal diapause in the tobacco hornworm, *Manduca sexta* (L.), and the inhibition of ovarian development in the adult house fly, *Musca domestica* L. Hydroxylation and conjugation were found to be major metabolic pathways for the synthetic ecdysone analog in both of these insects. In the tobacco hornworm the analog served as a precursor for the three insect ecdysones: a-ecdysone, 20-hydroxyecdysone, and 20, 26-dihydroxyecdysone. The two major ecdysones of insects and a small amount of unchanged 22,25-bisdeoxyecdysone were also found to be present as glucoside and sulfate conjugates, with the sulfate conjugates predominating. a-Ecdysone was present in far greater quantities than 20-hydroxyecdysone in the conjugated form, whereas 20-hydroxyecdysone was the major component in the free form. In the adult fly, the synthetic steroid was not metabolized to the ecdysones of insects, but instead the compound was converted into a number of unidentified tetrahydroxy and pentahydroxy steroids that occurred in the insect and feces principally as glucoside and sulfate conjugates.

Acknowledgement
The technical assistance of E. L. Lindquist, B. M. Bryce, and L. J. Fleming is acknowledged with gratitude.

References

1. CHERBAS, L. and CHERBAS, P. : Distribution and Metabolism of α-Ecdysone in Pupae of the Silkworm *Anteraea polyphemus.* Biol. Bull., *138*:115-128, 1970.
2. COLOWICK, S. P. and KAPLAN, N. O.: Methods in Enzymology. Preparation and and Assay of Enzymes. Vol. III, Academic Press, New York, 1955.
3. EARLE, N. W., PADOVANI, I., THOMPSON, M. J., and ROBBINS, W. E. : Inhibition of Larval Development and Egg Production in the Boll Weevil Following Ingestion of Ecdysone Analogues. J. Econ. Entomol., *63*:1064-1069, 1970.
4. GALBRAITH, M. N., HORN, D. H. S., MIDDLETON, E. J., and HACKNEY, R. J.: Moulting Hormones of Insects and Crustaceans: The Synthesis of 22-Deoxy-crustecdysone. Australian J. Chem., *22*:1517-1524, 1969.
5. HEINRICH, G. and HOFFMEISTER, H. : Bildung von Hormonglykosiden als Inaktivierungsmechanismus bei *Calliphora erythrocephala.* Z. Naturforsch. B, *25*: 358-361, 1970.
6. HOCKS, P., JAGER, A., KERB, U., WIECHERT, R., FURLEMEIER, A., FURST, A., LANGEMANN, A., and WALDVOGEL, G. : Synthetische Steroide mit Hautungshormonaktivitat. Angew. Chemie, *78*:680-681, 1966.
7. HUTCHINS, R. F. N. and KAPLANIS, J. N. : Sterol Sulfates in an Insect. Steroids, *13*:605-614, 1969.
8. KAPLANIS, J. N., ROBBINS, W. E., THOMPSON, M. J., and BAUMHOVER, A. H.: Ecdysone Analog: Conversion to Alpha Ecdysone and 20-Hydroxyecdysone by an Insect. Science, *166*:1540-1541, 1969.
9. KAPLANIS, J. N., TABOR, L. A., THOMPSON, M. J., ROBBINS, W. E., and SHORTINO, T. J. : Assay for Ecdysone (Molting Hormone) Activity Using the House Fly, *Musca domestica* L. Steroids, *8*:625-631, 1966.
10. KAPLANIS, J. N., THOMPSON, M. J., and ROBBINS, W. E. : The Effects of Ecdysones and Analogs on Ovarian Development and Reproduction in the House Fly *Musca domestica* (L.). XIII Intern. Congr. Entomol. Proc., 1972.
11. KAPLANIS, J. N., THOMPSON, M. J., YAMAMOTO, R. T., ROBBINS, W. E., and LOULOUDES, S. J.: Ecdysones from the Pupa of the Tobacco Hornworm, *Manduca sexta* (Johannson). Steroids, *8*:605-623, 1966.
12. KING, D. S. and SIDDALL, J. B.:Conversion of α-Ecdysone to β-Ecdysone by Crustaceans and Insects. Nature, *221*:955-956, 1969.
13. KRISHNAKUMARAN, A. and SCHNEIDERMAN, H. A. : Control of Molting in Mandibulate and Chelicerate Arthropods by Ecdysones. Biol. Bull., *139*:520-538, 1970.
14. LEBREQUE, G. C., ADCOCK, P. H., and SMITH, C. N. : Tests with Compounds Affecting House Fly Metabolism. J. Econ. Entomol., *53*:802-805, 1960.
15. LOULOUDES, S. J., SHORTINO, T. J., and BROWN, N. L. : Hydroxy Lecithin Emulsions for Treating Insects. J. Econ. Entomol., *55*:819, 1962.
16. MORIYAMA, H., NAKANISHI, K., KING, D. S., OKAUCHI, T., SIDDALL, J. B., and HAFFERL, W.: On the Origin and Metabolic Fate of α-Ecdysone in Insects. Gen. Comp. Endocrinol., *15*:80-87, 1970.
17. ROBBINS, W. E., KAPLANIS, J. N., THOMPSON, M. J., SHORTINO, T. J., COHEN, C. F., and JOYNER, S. C.: Ecdysones and Analogs: Effects on Development and Reproduction of Insects. Science, *161*:1158-1159, 1968.

18. ROBBINS, W. E., KAPLANIS, J. N., THOMPSÒN, M. J., SHORTINO, T. J., and JOY-NER, S. C. : Ecdysones and Synthetic Analogs: Molting Hormone Activity and Inhibitive Effects on Insect Growth, Metamorphosis and Reproduction. Steroids, *16*:105-125, 1970.

19. STAHL, E. : Thin-layer Chromatography. Academic Press, New York, p. 501, 1965.

20. THOMPSON, M. J., KAPLANIS, J. N., ROBBINS, W. E., and YAMAMOTO, R. T. : 20,26-Dihydroxyecdysone, a New Steroid with Moulting Hormone Activity from the Tobacco Hornworm, *Manduca sexta* (Johannson). Chem. Commun., *13*:650-653, 1967.

21. THOMPSON, M. J., ROBBINS, W. E., KAPLANIS, J. N., COHEN, C. F., and LAN-CASTER, S. M. : Synthesis of Analogs of α-Ecdysone. A Simplified Synthesis of 2β,3β,14α-trihydroxy-7-en-6-one-5β-steroids. Steroids, *16*:85-104, 1970.

22. WILLIAMS, C. M. : Ecdysone and Ecdysone-Analogues: Their Assay and Action on Diapausing Pupae of the Cynthia Silkworm. Biol. Bull., *134*:344-355, 1968.

23. WILLIAMS, C. M. and ROBBINS, W. E. : Conference on Insect-plant Interactions. BioScience, *18*:791-792, 797-799, 1968.

24. WRIGHT, J. E. : Hormonal Termination of Larval Diapause in *Dermacenter albipictus*. Science, *163*:390-391, 1969.

BIOSYNTHESIS and DEGRADATION of JUVENILE HORMONE

Manfred Metzler, Karl H. Dahm,
Dietrich Meyer, and Herbert Röller

The juvenile hormone [JH, Figure 1; (Röller *et al.*, 1967; Dahm *et al.*, 1968, 1967; Röller and Dahm, 1968)] and its lower homologue JH-II [Figure 2; (Meyer *et al.*, 1968)] have basic structures typical of acyclic sesquiterpenes, for example, farnesol (Figure 3). The most significant differences, however, are the ethyl groups at C7 and C11 or C11, respectively. This substitution poses an intriguing biochemical problem because no natural mevalonate-derived compound of this kind has been found before. Consequently, investigations of the biosynthesis of the hormone cannot be based on precedence.

The structural type of JH seems to indicate that its biosynthesis generally follows the route established for terpenoid compounds. The additional C-atoms may be introduced during a later stage of the biosynthesis, in which case mevalonate should be a key intermediate. Alternatively, the animal may produce homomevalonate from one C_3- and two C_2-units and combine one mevalonate and two homomevalonate residues to the juvenile hormone; in either case incorporation of mevalonate can be expected. L-Methionine may be considered a donor of C_1-units.

176

On the other hand, JH may not be a mevalonate derivative at all, but a product of the fatty-acid metabolism. In this case acetate, propionate, and butyrate might be the appropriate precursors in the biosynthesis. Finally, we should not overlook the possibility that the insect acquires a larger precursor with food and converts it by suitable transformations into the juvenile hormone.

The juvenile hormone homologue (Figure 2) exhibits variable biological activity — in one insect species it might have an activity similar to juvenile hormone, while in another species its specific activity tends to be relatively low. In all species investigated so far, the juvenile hormone is always accompanied by 10-30 per cent JH-II (Meyer *et al.,* 1968; Dahm and Röller, 1970; Metzler *et al.*, 1971; Meyer *et al.*, in preparation). Therefore, we cannot decide whether JH-II is a genuine hormone in its own right or whether it is a by-product of biosynthesis. Its presence, however, does not shed any light on the biosynthetic pathways involved.

The best source of JH still is the adult male of the giant silk moth *Hyalophora cecropia*. In order to investigate the biosynthesis of JH, we developed a purification prodecure which allows us to isolate and analyze the hormone starting with not more than 1-5 adult moths (Dahm and Röller, 1970). According to our most recent studies, freshly emerged male Cecropia contain little JH, but its titer increases rapidly up to 4-6 μg./moth between the first and fourth day of adult life (Metzler *et al.*, 1971). In contrast, Gilbert and Schneiderman (1961) found that the steepest increase of JH concentration occurs around the time of ecdysis. On the basis of our experiments, we decided to administer possible precursors to about 2-day-old moths and to incubate 10-30 hours, after which the JH was to be extracted.

In a series of experiments the incorporation of 5-^{3}H-mevalonate, L-[^{3}H-methyl]-methionine, 2-^{14}C-acetate, 1-^{14}C-acetate and ^{3}H-acetate was studied.

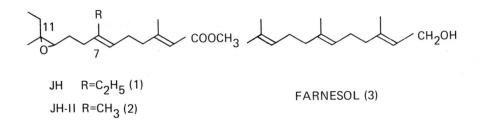

JH   R=C$_2$H$_5$ (1)

JH-II R=CH$_3$ (2)

FARNESOL (3)

5-^{3}H-Mevalonate

5-^{3}H-Mevalonate (spec. act. 7.77 x 10^9 d.p.m./μmole) in insect-Ringer-solution was injected into abdomens of four 2 to 3-day-old moths (58.7 x

10^6 d.p.m./moth). After an incubation period of 16 hours the juvenile hormone (14.4 μg.) was isolated. It did not contain a detectable amount of ^{3}H. The fraction containing *trans, trans*-farnesol, however, was highly labeled (1 x 10^6 d.p.m.). Repeating the experiment with 3 moths, we determined the amount of farnesol quantitatively by gas chromatography and also confirmed its identity. From three moths we recovered only 0.4 μg. [Good-fellow and Gilbert (1963) found amounts of 2 μg. farnesol/moth.] with a specific activity of about 500 x 10^6 d.p.m./μmole. About 0.5 per cent of the administered ^{3}H had been incorporated into the farnesol. The JH (10.5 μg.), in contrast, contained an insignificant amount of ^{3}H (161 d.p.m.). If the moth does not maintain separate pools of mevalonate, the experiments clearly indicate that, while terpenoid compounds are synthesized from mevalonate during the incubation period, JH is not produced *via* this pathway. It is possible, however, that the moth produces a JH-precursor from mevalonate during the larval or pupal stages which then is converted in the adult to JH by relatively minor transformations.

L-[^{3}H-methyl]-methionine

In three experiments using generally the same conditions as in the mevalonate experiments we injected the moths with L-methionine [^{3}H-methyl] (spec. act. 7.37 x 10^9 d.p.m./μmole, dose: 47.4 x 10^6 d.p.m./moth). The juvenile hormone (1.3, 1.2, and 1.4 μg./moth) had specific activities of 6.4 x 10^6, 5.0 x 10^6 and 9.4 x 10^6 d.p.m./μmole. Approximately 0.06, 0.04 and 0.1 per cent of the administered label had been incorporated into the hormone. A sample of the ^{3}H-hormone was hydrogenated (Metzler *et al.*, 1971), the resulting methyl 7-ethyl-3,11-dimethyl-tridecanoate purified by gas chromatography and, after addition of unlabeled ester, cleaved with lithium aluminum hydride. The gas chromatographically purified 7-ethyl-3,11-dimethyl-1-tridecanol was devoid of any radioactivity. The methanol from the methyl ester group was isolated as methyl 3,5-dinitrobenzoate (65 per cent overall yield starting with JH) and had retained the label (51 per cent recovery starting with JH). JH-II was isolated and degraded in the same manner; it also contained the label exclusively in the ester methyl group. The results of these experiments demonstrate that during the incubation period L-methionine is utilized for the synthesis of the methyl ester group but that the ethyl groups of C-7 and C-11 are not formed by a transfer of C_1-units from L-methionine.

2-^{14}C-Acetate

In a third series of experiments 2-^{14}C-acetate was administered as a possible precursor. Sixteen hours after application of the acetate (spec. act. 1.12 x 10^8 d.p.m./μmole, dose: 98 x 10^6 d.p.m./moth) to three two-day-old moths 3.3 μg. juvenile hormone were isolated with a specific activity of 0.35 x 10^6 d.p.m./μmole. In the same experiment 0.45 μg. *trans, trans*-farnesol with a specific activity of 0.34 x 10^6 d.p.m./μmole were isolated. Two additional experiments revealed similar results. After cleavage of the JH, as described above, the label was recovered with the 7-ethyl-3,11-dimethyl-1-tridecanol but not with the methanol from the carbomethoxy group. As a control, and in order to obtain more information about the utilization of acetate in the moth, we isolated also a series of saturated and unsaturated fatty acids after conversion to the methyl esters. Methyl palmitate (10.5 μg./moth) showed the highest incorporation (1.85 per cent of the dose) of $2\text{-}^{14}\text{C}$-acetate. Its specific activity (0.027 x 10^6 d.p.m./μmole) was about one-tenth that of JH. A result like this is to be expected, considering that all the juvenile hormone is synthesized during the adult stage of the moth while the bulk of the fatty acids is carried over unchanged from the pupal stage. A quantitative estimation, however, cannot be made.

$1\text{-}^{14}\text{C}$-acetate and $2\text{-}^{14}\text{C}$-acetate

Acetate is incorporated as a complete molecule. This is indicated by the fact that administration of $1\text{-}^{14}\text{C}$-acetate and $2\text{-}^{14}\text{C}$-acetate led to about equal incorporation.

^3H-Acetate

The incorporation of acetate into JH and JH-II was confirmed with ^3H-acetate of high specific activity (1Ci./mMole). Preliminary degradation experiments with these biosynthetically labeled hormones preclude that acetate provides the methyl group of the ethyl side chains only, since the levulinic aldehyde obtained by OsO_4/HJO_4 cleavage of JH and JH-II and purified by GLC contains significant radioactivity, comparable to the label located in homolevulinic aldehyde derived from JH. Furthermore, the C_{14}- and C_{13}-aldehydes obtained from JH and JH-II, respectively, after HJO_4 cleavage contained about equal radioactivity. Surprisingly, the other product of this cleavage reaction (2-butanone, isolated as 2.4-dinitrophenylhydrazone) was devoid of label.

Incorporation of Other Possible Precursors

We have experimented with a few other possible precursors of JH. Neither $2\text{-}^{14}\text{C}$-farnesol nor its pyrophosphate was incorporated. After application of $5\text{-}^3\text{H}$-isoleucin (spec. act. 75 x 10^9 d.p.m./μmole, dose: 33.2 x 10^6 d.p.m./moth) to four moths, 5.2 μg. JH were isolated with a specific activity (0.39 x 10^6 d.p.m./μmole) similar to that obtained in the acetate experiments (Metzler *et al.*, 1971). $2\text{-}^{14}\text{C}$-10-epoxy-7-ethyl-3,11-dimethyl-2.6-

tridecadienoic acid was converted in high yield (up to 10 per cent) to the hormone (Metzler *et al.*, 1971). In this case L-methionine was again utilized as a donor of the ester methyl group.

Summary

Biosynthesis

a. The juvenile hormone, which can be isolated from the fat body of adult male *Hyalophora cecropia,* is biosynthesized in the adult moth. The steepest increase in JH-concentration occurs between the second and fourth day after emergence.

b. L-Methionine provides the ester methyl group of both JH and JH-II, but it does not contribute to the ethyl groups at C-7 and C-11.

c. Mevalonate is not incorporated into JH but is used extensively during the experimental period for the synthesis of farnesol. With the additional assumption that the animal does not possess two separate pools of mevalonate for the biosynthesis of terpene-like compounds, this result proves conclusively, that in spite of the similarity of JH to terpenes, JH is not synthesized from mevalonate in the adult moth. Either a precursor with the carbon skeleton of JH is synthesized from mevalonate already during the larval or pupal stages, or the JH is not at all a product of the mevalonate metabolism.

d. Labeled acetate is incorporated into JH, JH-II and farnesol, giving products of similar specific activity. Preliminary degradation experiments with the labeled JH indicate that the label is distributed throughout the molecule. The overall incorporation of acetate into JH is very small ($\leqslant 0.003$ per cent). The limited amount of material we are dealing with in the acetate experiments (1-2μg. JH, 1,350 d.p.m./moth; 0.1-0.15 μg. farnesol, 230-660 d.p.m./moth) makes these studies extremely difficult and precludes a straight-forward interpretation of the results. The hypothesis that juvenile hormone is synthesized from acetate not following the mevalonate pathway is of such a radical nature that more detailed evidence, with refined techniques, has to be collected before it seriously can be advocated.

e. *H. cecropia* converts epoxy acid extensively into JH using the methyl group of L-methionine as a donor for the ester methyl group.

f. Incorporation experiments with propionate, farnesol and farnesyl pyrophosphate have been negative.

Degradation

The concentration of JH (Figure 1.) during the life cycle of an insect may be controlled through both the rate of its biosynthesis and degradation. In fifth-instar larvae of *Manduca sexta,* the degradation of JH starts with enzymatic hydrolysis to the acid, after which the oxirane-ring is cleaved to the diol (Slade *et al.,* in press). The ester group is hydrolized so smoothly by Manduca blood that we have used the reaction for synthesis of the labeled acid from 2-^{14}C-JH (Metzler *et al.,* 1972). In *Hyalophora cecropia* adults, exogenous JH is also rapidly degraded, and after 24 hours only 10 per cent can be recovered unchanged. We have characterized some of the products by their chromatographic properties but have not yet chemically identified them. Surprising is the finding that the acid does not seem to be the major degradation product in this species; on the contrary, it is incorporated in good yields into newly synthesized JH (Metzler *et al.,* 1972). It remains to be seen if the degradation of exogenous JH indeed reflects the metabolic fate of endogenous JH.

References

1. DAHM, K. H. and RÖLLER, H.: The Juvenile Hormone of the Giant Silk Moth *Hyalophora gloveri* (Strecker). Life Sci., 9:1397, 1970.
2. DAHM, K. H., RÖLLER, H., and TROST, B. M.: The Juvenile Hormone. IV. Stereochemistry of Juvenile Hormone and Biological Activity of Some of its Isomers and Related Compounds. Life Sci., 7:129, 1968.
3. DAHM, K. H., TROST, B. M., and RÖLLER, H.: The Juvenile Hormone. V. Synthesis of the Racemic Juvenile Hormone. J. Am. Chem. Soc., 89:5295, 1967.
4. GILBERT, L. I. and SCHNEIDERMAN, H. A.: The Content of Juvenile Hormone and Lipid in Lepidoptera: Sexual Differences and Developmental Changes. Gen. Comp. Endocr., 1:453-472, 1961.
5. GOODFELLOW, R. D. and GILBERT, L. I.: Sterols and Terpenes in the Cecropia Silkmoth. Amer. Zool., 3:508, 1963.
6. MEYER, A. S., SCHNEIDERMAN, H. A., HANZMANN, E., and KO, J. H.: The Two Juvenile Hormones from the Cecropia Silk Moth. Proc. Nat. Acad. Sci., U. S., 60:853, 1968.
7. MEYER, D., DAHM, K. H., and RÖLLER, H.: In preparation.
8. METZLER, M., DAHM, K. H., MEYER, D., and RÖLLER, H.: On the Biosynthesis of Juvenile Hormone in the Adult Cecropia Moth. Z. Naturforsch., in press.
9. METZLER, M., MEYER, D., DAHM, K. H., RÖLLER, H., and SIDDALL, J. B.: Biosynthesis of Juvenile Hormone from 10-Epoxy-7-Ethyl-3,11-Dimethyl-2,6-Tridecadienoic Acid in the Adult Cecropia Moth. Submitted for publication.
10. RÖLLER, H. and DAHM, K. H.: The Chemistry and Biology of Juvenile Hormone. Rec. Prog. Horm. Res., 24:651-680, 1968.
11. RÖLLER, H., DAHM, K. H., SWEELEY, C. C., and TROST, B. M.: The Structure of the Juvenile Hormone. Agnew. Chem. Int. Ed., 6:179, 1967.
12. SLADE, M., ZIBITT, C. H., and SIDDALL, J. B.: Proc. IUPAC Symposium, Tel Aviv (1971), in press.

PART II
ISOLATION, DISTRIBUTION, AND SUPPLY OF INVERTEBRATE HORMONES, PHYTOHORMONES, AND ANALOGS

Ecdysones

ECDYSONES of PLANT ORIGIN

H. Hikino and T. Takemoto

It is well known that the first insect molting hormone, a-ecdysone, was isolated from the silkworm, *Bombyx mori*, by Butenandt and Karlson in 1954 with a background of pioneering work performed by a number of researchers involved in the purification of the hormone. Since then six additional molting hormones (zooecdysones) have been isolated from a variety of arthropods, insects, and crustaceans. The content of these zooecdysones in animals is only $10^{-5}-10^{-9}$ per cent; the compound occurring most commonly is β-ecdysone. The structure of a-ecdysone was first elucidated in 1965, and the structures of another five zooecdysones were successively determined thereafter.

Until five years ago who would imagine that a plant might contain an insect-molting hormone? Had there been someone with such a fantastic idea, he would have been able to discover immediately that a number of botanical extracts showed insect-molting-hormone activity by means of a bioassay such as a Calliphora test already devised for assay of these hormones in animals. In fact, however, the discovery of substances that are the same as, or similar in structure to, insect-molting hormones from the plant kingdom (phytoecdysones) was made purely by chance. Thus Nakanishi *et al.*, during their chemical search for an anticancer component of *Podocarpus nakaii* leaves, isolated four compounds in 1964 and elucidated the structure of the main constituent, ponasterone A, in 1966. Since ponasterone A and its companions, ponasterone B and C, showed intense molting-hormone activity, this constitutes the first recognition of ecdysones in the plant kingdom. In the meantime, the chemical investigation for a diuretic principle in *Achyranthes fauriei* roots by Takemoto *et al.* yielded two related substances in 1965. Following the determination of structure for other zooecdysones (the 20-hydroxyecdysones) in 1966, one of the two substances was found to be identical with ecdysterone (β-ecdysone) and the other, inokosterone, was determined to be a position isomer.

Taking advantage of this discovery, it was realized that some substances (polypodine A and VT_1) which had already been isolated from other vegetable sources, *Polypodium vulgare* and *Vitex megapotamica,* respectively, were also identical with β-ecdysone. The discovery of phytoecdysones from a number of plant species that have no close taxonomic relationship, has stimulated extensive screening tests of plant materials for phytoecdysones with the aid of bioassays. As a result, it has been found that phytoecdysones are widely distributed in the plant kingdom. Some eighty families containing species exhibiting positive tests for molting hormone have so far been discovered (Table 1).

For extraction of phytoecdysones from botanical materials, polar solvents are commonly used. For purification of the extracts, a combination of solvent extraction, partition between various solvents including counter-current distribution, liquid chromotography, preparative thin-layer chromatography, and crystallization is employed. During the procedures for purification of phytoecdysones, thin-layer chromatography and bioassay have proved to be extremely useful techniques. While chemical knowledge of zoo-ecdysones has grown rather slowly, perhaps due to the much lower content of ecdysones and greater difficulty in isolation, chemical knowledge of phyto-ecdysones has expanded rapidly within a few years. Thus, 37 kinds of phyto-ecdysones have been isolated from plants. Among these phytoecdysones, 3 were identified as α-ecdysone, β-ecdysone, and deoxycrustecdysone already obtained from animal sources, and the remaining 34 were new substances whose structures now have been elucidated (Table 2). Inokosterone and makisterone A are ecdysones found in the plant kingdom first and discovered in the animal kingdom later.

The content of certain ecdysones in plants is sometimes over 1 per cent and therefore much higher than in animals. However, yields of most phyto-ecdysones are still very small. Therefore, elucidation of structures could not have been achieved successfully without the use of modern spectral techniques, such as ultraviolet, infrared, nuclear-magnetic-resonance, optical-rotary-dispersion, and circular-dichroism spectroscopy. The following phyto-ecdysones are the ones first reported to possess the significant features indicated, apart from differences in the positions of hydroxyl groups in the side-chains:

cyasterone	(C_{29} stigmastane skeleton, γ-lactone ring)
polypodine B	(5β-hydroxyl group)
ponasterone B	($2a$, $3a$-dihydroxyl groups)
rubrosterone	(C_{19} etiocholane skeleton, 17-oxo group)
makisterone A	(C_{28} ergostane skeleton)
ponasteroside A	(glycoside)
capitasterone	(δ-lactone ring)
shidasterone	(abnormal structure in side-chain)
ajugasterone B	(double bond in the side-chain)
viticosterone E	(acetoxyl group)
podecdysone B	(addition double bond in nucleus)
ajugasterone C	($11a$-hydroxyl group)
stachysterone A	(rearranged nucleus)
stachysterone D	(ether linkage)
poststerone	(C_{21} pregnane skeleton)
deoxycrustecdysone	(no 2-hydroxyl)
epicyasterone	($5a$-hydrogen)
2-cinnamoyl crustecdysone	(cinnamoyl group)

Because investigations on the mode of their action in higher animals as well as in arthropods have been limited by the small supply of ecdysones from animal sources, chemical syntheses of ecdysones have been carried out even though they are tedious and expensive. Now the discovery of phyto-ecdysones has opened the door to an ample supply of material for such studies.

The occurrence of phytoecdysones in plants raises the question whether they have any beneficial or adverse effects on the plants themselves or on phytophagous animals in their natural habitat. However, no definite answers to these questions have been found at this time. It has been said that the presence of phytoecdysones in plants may provide some way of protection against attack by insects. Although it may be true in some cases, it cannot always be true, since the leaves of *Morus* species and *Podocarpus macrophyllus* which are known to contain considerable amounts of phytoecdysones, are food of the larvae of the moths, *Bombyx mori* and *Milionia vasalis pryeri*, respectively.

Tissue cultures of plants are now expected to be an effective tool in studying the production and the metabolic pathway of constituents in plants. Therefore, in the hope that this technique may provide useful information about biosynthesis of phytoecdysones, callus tissues were induced in

Achyranthes plants and growth of the induced callus observed. Extracts of the callus tissue grown under various conditions were found to exhibit strong insect-molting-hormone activity, indicating the occurrence of ecdysones identified as β-ecdysone and inokosterone. However, the content of ecdysones in the callus tissues was very small (less than 0.002 per cent) when compared to concentration of hormones in normal plants. If an increase in the amount of ecdysones in callus tissues can be achieved by modification of components in the medium, it will be a useful technique in investigating biosynthesis of phytoecdysones.

TABLE 1

FAMILIES OF PLANTS CONTAINING ECDYSONES

Pteridophyta	Gramineae	-	-
-	Cyperaceae	-	-
Lycopodiaceae	-	Ranunculaceae	Tamaricaceae
Selaginellaceae	-	Lardizabalaceae	Cistaceae
Psilotaceae	-	Berberidaceae	Violaceae
-	-	-	Flacourtiaceae
-	-	Magnoliaceae	Stachyuraceae
Marattiaceae	-	-	Passifloraceae
Osmundaceae	Commelinaceae	-	-
Schixaeaceae	-	-	-
Gleicheniaceae	-	-	-
Hymenophyllaceae	Stemonaceae	-	-
Cyatheaceae	Liliaceae	Papaveraceae	-
-	Amaryllidaceae	Capparidaceae	-
-	-	Cruciferae	-
Polypodiaceae	Dioscoreaceae	-	-
Aspidiaceae	Iridaceae	-	-
-	Musaceae	-	-
Blechnaceae	Zingiberaceae	-	-
-	-	-	-
-	-	-	-
Plagiogyriaceae	-	-	Sympetalae
Pteridaceae	-	Platanaceae	-
-	Dicotyledoneae	Rosaceae	-
Parkeriaceae	Archichlamydeae	Leguminosae	-
-	-	-	-
-	-	Oxalidaceae	-
-	-	-	-
Gymnospermae	-	-	-
Cycadaceae	-	-	-
Ginkgoaceae	-	Zygophyllaceae	-
Podocarpaceae	-	Rutaceae	-
Cephalotaxaceae	Ulmaceae	Simaroubaceae	-
Taxaceae	Moraceae	-	Polemoniaceae
-	Urticaceae	-	-
-	-	-	Boraginaceae
Cupressaceae	-	-	Verbenaceae
-	-	-	Labiatae
Taxodiaceae	-	-	Solanaceae
Pinaceae	-	-	Scrophulariaceae
Ephedraceae	-	-	-
-	Polygonaceae	-	-
-	Chenopodiaceae	-	-
Angiospermae	Amaranthaceae	-	-
Monocotyledoneae	Nyctaginaceae	-	-
-	Cynocrambaceae	-	-
-	Phytolaccaceae	-	-
-	Aizoaceae	Tiliaceae	-
-	Portulacaceae	Malvaceae	-
-	Basellaceae	-	-
-	Caryophyllaceae	Stercuriaceae	Cucurbitaceae
-	-	-	Campanulaceae
-	Ceratophyllaceae	-	-
Triuridaceae	-	-	Compositae

TABLE 2

ECDYSONES OF PLANT ORIGIN

Phytoecdysones

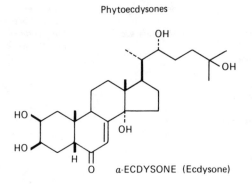

a-ECDYSONE (Ecdysone)

Plant Sources	References
Pteridium aquilinum	20
Polypodium vulgare	5
Lemmaphyllum microphyllum	32
Osmunda asiatica	36
Osmunda japonica	26
Neocheiropteris ensata	48
Blechnum minus	28

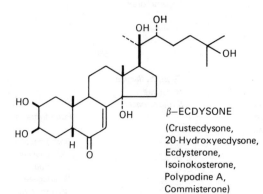

β—ECDYSONE

(Crustecdysone,
20-Hydroxyecdysone,
Ecdysterone,
Isoinokosterone,
Polypodine A,
Commisterone)

Osmunda asiatica	36
Osmunda japonica	36
Cryosinus hastatus	48
Lemmaphyllum microphyllum	34
Neocheiropteris ensata	34
Pleopeltis thunbergiana	34
Polypodium japonicum	17
Polypodium vulgare	18
Athyrium niponicum	48
Athyrium yokoscence	48
Lastrea japonica	48
Lastrea thelypteris	48
Matteucia struthiopteris	33
Onoclea sensibilis	48

Blechnum amabile	47
Blechnum niponicum	47
Pteridium aquilinum	26
Dacrydium intermedium	28
Podocarpus elatus	2
Podocarpus macrophyllus	12
Taxus baccata	10
Taxus cuspidata	12
Cyanotis vaga	29
Trillium smallii	19
Trillium tschonoskii	17
Morus spp.	43
Achyranthes bidentata	42
Achyranthes fauriei	41
Achyranthes japonica	42
Achyranthes japonica var. hachijoensis	24
Achyranthes longifolia	44
Achyranthes mollicula	24
Achyranthes obtusifolia	46
Achyranthes ogatai	24
Achyranthes rubrofusca	45
Bosea yervamora	44
Cyathula prostrata	42
Stachyurus praecox	17
Vitex megapotamica	27
Ajuga decumbens	17
Ajuga incisa	17
Ajuga japonica	14
Ajuga nipponensis	17

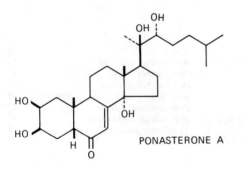

PONASTERONE A

Osmunda asiatica	*36*
Osmunda japonica	*36*
Gleichenia glauca	*48*
Athyrium niponicum	*48*
Lastrea thelypteris	*48*
Matteucia struthiopteris	*48*
Onoclea sensibilis	*33*
Blechnum amabile	*47*
Blechnum niponicum	*47*
Pteridium aquilinum var. *latiusculum*	*31*
Podocarpus macrophyllus var. *maki*	*12*
Podocarpus nakaii	*23*
Podocarpus neriifolius	*49*
Taxus cuspidata	*12*
Taxus cuspidata var. *nana*	*37*

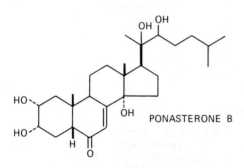

PONASTERONE B

Podocarpus nakaii 22,23

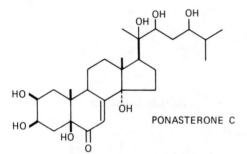

PONASTERONE C

Podocarpus nakaii 21,22

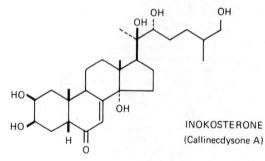

INOKOSTERONE
(Callinecdysone A)

Morus sp.	43
Achyranthes bidentata	42
Achyranthes fauriei	41
Achyranthes japonica	42
Achyranthes japonica var. hachijoensis	24
Achyranthes longifolia	42
Achyranthes rubrofusca	42
Vitex megapotamica	25

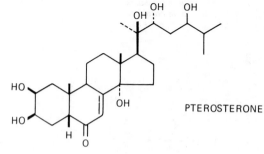

PTEROSTERONE

Lemmaphyllum microphyllum	32
Athyrium niponicum	48
Lastrea thelypteris	33
Onoclea sensibilis	33
Pteridium aquilinum var. latiusculum	31
Vitex megapotamica	26

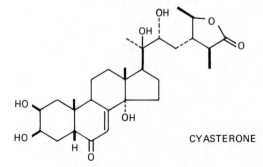

CYASTERONE

Cyathula capitata	38
Ajuga decumbens	17
Ajuga incisa	17
Ajuga japonica	14
Ajuga nipponensis	17

ISOCYASTERONE

Cyathula capitata	9

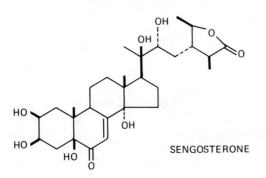

SENGOSTERONE

Cyathula capitata   7

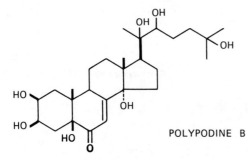

POLYPODINE B

Polypodium vulgare   19
Dacrydium intermedium   28
Vitex megapotamica   26
Ajuga incisa   17

CAPITASTERONE

Cyathula capitata   40

PRECYASTERONE

Cyathula capitata   6

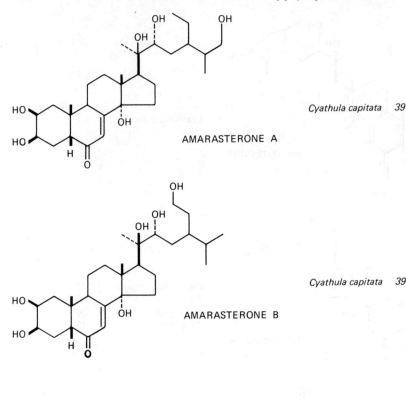

AMARASTERONE A

Cyathula capitata   *39*

AMARASTERONE B

Cyathula capitata   *39*

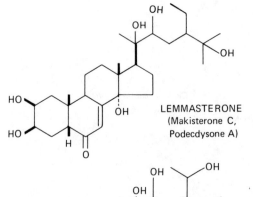

LEMMASTERONE
(Makisterone C,
Podecdysone A)

Lemmaphyllum microphyllum   *32*
Podocarpus elatus   *4*
Podocarpus macrophyllus   *13*

MAKISTERONE D

Podocarpus macrophyllus   *13*

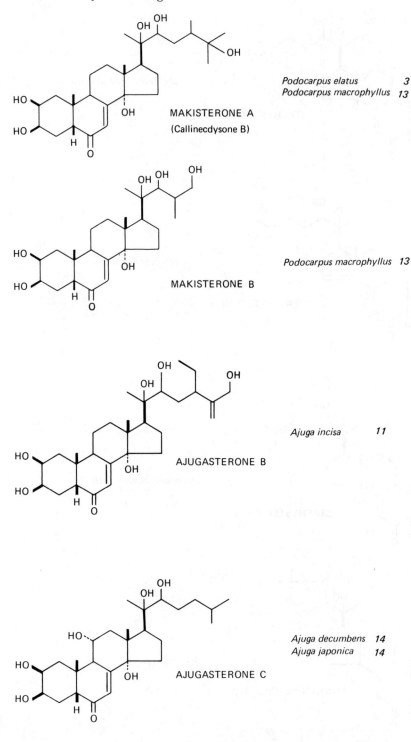

MAKISTERONE A
(Callinecdysone B)

Podocarpus elatus   *3*
Podocarpus macrophyllus *13*

MAKISTERONE B

Podocarpus macrophyllus *13*

AJUGASTERONE B

Ajuga incisa   *11*

AJUGASTERONE C

Ajuga decumbens *14*
Ajuga japonica   *14*

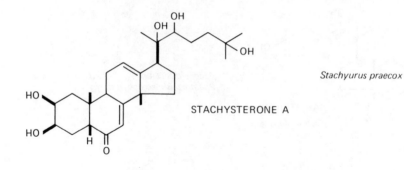

STACHYSTERONE A

Stachyurus praecox   **15**

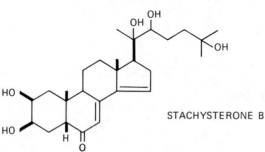

STACHYSTERONE B

Stachyurus praecox   **15**

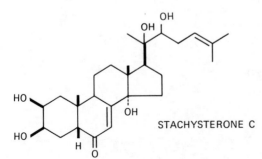

STACHYSTERONE C

Stachyurus praecox   **16**

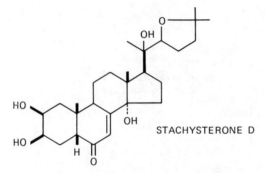

STACHYSTERONE D

Stachyurus praecox   **16**

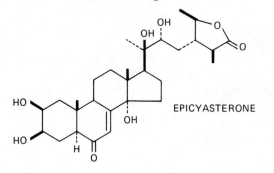

Cyathula capitata   *9*

EPICYASTERONE

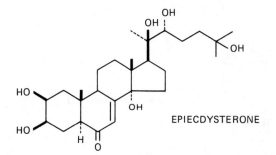

Achyranthes fauriei   24

EPIECDYSTERONE

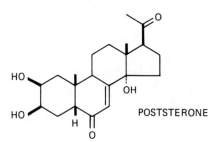

Cyathula capitata   *8*

POSTSTERONE

Achyranthes fauriei   *24*
Achyranthes obtusifolia *24*
Achyranthes rubrofusca *35*

RUBROSTERONE

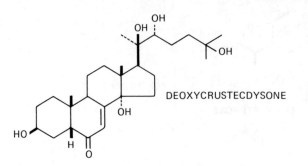

DEOXYCRUSTECDYSONE

Blechnum minus   *1*

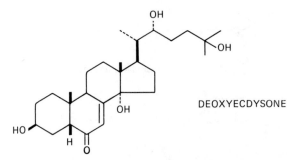

DEOXYECDYSONE

Blechnum minus   *1*

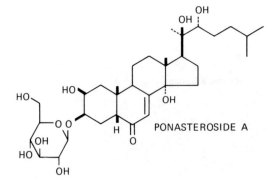

PONASTEROSIDE A

Pteridium aquilinum
var. *latiusculum*   *30,31*

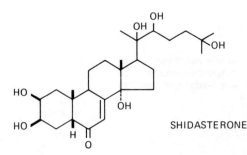

SHIDASTERONE

Blechnum niponicum   *47*

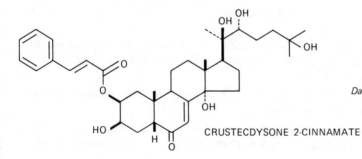

Dacrydium intermedium   **28**

CRUSTECDYSONE 2-CINNAMATE

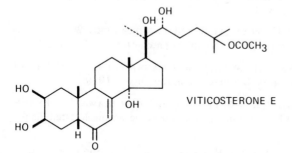

Dacrydium intermedium   **28**

POLYPODINE B 2-CINNAMATE

Vitex megapotamica   **26**

VITICOSTERONE E

Podocarpus elatus   **3**

PODECDYSONE B

References

1. CHONG, Y. K., GALBRAITH, M. N., and HORN, D. H. S.:Isolation of Deoxycrustecdysone, Deoxyecdysone, and α-Ecdysone from the Fern *Blechnum minus.* Chem. Commun., p. 1217, 1970.

2. GALBRAITH, M. N. and HORN, D. H. S.: An Insect-molting Hormone from a Plant. Chem. Commun., p. 905, 1966.

3. GALBRAITH, M. N., HORN, D. H. S., MIDDLETON, E. J., and HACKNEY, R. J.:   The Structure of Podecdysone B, a New Phytoecdysone. Chem. Commun., p. 402, 1969.

4. GALBRAITH, M. N., HORN, D. H. S., PORTER, Q. N., and HACKNEY, R. J.:   Structure of Podecdysone A, a Steroid with Molting Hormone Activity from the Bark of *Podocarpus elatus* R. Br. Chem. Commun., p. 971, 1968.

5. HEINRICH, G. and HOFFMEISTER, H.: Ecdyson als Begleitsubstanz des Ecdysterons in *Polypodium vulgare* L. Experientia, *23*:995, 1967.

6. HIKINO, H., NOMOTO, K., INO, R., and TAKEMOTO, T.: Structure of Precyasterone, a Novel C_{29} Insect-molting Substance from *Cyathula capitata.* Chem. Pharm. Bull. (Japan), *18*:1078, 1970.

7. HIKINO, H., NOMOTO, K., and TAKEMOTO, T. : Structure of Sengosterone, a Novel C_{29} Insect-molting Substance from *Cyathula capitata.* Tetrahedron Letters, p. 1417, 1969.

8. HIKINO, H., NOMOTO, K., and TAKEMOTO, T.: Posterone, a Metabolite of Insect-metamorphosing Substances from *Cyathula capitata.*Steroids, *16*:393,1970.

9. HIKINO, H., NOMOTO, K., and TAKEMOTO, T.:Structure of Isocyasterone and Epicyasterone, Novel C_{29} Insect-molting Substances from *Cyathula capitata.* Chem. Pharm. Bull. (Japan), *19*:433, 1971.

10. HOFFMEISTER, H., HEINRICH, G., STAAL, G. B., and VAN DER BERG, W. J.: Uber das Vorkommem von Ecdysteron in Eiben. Naturwissenschaften, *54*:471, 1967.

11. IMAI, S., FUJIOKA, S., MURATA, E., OTSUKA, K., and NAKANISHI, K.: Structure of the Phytoecdysone, Ajugasterone B. Chem. Commun., p. 82, 1969.

12. IMAI, S., FUJIOKA, S., NAKANISHI, K., KOREEDA, M., and KUROKAWA, T.:   Extraction of Ponasterone A and Ecdysterone from Podocarpaceae and Related Plants. Steroids, *10:*557, 1967.

13. IMAI, S., HORI, M., FUJIOKA, S., MURATA, E., GOTO, M., and NAKANISHI, K.:   Isolation of Four New Phytoecdysones, Makisterone A, B, C, D and the Structure of Makisterone A, a C_{28} Steroid. Tetrahedron Letters, p. 3883, 1968.

14. IMAI, S., MURATA, E., FUJIOKA, S., KOREEDA, M., and NAKANISHI, K.:Structure of Ajugasterone C, a Phytoecdysone with an 11-Hydroxy Group.Chem. Commun., p. 546, 1969.

15. IMAI, S., MURATA, E., FUJIOKA, S., MATSUOKA, T., KOREEDA, M., and NAKANISHI, K.: Structures of Stachysterone A, the First Natural 27-Carbon Steroid with a Rearranged Methyl Group, and Stachysterone B. J. Amer. Chem. Soc., *92*:7510, 1970.

16. IMAI, S., MURATA, E., FUJIOKA, S., MATSUOKA, T., KOREEDA, M., and NAKANISHI, K.: Structure of Stachysterones C and D. Chem. Commun., p. 352, 1970.

17. IMAI, S., TOYOSATO, T., SAKAI, M., SATO, Y., FUJIOKA, S., MURATA, E., and GOTO, M. : Isolation of Cyasterone and Ecdysterone from Plant Materials. Chem. Pharm. Bull. (Japan), *17:*335, 1969.

18. JIZBA, J., HEROUT, V., and SORM, F.: Isolation of Ecdysterone (Crustecdysone) from *Polypodium vulgare* L. Rhizomes. Tetrahedron Letters, p. 1689, 1967.

19. JIZBA, J., HEROUT, V., and SORM, F.: Polypodine B - a Novel Ecdysone-like Substance from Plant Material. Tetrahedron Letters, p. 5139, 1967.

20. KAPLANIS, J. N., THOMPSON, M. J., ROBBINS, W. E., and BRYCE, B. M.: Insect Hormones: α-Ecdysone and 20-Hydroxyecdysone in Bracken Fern. Science, *157:* 1436, 1967.

21. KOREEDA, M. and NAKANISHI, K.: 5β-Hydroxy-ecdysones and a Revision of the Structure of Ponasterone C. Chem. Commun., p. 351, 1970.

22. NAKANISHI, K., KOREEDA, M., CHANG, M. L., and HSU, H. Y.: Insect Hormones. V. The Structures of Ponasterones B and C. Tetrahedron Letters, p. 1105, 1968.

23. NAKANISHI, K., KOREEDA, M., SASAKI, S., CHANG, M. L., and HSU, H. Y.: Insect Hormones. I. The Structure of Ponasterone A, an Insect-molting Hormone from the Leaves of *Podocarpus nakaii* Hay. Chem. Commun., p. 915, 1966.

24. OGAWA, S., NISHIMOTO, N., OKAMOTO, N., and TAKEMOTO, T.: Studies on the Constituents of *Achyranthes* Radix. VIII. The Insect-molting Substances in Achyranthes Genus. (Supplement 2), Yakugaku Zasshi, *91:*916, 1971.

25. RIMPLER, H.: Steroide mit ecdysonartiger Wirkung aus *Vitex megapotamica.* Pharmaz. Ztg., *48:*1799, 1967.

26. RIMPLER, H.: Pterosteron, Polypodin B und ein neues ecdysonartiges Steroid (Viticosteron E) aus *Vitex megapotamica* (Verbenaceae). Tetrahedron Letters, p. 329, 1969.

27. RIMPLER, H. and SCHULZ, G.:Vorkommen von 20-Hydroxy-ecdyson in *Vitex megapotamica.* Tetrahedron Letters, p. 2033, 1967.

28. RUSSELL, G. B., HORN, D. H. S., and MIDDLETON, E. J.: New Phytoecdysones from *Dacrydium intermedium.* Chem. Commun., p. 71, 1971.

29. SANTOS, A. C., CHUA, M. T., EUFEMIO, N., and ABELA, C.: Isolation of Commisterone, a New Phytoecdysone from *Cyanotics vaga.* Experientia, *26:*1053,1970.

30. TAKEMOTO, T., ARIHARA, S., and HIKINO, H.:Structure of Ponasteroside A, a Novel Glycoside of Insect-molting Substance from *Pteridium aquilinum* var. *latiusculum.* Tetrahedron Letters, p. 4199, 1968.

31. TAKEMOTO, T., ARIHARA, S., HIKINO, Y., and HIKINO, H.: Isolation of Insect Molting Substances from *Pteridium aquilinum* var. *latiusculum.* Chem. Pharm. Bull. (Japan), *16:*762, 1968.

32. TAKEMOTO, T., HIKINO, Y., ARAI, T.,and HIKINO, H.:Structure of Lemmasterone, a Novel C_{29} Insect-molting Substance from *Lemmaphyllum microphyllum.* Tetrahedron Letters, p. 4061, 1968.

33. TAKEMOTO, T., HIKINO, Y., ARAI, T., KAWAHARA, M., KONNO, C., ARIHARA, S.,and HIKINO, H.:Isolation of Insect-molting Substances from *Matteuccia struthiopteris, Lastrea thelypteris,* and *Onoclea sensibilis.* Chem. Pharm. Bull. (Japan), *15*:1816, 1967.

34. TAKEMOTO, T., HIKINO, Y., ARAI, T., KONNO, C., NABETANI, S., and HIKINO, H.: Isolation of Insect-molting Substances from *Pleopeltis thunbergiana, Neocheiropteris ensata,* and *Lemmaphyllum microphyllum.* Chem. Pharm. Bull. (Japan), *16*:759, 1968.

35. TAKEMOTO, T., HIKINO, Y., HIKINO, H., OGAWA, S., and NISHIMOTO, N.: Structure of Rubrosterone, a Novel C_{19} Metabolite of Insect-molting Substances from *Achyranthes rubrofusca.* Tetrahedron Letters, p. 3053, 1968.

36. TAKEMOTO, T., HIKINO, Y., JIN, H., ARAI, T., and HIKINO, H.: Isolation of Insect-molting Substances from *Osmunda japonica* and *Osmunda asiatica.* Chem. Pharm. Bull. (Japan), *16*:1636, 1968.

37. TAKEMOTO, T., HIKINO, Y., JIN, H., and HIKINO, H.: Isolation of Ponasterone A from *Taxus cuspidata* var. *nana.* Yakugaku Zasshi, *88*:359, 1968.

38. TAKEMOTO, T., HIKINO, Y., NOMOTO, K., and HIKINO, H.: Structure of Cyasterone, a Novel C_{29} Insect-molting Substance from *Cyathula capitata.* Tetrahedron Letters, p. 3191, 1967.

39. TAKEMOTO, T., NOMOTO, K., and HIKINO, H.: Structure of Amarasterone A and B, Novel C_{29} Insect-molting Substances from *Cyathula capitata.* Tetrahedron Letters, p. 4953, 1968.

40. TAKEMOTO, T., NOMOTO, K., HIKINO, Y., and HIKINO,H.: Structure of Capitasterone, a Novel C_{29} Insect-molting Substance from *Cyathula capitata.* Tetrahedron Letters, p. 4929, 1968.

41. TAKEMOTO, T., OGAWA, S., and NISHIMOTO, N.: Isolation of Molting Hormones of Insects from Achyranthes Radix. Yakugaku Zasshi, *87*:325, 1967.

42. TAKEMOTO, T., OGAWA, S., NISHIMOTO, N., HIRAYAMA, H., and TANIGUCHI, S.: Studies on the Constituents of Achyranthes Radix. VII. The Insect-molting Substances of Achyranthes and Cyathula Supplement. Yakugaku Zasshi, *88*: 1293, 1968.

43. TAKEMOTO, T., OGAWA, S., NISHIMOTO, N., HIRAYAMA, H., and TANIGUCHI, S.: Isolation of the Insect-molting Hormones from Mulberry Leaves. Yakugaku Zasshi, *87*:748, 1967.

44. TAKEMOTO, T., OGAWA, S., NISHIMOTO, N., and HOFFMEISTER, H.: Steroide mit Häutungshormon-Aktivität aus Tieren und Pflanzen. Z. Naturforsch., *22b*: 681, 1967.

45. TAKEMOTO, T., OGAWA, S., NISHIMOTO, N., and TANIGUCHI, S.: Studies on the Constituent of Achyranthes Radix. IV. Isolation of the Insect-molting Hormones from Formosan *Achyranthes* spp. Yakugaku Zasshi, *87:*1478, 1967.

46. TAKEMOTO, T., OGAWA, S., NISHIMOTO, N., YEN, K.-Y., ABE, K., SATO, T., OSAWA, K., andTAKAHASKI, M.: The Isolation of Ecdysterone from the Radix of *Achyranthes obtusifolia* Lam. Yakugaku Zasshi, *87:*1521, 1967.

47. TAKEMOTO, T., OKUYAMA, T., ARIHARA, S., HIKINO, Y., and HIKINO, H.: Isolation of Insect-molting Substances from *Blechnum amabile* and *Blechnum niponicum.* Chem. Pharm. Bull. (Japan), *17:*1973, 1969.

48. Unpublished results in our laboratory.

49. Unpublished results, M. N. GALBRAITH and D. H. S. HORN.

RECENT STUDIES on ECDYSONES

Koji Nakanishi, M. Koreeda,
and D. A. Schooley

I. THE OCCURRENCE OF VARIOUS ECDYSONES IN A SINGLE PLANT

Progress in physico-chemical methods has made it feasible to determine the structure of minor congeners, and a natural consequence of this is that a particular natural product found in a plant is usually accompanied by several other products having closely related structures.

The phytoecdysones, which are polyhydroxylated phytosteroids, are not exceptions as depicted in Figures 1 to 4. As a result of this, the numbers of phytoecdysones have rapidly increased since their discovery in late 1966 to a total of forty at this time (Nakanishi, 1971). On the other hand, six zooecdysones are known to date (Nakanishi, 1971) only one of which, 20, 26-dihydroxy-a-ecdysone (Thompson *et al.*, 1967), has as yet not been isolated from plants.

This plant,*Podocarpus nakaii* Hay, we studied (Nakanishi *et al.*, 1966) and *Achyranthes fauriei* studied by Takemoto and coworkers (Takemoto *et al.*, 1967) were the first two sources of phytoecdysones. *P. nakaii* is rather unique in that it contains ponasterone B (Nakanishi *et al.*, 1968), the only naturally occurring 2*a*, 3*a*-dihydroxyecdysone. Ponasterone C (Koreeda *et al.*, 1970 a) is a 5β-hydroxyecdysone, which is represented by the first member to be structurally elucidated, polypodine B (Jizba *et al.*, 1967). Another phytoecdysone, ponasterone D, is present in this plant, but the structure remains to be clarified; PN-D appears not to contain the enone chromophore.

Figure 1

Ecdysones from *Podocarpus nakaii* Hay

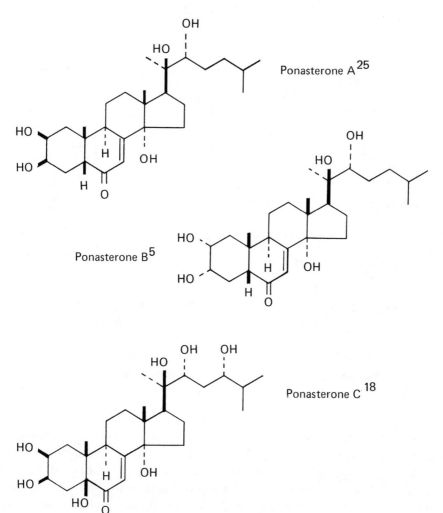

In spite of the extremely wide occurrence of β-ecdysone in plants, it is interesting that the distribution of *a*-ecdysone, which incidentally is the only ecdysone lacking the C-20 hydroxyl group and which has so far not been detected in crustaceans, is limited and it was first isolated (Kaplanis *et al.*, 1967) from the common fern, *Pteridium aquilinum* Kuhn. It is worthwhile mentioning that, in conjunction with our studies on the fern antheridia-inducing hormones, *i.e.*, antheridiogen-A_{AN}, (Endo *et al.*, 1972; Nakanishi *et al.*, 1971), we have isolated ponasterone A from the culture of liquid of *P. aluilinum* (Endo *et al.*, to be published).

Figure 2

Ecdysones from the fern *Pteridium aquilinum* Kuhn

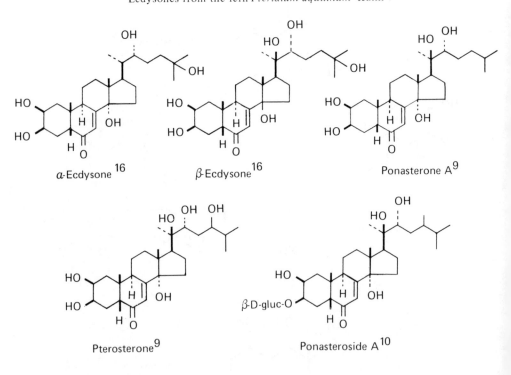

a-Ecdysone [16]   β-Ecdysone [16]   Ponasterone A [9]

Pterosterone [9]   Ponasteroside A [10]

All six ecdysones isolated from *Stachyrux praecox* and C_{27} steroids, and furthermore, stachysterones A, B, C, and D all have the same molecular formula of $C_{27}H_{42}O_6$. Stachysterone B (Imai *et al.*, 1970 b) containing the conjugated dienone system can be equilibrated with the deconjugated dienone (8, 14-dien-6-one), i.e., podecdysone B, (Galbraith *et al.*, 1969) upon treatment with mild acid. Although the ecdysone chromophore gives an equilibrium mixture of the two dienones when heated briefly in acidic methanol (Karlson *et al.*, 1965), the two dienones mentioned are not artifacts (Imai *et al.*, 1970 b; Galbraith *et al.*, 1969). Stachysterone A is very unique because of its rearranged steroid skeleton (the first naturally-occurring skeleton of this type); but, in spite of the rearranged nucleus, it still exhibits bioactivity. It is intriguing to speculate that its molting-hormone activity is the result of a reversed rearrangement of β-ecdysone in the insect.

Figure 3
Ecdysones from *Stachyrus praecox* Sieb. *et* Zucc.

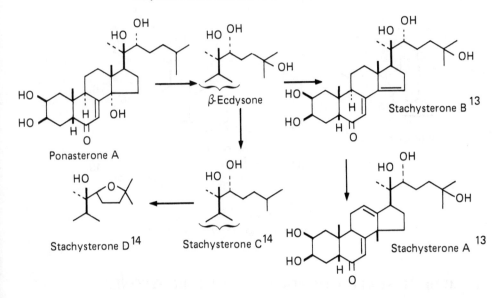

Ajuga decumbens contains a mixture of C_{27} and C_{29} phytosteroids. The most interesting compound from an activity viewpoint is ajugalactone (Koreeda *et al.*, 1970 b). This is the first naturally occurring compound structurally characterized which shows an inhibitory action against ponasterone A (Koreeda *et al.*, 1970 b). However, we do not claim it to be a genuine "antihormone" as the antagonistic effect is only manifested in the dipping test utilizing *Chilo suppressalis* (the rice-stem borer) at the level of 250 p.p.m. of ajugalactone versus 50 p.p.m. of ponasterone A. Surprisingly, it does not inhibit the activity of β-ecdysone in the dipping test, nor does it have any inhibitory action when injected. In fact, when injected into diapausing pupae of *Manduca sexta*, the tobacco hornworm, ecdysone activity was observed instead (Williams, private communication). Nevertheless, the existence of such a compound is encouraging, since it indicates the possible existence of real antihormones.

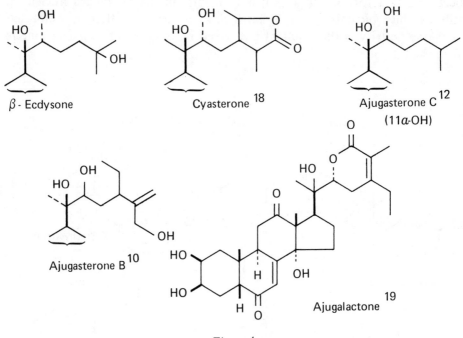

Figure 4

Ecdysones from *Ajuga decumbens* Thunb

II. MEDIUM–SCALE ISOLATION OF PHYTOECDYSONES

Plants are obviously the best sources for securing large supplies of ecdysones for various studies. However, owing to the rather hydrophilic nature of ecdysones and the fact that they occur frequently as mixtures, there has been no well-defined method in spite of a few attempts (Imai *et al.*, 1967). In fact, the hydrophilicity has been one of the major reasons for the delay in their discovery.

The ingenious application of high-pressure liquid chromatography to the separation of phytoecdysones (Hori, 1969) and an understanding of the behavior of available column-packing materials (Schooley *et al.*, in press) has led to a simplified procedure (Schooley *et al.*, 1972) outlined in Figure 5. With minor modification, we trust that the method is generally applicable to the gram-quality isolation and separation of phytoecdysones from crude extracts of leaves, barks, etc.

The Rohm and Haas resin XAD-2 is a cross-linked styrene divinylbenzene copolymer and functions by reverse-phase absorption chromatography, namely, the less polar methanol becomes a solvent with stronger eluting power than the more polar water, and in addition the polar substrates are eluted earlier. The present method employs both the batch process and column chromatography; under circumstances where further separation of several ecdysones becomes necessary, the appropriate fraction can be submitted to the pressurized liquid-chromatography technique. Of the known ecdysones, ponasterone A turns out to be one of the least polar judging from its behaviour on XAD-2 columns, and consequently more polar material is expected to be eluted before ponasterone A; in contrast, β-ecdysone is one of the most polar ecdysones.

Figure 5

Ponasterones A and C from crude *P. nakaii* extracts

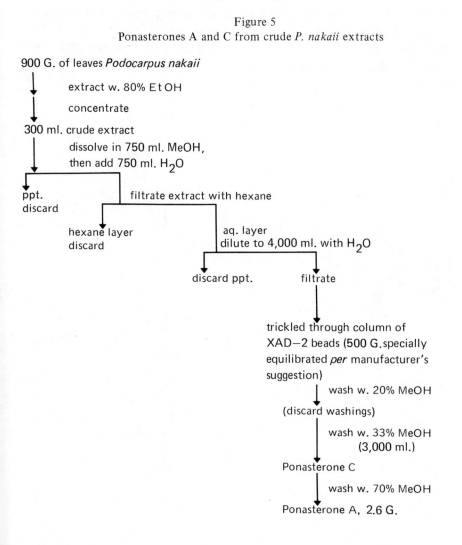

900 G. of leaves *Podocarpus nakaii*

  extract w. 80% EtOH

  concentrate

300 ml. crude extract

  dissolve in 750 ml. MeOH,
  then add 750 ml. H₂O

ppt.
discard   filtrate extract with hexane

        hexane layer   aq. layer
        discard   dilute to 4,000 ml. with H₂O

            discard ppt.   filtrate

                          trickled through column of
                          XAD–2 beads (500 G. specially
                          equilibrated *per* manufacturer's
                          suggestion)
                                    wash w. 20% MeOH
                          (discard washings)
                                    wash w. 33% MeOH
                                       (3,000 ml.)
                          Ponasterone C
                                    wash w. 70% MeOH
                          Ponasterone A, 2.6 G.

III. ABSOLUTE CONFIGURATIONS AT C-20 AND C-22 22

Until recently, *a*-ecdysone   was the only ecdysone in which the full side-chain stereochemistry had been elucidated   by x-ray (Huber *et al.*, 1965); as this is the sole ecdysone lacking a C-20 hydroxyl group, physical data such as those obtained by nuclear magnetic resonance (n.m.r.) are not applicable for deducing the configurations at C-20 and C-22 in other ecdysones. On the other hand, comparisons of NMR data pertaining to the 13-Me, 20-Me, and 22-H signals of the various ecdysones, excepting shidasterone which is epimeric at C-20 and/or C-22, (Takemoto *et al.*, 1968) clearly show that they all belong to the same stereochemical series.

The C-20 and C-22 configurations do play an important role in determining the biological activity, since ecdysone is devoid of activity (Siddall, 1970; Robbins *et al.*, 1970; Harrison *et al.*, 1966) in spite of the variations in the side-chain hydroxylation pattern of natural ecdysones which more or less have similar activities.

Figure 6
The side-chain configurations

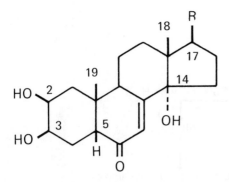

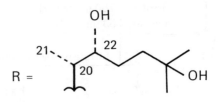

1   R =

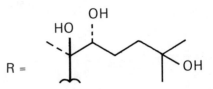

2   R =

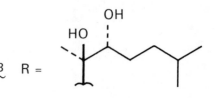

3   R =

Vigorous acetylation of ponasterone A 2, 3, 22-triacetate gave the dehydro-triacetate 4 which upon ozonolysis furnished rubrosterone 2, 3-diacetate 5 and the methyl ketone 6; the *a*-acetoxy ketone 6 had an ord curve with a negative Cotton effect at 293 nm. The *a*-acetoxy ketone 9 of known configuration was prepared from S-(-)-leucic acid; the Cotton effect of 9 was at 296 nm and positive. Since a difference of one methylene group would not effect the sign of the Cotton effect, the configuration of 6 is opposite to that of 9 and hence is R.

Figure 7

The C-22 configuration

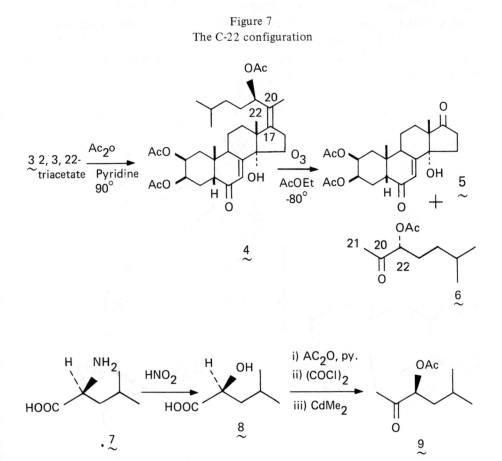

This was determined on the basis of an n.m.r. method which enables threo- and erythro-isomers to be differentiated in a facile and rigorous manner (Figure 9). Thus irradiation of the 20-Me n.m.r. signal of ponasterone A 2, 3-diacetate 20, 22-acetonide resulted in a 12 per cent increase in the height of the 22-H signal but no increase in the integrated area. This meant that the 22-H peak was subject to a W-type coupling with the 20-Me protons but was not subject to an intramolecular nuclear Overhauser effect (NOE). The 20-Me and 22-H should thus be *trans* with respect to the acetonide ring. Since the C-22 configuration has already been established, the C-20 configuration is also established and should be R.

In summary, the C-20/C-22 configurations in naturally-occurring ecdysones are both R, as depicted in Figure 6 (Koreeda *et al.*, 1971). A study with x-rays carried out independently on β-ecdysone has justified the same conclusion (Dammeier *et al.*, 1971).

Figure 8

The C-20 configuration

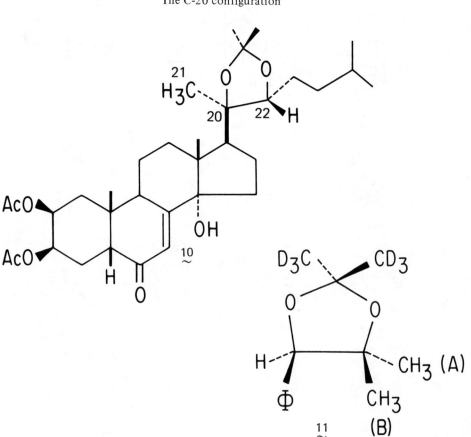

As shown in Figure 9b, a five-membered derivative of the erythro-isomer, such as that obtained by reaching with acetone, acetone-d_6 (preferable for reasons of having two less n.m.r. Me signals), benzaldehyde, etc., will give an NOE but no W-type coupling when the CH_3 group is irradiated and the methine proton is observed. For threo-isomers, the reverse relation holds. This method is not confined to a-glycols but also applies to a-amino alcohols, a-amino thiols, etc. (Nakanishi *et al.*, 1972b). The first example in Figure 9a, squalene-6, 7-erythro diol and other cases indicated that this simple technique is applicable to methine protons which are already subject to considerable intramolecular relaxation through coupling to geminal C-H groups. The preferred solvent is DMSO-d_6.

Figure 9a

Differentiation between threo- and erythro-isomers

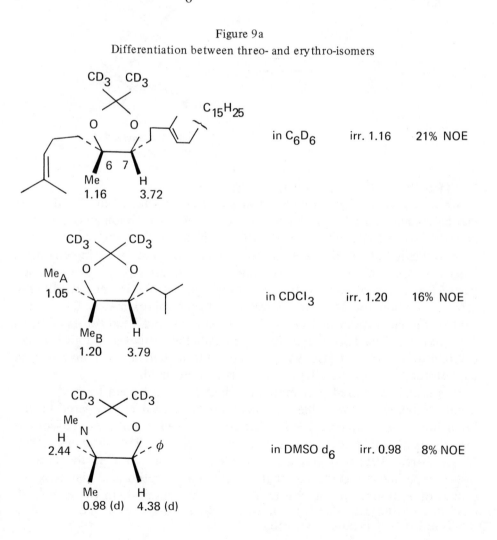

in C_6D_6 irr. 1.16   21% NOE

in $CDCl_3$ irr. 1.20   16% NOE

in DMSO d_6 irr. 0.98   8% NOE

Figure 9b
Differentiation between threo- and erythro-isomers

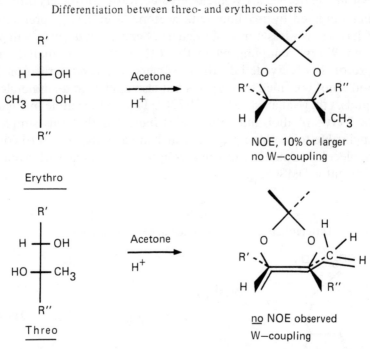

IV. THE SITE OF ECDYSONE SYNTHESIS

We have recently been able to show conclusively that α- and β-ecdysones can be biosynthesized from cholesterol in the isolated abdomen of *Bombyx mori* (silkworm) (Nakanishi *et al.*, 1972a). Namely, fifth instar larvae (day 6) were ligated at the first abdominal segment, and they were injected with labeled 4-^{14}C-cholesterol after cutting off the anterior parts. The anterior parts clearly do not contain the prothoracic glands (PTG) but nevertheless, after incubation for 24 hours, it was found that approximately 0.0016 per cent of the cholesterol had been converted into α- and β-ecdysones (about a 1:1 mixture). The two ecdysones were characterized beyond doubt by co-crystallization. In contrast, we were not able to detect the conversion of cholesterol to ecdysone when day-2 larvae were used.

It is usually accepted that molting in insects is controlled by prothoracic glands (Fukuda, 1949; Williams, 1947) which in turn are triggered by the brain hormone (Williams, 1952; Wigglesworth, 1951) and that ecdysone is directly responsible for molting (Butenandt *et al.*, 1954; Williams, 1954; Wigglesworth, 1955). It has also been accepted, in spite of the lack of direct experimental evidence, that secretion by prothoracic glands is the source of ecdysone or the site of ecdysone biosynthesis. In the case of *B. mori*, the prothoracic glands are known to be resting, *i. e.*, inactive, around day 2 and that it becomes activated after day 3.

In view of this evidence, our present results would appear to be best accomodated by assuming that the prothoracic gland is involved in ecdysone synthesis in the sense that it produces a synthetase involved in some step in the conversion of cholesterol to ecdysone, and that the actual synthetic site is not the prothoracic gland. Although it would be extremely difficult to prove that no ecdysone is biosynthesized in the prothoracic gland, the results described are the first experimental evidence showing clearly that cholesterol can at least be converted into ecdysones at a site totally outside the glands.

Acknowledgement

This work was supported by PHS Grants CA-11572 and AI-10187.

References

1. BUTENANDT, A. and KARLSON, P.: Über die Isolierung eines Metamorphose-Hormons der Insekten in Kristallisierten Form. Z. Naturforsch., *9*:389, 1954.

2. DAMMEIER, B. and HOPPE, W.: Crystal and Molecular Structure Analysis of the Insect-molting Hormone 20-Hydroxyecdysone (Ecdysterone). Chem. Ber., *104*: 1660, 1971.

3. ENDO, M., NAKANISHI, K., NÄF, U., McKEON, W., and WALKER, R.: Antheridiogen of *Anemia phyllitidis:* Its Isolation. Physiol. Plant, *26*:183, 1972.

4. ENDO, M., ZANNO, P., NAKANISHI, K., and NÄF, U.: Occurrence of Ponasterone A in the Culture Medium of *Anemia phyllitidis*. To be published.

5. FUKUDA, S.: The Hormonal Mechanism of Larval Molting and Metamorphosis in the Silkworm. J. Fac. Sci., Univ. Tokyo, Sect. IV, *6*:477, 1949.

6. GALBRAITH, M. N., HORN, D. H. S., MIDDLETON, E. J., and HACKNEY, R. J.: The Structure of Polypodine B, a New Phytoecdysone. Chem. Commun., 402, 1969.

7. HARRISON, I. T., SIDDALL, J. B., and FRIED, J. H.: Steroids CCXCVII, Synthetic Studies on Insect Hormones. Part III. An Alternative Synthesis of Ecdysone and 22-Isoecdysone. Tetrahedron Letters, 3457, 1966.

8. HORI, M.: Automatic Column Chromatographic Method for Insect-molting Steroids. Steroids, *14*:33, 1969.

9. HUBER, R. and HOPPE, W.: Zur Chemie des Ecdysones. VII. Die Kristallund Molekülstrukturanalyse des Insektenverpuppungshormons Ecdyson mit der Automatisierten Faltmolekülmethode. Chem. Ber., *98*:2043, 1965,

10. IMAI, S., FUJIOKA, S., MURATA, E., OTSUKA, K., and NAKANISHI, K.: Structure of the Phytoecdysone, Ajugasterone B. Chem. Commun., 82, 1969a.

11. IMAI, S., FUJIOKA, S., NAKANISHI, K., KOREEDA, M., and KUROKAWA, T.: Extraction of Ponasterone A and Ecdysterone from *Podocarpaceae* and Related Plants. Steroids, *10*:557, 1967.

12. IMAI, S., MURATA, E., FUFIOKA, S., KOREEDA, M., and NAKANISHI, K.: Structure of Ajugasterone C, a Phytoecdysone with an 11-Hydroxy Group. Chem. Commun., 546, 1969b.

13. IMAI, S., MURATA, E., FUJIOKA, S., MATSUOKA, T., KOREEDA, M., and NAKANISHI, Structures of Stachysterone A, the First Natural 27-Carbon Steroid with a Rearranged Methyl Group, and Stachysteroid B. J. Am. Chem. Soc., *92*:7510, 1970a.

14. IMAI, S., MURATA, E., FUJIOKA, S., MATSUOKA, T., KOREEDA, M.,and NAKANISHI, K.: Structures of Stachysterones C and D. Chem. Commun., 352, 1970b.

15. JIZBA, J., HEROUT, V., and SORM, F.: Polypodine B—a Novel Ecdysone-like Substance from Plant Material. Tetrahedron Letters, 5139, 1967.

16. KAPLANIS, J. N., THOMPSON, M. J., ROBBINS, W. E., and BRYCE, B. M.: Insect Hormones: Alpha Ecdysone and 20-Hydroxyecdysone in Bracken Fern. Science, *157*:1436, 1967.

17. KARLSON, P., HOFFMEISTER, H., HUMMEL, H., HOCKS, P., and SPITELLER, G.: Zur Chemie des Ecdysons. VI. Reaktionen des Ecdysonmoleküls. Chem. Ber., *98*: 2394, 1965.

18. KOREEDA, M. and NAKANISHI, K.: 5β-Hydroxy-ecdysones and a Revision of the Structure of Ponasterone C. Chem. Commun., 351, 1970a.

19. KOREEDA, M., NAKANISHI, K., and GOTO, M.: Ajugalactone, an Insect Molting Inhibitor as Tested by the Chilo Dipping Method. J. Am. Chem. Soc., *92*:7512, 1970b.

20. KOREEDA, M., SCHOOLEY, D. A., NAKANISHI, K., and HAGIWARA, H.: The Absolute Configurations at C-20 and C-22 in Ecdysones. J. Am. Chem. Soc., *93*:4084, 1971.

21. NAKANISHI, K.: Recent Studies on Insect Hormones. IUPAC XXIII Congress, Boston, *3*:27, Butterworths, London, 1971.

22. NAKANISHI, K.: The Ecdysones. Pure and Applied Chemistry, *25*:167, 1971.

23. NAKANISHI, K., ENDO, M., NÄF, U., and JOHNSON, L. F.: Structure of the Fern *Anemia phyllitidis*. J. Am. Chem. Soc., *93*:5571, 1971.

24. NAKANISHI, K., KOREEDA, M., CHANG, M. L., and HSU, H. Y.: Insect Hormones. V. The Structure of Ponasterone B and C. Tetrahedron Letters, p. 1105, 1968

25. NAKANISHI, K., KOREEDA, M., SASAKI, S., CHANG, M. L., and HSU, H. Y.:   Insect Hormones. I. The Structure of Ponasterone A, an Insect-molting Hormone from the Leaves of *Podocarpus nakaii* Hay. Chem. Commun., 915, 1966.

26. NAKANISHI, K., MORIYAMA, H., OKAUCHI, T., FUJIOKA, S., and KOREEDA, M.: Biosynthesis of α- and β-ecdysones from Cholesterol outside the Prothoracic Gland in *Bombyx mori*. Science, *176*:51, 1972a.

27. NAKANISHI, K., SCHOOLEY, D. A., KOREEDA, M., and MIURA, I.: A General Method for Distinguishing *threo* and *erythro* Isomers of Certain Glycols and Similar Compounds. J. Am. Chem. Soc., *94*:2865, 1972b.

28. ROBBINS, W. E., KAPLANIS, J. N., THOMPSON, M. J., SHORTINO, T. J., and JOYNER, S. C.: Ecdysones and Synthetic Analogs: Molting Hormone Activity and Inhibitive Effects on Insect Growth, Metamorphosis and Reproduction. Steroids, *16*:105, 1970.

29. SATO, Y., SAKAI, M., IMAI, S., and FUJIOKA, S.:Ecdysone Activity of Plant-origin-

ated Molting Hormones Applied on the Body Surface of *Lepidopterous* Larvae. Appl. Ent. Zool. (Japan), *3*:49, 1968.

30. SCHOOLEY, D. A. and NAKANISHI, K.:Application of High Pressure Liquid Chromatography to the Separation of Insect Molting and Juvenile Hormone. *In*: E. Heftmann (ed.), Modern Methods of Steroid Analysis. New York: Academic Press, in press.

31. SCHOOLEY, D. A., WEISS, G., and NAKANISHI, K.: A Simple and General Extraction Procedure for Phytoecdysones Based on Reversed-phase Absorption Chromatography. Steroids, *19*:377, 1972.

32. SIDDALL, J. B.: Chemical Aspects of Hormonal Interactions. *In*: E. Sondheimer and J. B. Simeone (ed.), Chemical Ecology. p. 281. New York: Academic Press, 1970.

33. TAKEMOTO, T., ARIHARA, S., and HIKINO, H.: Structure of Ponasteroside A, a Novel Glucoside of Insect-molting Substance from *Pteridium aquilinum* var. *latisculum.* Tetrahedron Letters, p. 4199, 1968.

34. TAKEMOTO, T., ARIHARA, S., HIKINO, Y., and HIKINO, K.: Isolation of Insect Molting Substances from *Pteridium aquilinum* var. *latiusculum.* Chem. Pharm. Bull., *16*:762, 1968.

35. TAKEMOTO, T., HIKINO, Y., NOMOTO, K., and HIKINO, H.: Structure of Cyasterone, a Novel C29 Insect-molting Substance from *Cyathula capitata.* Tetrahedron Letters, p. 3191, 1967.

36. TAKEMOTO, T., HIKINO, Y., OKUYAMA, T., ARIHARA, S., and HIKINO, H.: A Novel Insect-molting Substance from *Blechnum niponicum.* Tetrahedron Letters, p. 6095, 1968.

37. TAKEMOTO, T., OGAWA, S., and NISHIMOTO, N.: Isolation of the Molting Hormones of Insects from *Achyranthes* Radix. Yakugaku Zasshi, *87*:325, 1967.

38. THOMPSON, M. J., KAPLANIS, J. N., ROBBINS, W. E., and YAMAMOTO, R. T.: 20, 26-Dihydroxyecdysone, a New Steroid with Molting Hormone Activity from the Tobacco Hornworm, *Manduca sexta* (Johannson). Chem. Commun., p. 650, 1967.

40. WIGGLESWORTH, V. B.: High Temperature and Arrested Growth in *Rhodnius:* Quantitative Requirements for Ecdysones. J. Exp. Biol., *32*:649, 1955.

39. WIGGLESWORTH, V. B.: Source of Molting Hormones in *Rhodnius.* Nature, *168*:558, 1951.

41. WILLIAMS, C. M.: Physiology of Insect Diapause. II. Interaction Between the Pupal Brain and Prothoracic Glands in the Metamorphosis of the Giant Silkworm, *Platysamia cecropia.* Biol. Bull., *93*:89, 1947.

42. WILLIAMS, C. M.: Physiology of Insect Diapause. IV. The Brain and Prothoracic Glands as an Endocrine System in the *Cecropia* Silkworm. Biol. Bull., *103*:120, 1952.

43. WILLIAMS, C. M.: Isolation and Identification of the Prothoracic Gland Hormone of Insects. Anat. Rec., *120*:743, 1954.

44. WILLIAMS, C. M.: Harvard University, private communication.

45. Part XXIX of Insect Hormones. For Part XXVIII see ref. 31. The studies were supported by PHS Grants CA-11572 AI-10187.

SOURCE and AVAILABILITY
of ECDYSTERONES

*Shuntaro Ogawa, Nobushige Nishimoto,
and Hiroyuki Matsuda*

Achyranthes radix, a source of the phytoecdysones, ecdysterone (I) and inokosterone (II), is an important crude drug that has been used for diuretic, tonic, and analgesic purposes in East Asia from ancient times. The components of this crude drug have been reported by many chemists to be a saponin with oleanolic acid as a sapogenin, achyrantin, inorganic salts, and a glucuronic acid-like substance. However, we thought that the effective principle of the crude drug might not be attributed to these compounds. Therefore a study was carried out in order to elucidate the effective principle under the direction of Professor Takemoto at Tohoku University. The roots used in the study were obtained from *Achyranthes fauriei*, one of the original plants from which the crude drugs has been obtained. It is seen everywhere in Japan along roadsides, in fields, and elsewhere.

During the investigation the following substances were identified: β-sitosterol, stigmasterol, a mixed crystal of β-sitosterylglucoside and stigmasteryl-

uracil, etc. as the components of *Achyranthes radix* (Takemoto *et al.,* 1967b). Furthermore, two unknown substances (Takemoto *et al.,* 1967a) named inokosterone (II) and isoinokosterone (I) were isolated by means of the method shown in Figure 1.

Figure 1

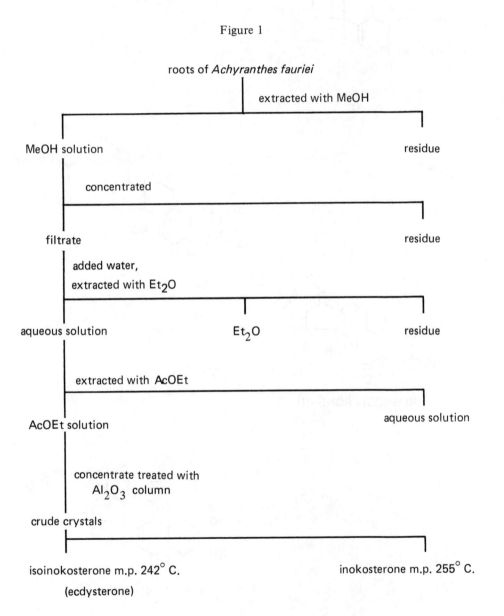

roots of *Achyranthes fauriei*

extracted with MeOH

MeOH solution — residue

concentrated

filtrate — residue

added water,
extracted with Et$_2$O

aqueous solution — Et$_2$O — residue

extracted with AcOEt

AcOEt solution — aqueous solution

concentrate treated with
Al$_2$O$_3$ column

crude crystals

isoinokosterone m.p. 242° C. — inokosterone m.p. 255° C.

(ecdysterone)

Figure 2

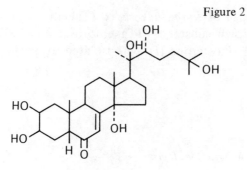

ECDYSTERONE (I)

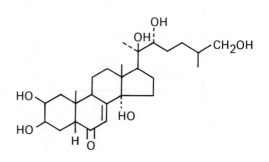

INOKOSTERONE (II)

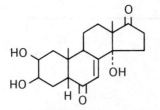

RUBROSTERONE (III)

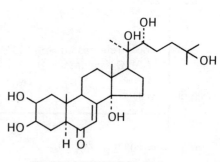

EPIECDYSTERONE (IV)

TABLE 1

PROPERTIES OF PHYTOECDYSONES EXTRACTED
FROM PLANTS IN THE GENUS, ACHYRANTHES

Property	Ecdysterone[*] (I)	Isoinokosterone (I)	Inokosterone (II)	Rubrosterone (III)	Epiecdysterone (IV)
Formula	$C_{27}H_{44}O_7$	$C_{27}H_{44}O_7$	$C_{27}H_{44}O_7$	$C_{19}H_{26}O_5$	$C_{27}H_{44}O_7$
M.P.($^\circ$C.)	234	242	255	245	278
IR cm.$^{-1}$	1645	1650	1645	1741, 1646	1655
UV mμ.	240	243	243	240	242

[*] H. Hoffmeister and H. F. Grützmacher; Tetrahedron Letters, 4017 (1966).

Isoinokosterone has positive steroidal color reactions. The formula of isoinokosterone was concluded to be $C_{27}H_{44}O_7$ from the elemental analysis, the mass spectrum, and the properties of the derivatives. The infrared (IR) spectrum shows the presence of hydroxyl groups and an α, β-unsaturated carbonyl group. The ultraviolet (UV) spectrum also shows the presence of the carbonyl group. This UV absorption is shifted from 243 nm. to 294 nm. and 241 nm. with HCl, suggesting the presence of 14-hydroxy-7-ene-6-one in the steroidal skeleton. The nuclear-magnetic-resonance (NMR) spectrum demonstrates the presence of 5 steroidal methyl groups.

When the structure of isoinokosterone was being contemplated on the basis of these results in the summer of 1966, a paper (Hoffmeister and Grütz - macher, 1966) was read reporting that Hoffmeister and Grützmacher had isolated a new insect molting hormone, ecdysterone, from the pupae of silkworms that was more effective than ecdysone. The properties they reported for ecdysterone were so similar to those of isoinokosterone that both compounds were considered to be the same. When a sample of iso- inokosterone was sent to Dr. Hoffmeister to compare with ecdysterone, he confirmed the view that the compounds were identical.

Since the properties of inokosterone (II) are very similar to those of ecdysterone (I), it is logical to think that the structure of both substances may be very similar. However, a significant difference between inokosterone

TABLE 2

METHYL CHEMICAL SHIFTS OF PHYTOECDYSONES
(P. P. M. IN PYRIDINE)

Substance	C – 18	C – 19	C – 21	C – 26	C – 27
Ecdysterone (I)[*]	1.19	1.06	1.55	1.34	1.34
Isoinokosterone (I)	1.20	1.07	1.57	1.37	1.37
Inokosterone (II)	1.19	1.07	1.52	–	1.03 (D)
Rubrosterone (III)	0.85	1.06	–	–	–
Epiecdysterone (IV)	1.21	1.41	1.59	1.39	1.39

[*] H. Hoffmeister and H. F. Grützmacher; Tetrahedron Letters, 4017 (1966).

and ecdysterone is that inokosterone has no methyl signal based on C-26 and a methyl signal splitting to a doublet on C-27. This suggests the presence of $-\underset{\underset{CH_2}{|}}{CH}-CH_2OH$ at the side chain of inokosterone. The periodate oxidation of inokosterone (II) gave a methylketone (V) that was identified as the substance derived from ecdysterone (I) and an hydroxyaldehyde (VI). The oxidation of compound VI with $KMnO_4$ gave (±)-a-methylglutaric acid (VII) which was identified with the authentic sample (Takemoto *et al.*, 1967c). The asymmetric carbon next to the carbonyl group may be racemized by the oxidation under an alkaline condition. However, direct oxidation of inokosterone (II) with chromic acid under an acidic condition gave the racemic compound (VII) too. Furthermore periodate oxidation of inokosterone diacetate (VIII) gave an acetoxyaldehyde (IX) and methylketone (X) which was identified with the compound derived from ponasterone A. The oxidation of the acetoxyaldehyde (IX) with chromic acid gave an acetocarboxylic acid (XI), and the methylate of this carboxylic acid, methyl a-methyl-δ-acetoxyvalerate, was optically inactive also. In this case, racemization at C-25 is impossible; therefore inokosterone was concluded to be a mixture of the epimers at C-25 (Takemoto *et al.*, 1968). The biological activity of inokosterone has been assayed by many biologists and found to be very remarkable.

When we isolated inokosterone and ecdysterone, Nakanishi and co-workers isolated ponasterones from *Podocarpus nakaii* independently (Nakanishi *et al.*, 1966). These facts suggested that such compounds may be widely distributed in the plant kingdom. Now at least 40 phytoecdysones or related compounds have been isolated and reported by many scientists. We have examined the distribution of phytoecdysones in plants included in the Achyranthes genus and have isolated a crystalline substance (III) from the roots of *Achyranthes rubrofusca* growing in Formosa (Takemoto *et al.*, 1969). This substance was less polar than ecdysterone or inokosterone and was named rubrosterone. The molecular formula was estimated to be $C_{19}H_{26}O_5$ from the mass spectrum and elemental analysis. The IR spectrum indicates the presence of hydroxy groups and two carbonyl groups, a cyclopentanone, and an a,β-unsaturated cyclohexanone, and the NMR spectrum demonstrates the presence of 2 methyl groups in the steroidal skeleton. Differing from other phytoecdysones, the structure of rubrosterone was concluded to be $2\beta,3\beta,14a$-trihydroxy-5β-androst-7-en-6,17-dione by these results, properties brought out by HCl, the ORD and CD spectra, the properties of derivatives, *etc.*

Figure 3

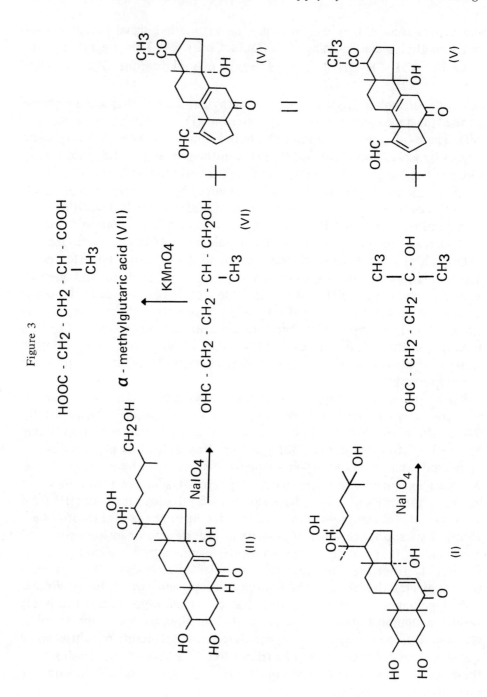

Figure 4

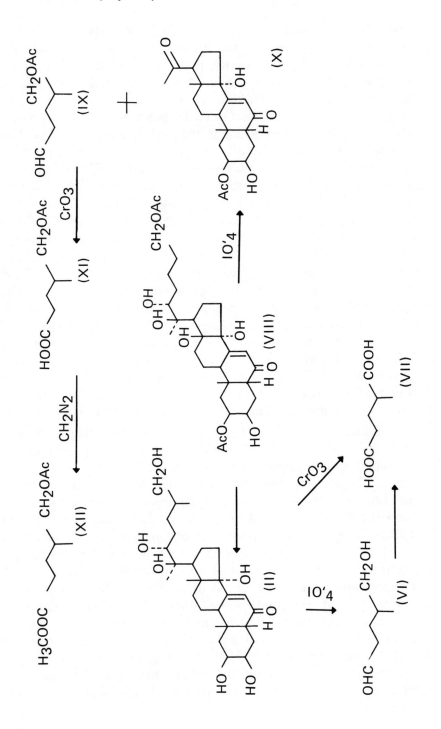

Rubrosterone is the first compound with 5β-androstan skeleton to be isolated from the plant kingdom, and it possibly represents a metabolite from phytoecdysones in plants. Recently, poststerone, which is thought to be an intermediate metabolite from phytoecdysones to rubrosterone, was isolated from *Cyathula capitata* by Hikino (Hikino *et al.*, 1970). The structure of rubrosterone has also been confirmed by syntheses *via* various routes. The biological activity of rubrosterone in the fleshfly-test is very low. However, according to Otaka (Otaka *et al.*, 1968), the activity of rubrosterone in affecting protein synthesis in murine liver is nearly equal to ecdysterone or inokosterone. Also Kuroda (Kuroda, 1969) demonstrated that rubrosterone accelerated the differentiation of the eye-antennal discs of *Drosophila melanogaster* in organ culture at very low concentration, 1 x 10^{-8} mg./ml.

Recently we isolated a minor substance (IV) from the roots of *Achyranthes fauriei* (Ogawa *et al.*, 1971). This substance has nearly the same properties as ecdysterone, but the NMR methyl signal based on C-19 shifts 0.35 p.p.m. to the low field in comparison with ecdysterone. This fact suggests an A/B *trans* ring-junction, which also differs from ecdysterone. Therefore, this compound was considered to be the epimer at C-5 of ecdysterone and was named epiecdysterone. The structure was confirmed by the identification of epiecdysterone with the substance derived from ecdysterone by treatment with K_2CO_3. The ORD spectrum also demonstrates that the A/B ring-junction is *trans*. It is not certain whether epiecdysterone is an artifact or a natural product. Epiecdysterone has no activity in the fleshfly-test.

The distribution of the phytoecdysones in Achyranthes-genus plants growing in various areas is of considerable interest. Japanese and Chinese Achyranthes species usually contain both inokosterone and ecdysterone. However, the Achyranthes species growing in the areas south of northern Formosa or the Ryukyu islands contained only ecdysterone.

Both the fleshfly-test (Takemoto *et al.*, 1967) and the Chilo dipping-test (Sato *et al.*, 1968) are useful for screening of the phytoecdysones in plants, but these tests are not entirely reliable indicators for the presence of phytoecdysones because some plants may contain antiecdysones. Phytoecdysones were determined in plants of the Achyranthes genus by the following method (Takemoto *et al.*, 1968). The methanol extract of the sample was treated by preparative thin-layer chromatography, then the isolated phytoecdysones were reduced by $NaBH_4$, and the reduced amount was determined photometrically at 250 nm. in aqueous solution. This method does not separate ecdysterone and inokosterone quantitatively, since both substances have nearly similar properties on thin-layer chromatography, but

Figure 5

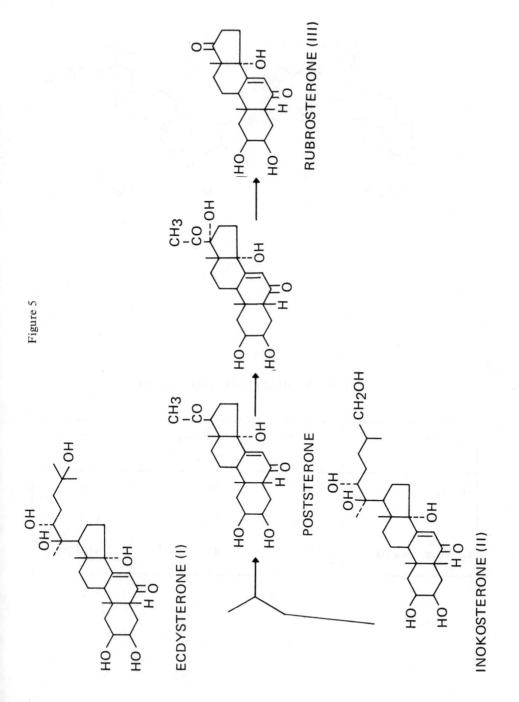

ECDYSTERONE (I)

POSTSTERONE

RUBROSTERONE (III)

INOKOSTERONE (II)

Figure 6

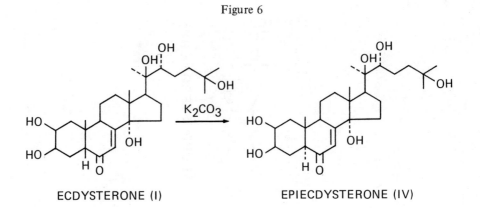

ECDYSTERONE (I)   EPIECDYSTERONE (IV)

TABLE 3

AMPLITUDES OF COTTON EFFECT (IN DIOXANE)

Substance	A / B	240 mμ. $\pi \longrightarrow \pi^*$	340 mμ. $n \longrightarrow \pi^*$
General	cis	-240	+60
	trans	-520	+140
Epiecdysterone (IV)	trans	-475(242)	+134(342)

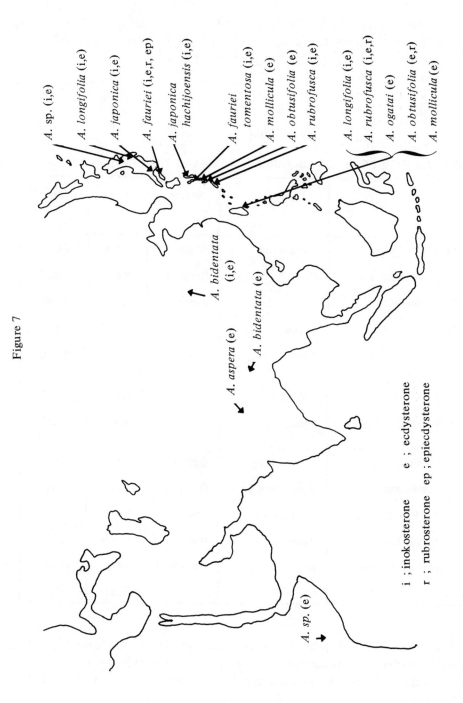

Figure 7

A. sp. (i,e)
A. longifolia (i,e)
A. japonica (i,e)
A. fauriei (i,e,r, ep)
A. japonica hachijoensis (i,e)
A. fauriei tomentosa (i,e)
A. mollicula (e)
A. obtusifolia (e)
A. rubrofusca (i,e)
A. longifolia (i,e)
A. rubrofusca (i,e,r)
A. ogatai (e)
A. obtusifolia (e,r)
A. mollicula (e)

A. bidentata (i,e)
A. bidentata (e)
A. aspera (e)

A. sp. (e)

i ; inokosterone   e ; ecdysterone
r ; rubrosterone   ep ; epiecdysterone

it constitutes a useful and simple method for determining total phytoecdysones. Table 4 shows the content of total phytoecdysones, calculated as
ecdysterone, in plants of the Achyranthes genus.

TABLE 4

DETERMINATION OF INSECT MOLTING SUBSTANCES IN THE GENUS, ACHYRANTHES

Species	Location	Season	Part	Per Cent of Molting Substances
Achyranthes fauriei	Tokushima	Winter	Roots	0.041
Achyranthes fauriei	Osaka	October	Roots	0.052
Achyranthes fauriei	Osaka	October	Stems	0.048
Achyranthes fauriei	Osaka	October	Leaves	0.078
Achyranthes fauriei	Tanegashima	October	Whole	0.120
Achyranthes fauriei var. tomentosa	Yakushima	October	Whole	0.102
Achyranthes japonica	Tanegashima	October	Whole	0.145
Achyranthes japonica var. hachijoensis	Okinoerabujima	October	Whole	0.054
Achyranthes mollicula	Amamioshima	October	Whole	0.043
Achyranthes rubrofusca	Formosa	Spring	Roots	0.049
Achyranthes longifolia	Formosa	March	Whole	0.047
Achyranthes obtusifolia	Formosa	November	Whole	0.045
Achyranthes bidentata	China		Roots	0.082

Since the phytoecdysones in Achyranthes species are the same substances
as ecdysterone and callinecdysone A (Faux *et al.*, 1969) in invertebrates, and
Achyranthes species contain no antiecdysones, crude extract of Achyranthes

species may be used in a practical way. For example, when crude extract of *Achyranthes fauriei* is added to the diet of fifth-stage silkworms, the period for the appearance of pupae is shortened and synchronized and thus of possible economic importance in sericulture (Okauchi, 1969).

References

1. FAUX, A., HORN, D. H. S., MIDDLETON, E. J., FALES, H. M., and LOWE, M. E. :
    Moulting Hormones of a Crab during Ecdysis. Chem. Commun., 175-176, 1969,
2. HIKINO, H., NOMOTO, K., and TAKEMOTO, T. : Poststerone, a Metabolite of Insect
    Metamorphosing Substances from *Cyathyla capitata*. Steroids, *16*:393-400, 1970.
3. HOFFMEISTER, H. and GRUTZMACHER, H. F. : Zur Chemie des Ecdysterons. Tet-
    rahedron Letters, 4017-4023, 1966.
4. KURODA, Y. : Growth and Differentiation of Embryonic Cells of *Drosophila
    melanogaster in Vitro*. Japan. J. Genetics, *44*:42-50, 1969.
5. NAKANISHI, K., KOREEDA, M., SASAKI, S., CHANG, M. L., and HSU, H. Y. :Insect
    Hormones. The Structure of Ponasterone A, an Insect-moulting Hormone from
    the Leaves of *Podocarpus nakaii* Hay. Chem. Commun., 915, 1966.
6. OGAWA, S., NISHIMOTO, N., OKAMOTO, N., and TAKEMOTO, T. : Studies on the
    Constituents of *Achyranthis radix*. VIII. Insect-moulting Substances in Achy-
    ranthis Genus. (Supplement to) Yakugaku Zasshi, *91*:916-920, 1971.
7. OKAUCHI, T. : Recent Studies on Phytoecdysones, Bochukagaku.,*34*:140-156, 1969.
8. OTAKA, T., UCHIYAMA, M., OKUI, S., TAKEMOTO, T., HIKINO, H., OGAWA, S.,
    and NISHIMOTO, N. : Stimulatory Effect of Insect-metamorphosing Steroids from
    Achyranthes and Cyathula on Protein Synthesis in Mouse Liver. Chem. Pharm.
    Bull., *16*:2426-2429, 1968.
9. SATO, Y., SAKAI, M., IMAI, S., and FUJIOKA, S. : Ecdysone Activity of Plant-origi-
    nated Molting Hormones Applied on the Body Surface of Lepidopterous Larvae.
    Appl. Ent. Zool., *3*:49-51, 1968.
10. TAKEMOTO, T., HIKINO, Y., ARIHARA, S., HIKINO, H., OGAWA, S., and NISHI-
    MOTO, N.: Absolute Configuration of Inokosterone, an Insect-moulting Sub-
    stance from *Achyranthes fauriei*. Tetrahedron Letters, 2475-2478, 1968.
11. TAKEMOTO, T., HIKINO, Y., HIKINO, H., OGAWA, S., and NISHIMOTO, N. : Rub-
    rosterone, a Metabolite of Insect Metamorphosing Substance from *Achyranthes
    rubrofusca:* Structure and Absolute Configuration. Tetrahedron Letters, 1241-
    1248, 1969.
12. TAKEMOTO, T., OGAWA, S., MORITA, M., NISHIMOTO, N., DOME, K., and MORI-
    SHIMA, K. : Studies on the Constituents of *Achyranthis radix*. VI. Determina-
    tion of Insect-moulting Hormones. Yakugaku Zasshi, *88*:39-43, 1968.
13. TAKEMOTO, T., OGAWA, S., and NISHIMOTO, N.: Isolation of the Moulting Hor-
    mones of Insects from *Achyranthis radix*. Yakugaku Zasshi, *87*:325-327, 1967.
14. TAKEMOTO, T., OGAWA, S., and NISHIMOTO, N. : Studies on the Constituents of
    Achyranthis radix. I. Yakugaku Zasshi, *87*:1463-1468, 1967.
15. TAKEMOTO, T., OGAWA, S., and NISHIMOTO, N. : Studies on the Constituents of
    Achyranthis radix. III. Structure of Inokosterone. Yakugaku Zasshi, *87*:1474-
    1477, 1967.
16. TAKEMOTO, T., OGAWA, S., NISHIMOTO, N., ARIHARA, S., and BUE, K. : Insect
    Moulting Activity of Crude Drugs and Plants. Yakugaku Zasshi, *87*:1414-1418,
    1967.
17. TAKEMOTO, T., OGAWA, S., NISHIMOTO, N., HIRAYAMA, H., and TANIGUCHI, S.:
    Studies on the Constituents of *Achyranthis radix*. VII. The Insect-moulting Sub-
    stances in Achyranthis and Cyathula Genera. Yakugaku Zasshi, *88*:1293-1297,
    1968.

Juvenile Hormones

ISOLATION of JUVENILE HORMONE in DIFFERENT SPECIES

Herbert Röller and Karl H. Dahm

F ollowing isolation (Röller *et al.*, 1965; Röller *et al.*, 1969), identification (Röller *et al.*, 1967; Dahm *et al.*, 1968), and the first synthesis (racemic form) of the juvenile hormone [JH (Dahm *et al.*, 1967)] of the giant silk moth,*Hyalophora cecropia*, we started investigating the biosyn thesis of the hormone. In order to study this question successfully, our original purification procedure for JH has been refined, and the new method has been tested for the first time in *Hyalophora gloveri* [(Dahm and Röller, 1970) and Table 1]. Its efficiency was determined through addition of synthetic $2\text{-}^{14}C$ JH to the crude oil, and the recovery of JH in all cases was found to be 50-60 per cent. The major loss of hormone occurs during the cold precipitation, when 30 per cent of the JH remains as part of the precipitate. The hormone can be recovered, only at the cost of a substantially decreased purification factor, by a change of the ratio of solvent and its amount. Precipitation at low temperature is an essential step in the process for isolation since this procedure eliminates lipoidal material that would interfere with the final separation of JH by gas chromatography.

PURIFICATION OF JUVENILE HORMONE

213 Abdomens of 6-7 day-old male *H. gloveri*
    | addition of sodium sulfate
    ↓   homogenization and extraction with ether 3x

37.9 G. Crude Oil
    ↓   cold precipitation at $-78°C.$ in 760 ml. ether-methanol (1:1)

3.7 G. Filtrate
    ↓   column chromatography on Sephadex LH-20 in benzene-methanol (1:1)

270 mg. Fraction containing juvenile hormone
    ↓   thin layer chromatography on Silica Gel H; chloroform-ethyl acetate (2:1)

Zone R_F 0.77-0.92
    | thin layer chromatography on silica gel H; 5 per cent ethyl acetate in
    ↓   benzene

Zone R_F 0.22-0.33
    ↓   gas chromatography on XE-60

JH, JH-II

Despite great interest and many efforts, very little is known about the occurrence and levels of JH in other species. Although JH activity has been detected in quite a few insect species, it has, with the exception of three saturniid species examined by us, not been possible to determine whether this activity is associated with the Cecropia hormone or another substance. In addition to obtaining the hormone from *Hyalophora cecropia,* we have isolated and analyzed the juvenile hormone from *Hyalophora gloveri* (Dahm and Röller, 1970), *Samia cynthia* (Meyer *et al.,* in preparation), and from organ cultures of corpora allata from male *H. cecropia* [the medium contained the hormone released by the corpora allata *in vitro* (Röller and Dahm, 1970)]. The following data are pertinent:

Species	Age (in Days)	μg. JH/Abdomen
♂ . *Hyalophora cecropia*	6–7	2–6
♂ *Hyalophora gloveri*	6–7	0.2–0.5
♂ *Samia cynthia*	4–5	0.05–0.005

We recovered 0.04-0.12 µg. of JH, released *in vitro* by one pair of corpora allata (from Cecropia males) into the medium during a 7-day period. In all three saturniid species, JH was always accompanied by 10-30 per cent of its lower homologue, JH-II. An age-dependent change in this ratio was never detected. JH-II was isolated and identified for the first time from *H. cecropia* by Meyer *et al.* (1968).

The lack of information about the identity of JH in insects of other orders is due to the minute amounts of hormone present in these species (as determined in some cases by highly sensitive bioassays) and to the shortcomings of methods with a suitable range of sensitivity for identification of the hormone. Therefore the question about the possible occurrence of a structural diversification of JH during insect evolution remains open, since it requires direct proof in chemical terms. At present, however, no experimental data (in addition to results of various transplantation experiments with corpora allata, the biological activity of Cecropia JH has been intensively investigated in many species of different orders) oblige us to assume that such an evolutionary process has occurred.

References

1. DAHM, K. H. and RÖLLER, H.: The Juvenile Hormone of the Giant Silk Moth *Hyalophora gloveri* (Strecker). Life Sci., 9:1397, 1970.

2. DAHM, K. H., RÖLLER, H., and TROST, B. M.: The Juvenile Hormone. IV. Stereochemistry of Juvenile Hormone and Biological Activity of Some of Its Isomers and Related Compounds. Life Sci., 7:129, 1968.

3. DAHM, K. H., TROST, B. M., and RÖLLER, H.: The Juvenile Hormone. V. Synthesis of the Racemic Juvenile Hormone. J. Am. Chem. Soc., 89:5295, 1967.

4. MEYER, A. S., SCHNEIDERMAN, H. A., HANZMANN, E., and KO, J. H.: The Two Juvenile Hormones from the Cecropia Silk Moth. Proc. Nat. Acad. Sci., U. S., 60: 853, 1968.

5. MEYER, D., DAHM, K. H., and RÖLLER, H.: In preparation.

6. RÖLLER, H., BJERKE, J. S., HOLTAUS, L. M., NORGARD, D. W., and McSHAN, W. H.: Isolation and Biological Properties of the Juvenile Hormone. J. Insect. Physiol., 15:379, 1969.

7. RÖLLER, H., BJERKE, J. S., and McSHAN, W. H.: The Juvenile Hormone. I. Methods of Purification and Isolation. J. Insect Physiol., 11:1185, 1965.

8. RÖLLER, H. and DAHM, K. H.: The Identity of Juvenile Hormone Produced by Corpora Allata *in Vitro.* Naturw., 57:454, 1970.

9. RÖLLER, H., DAHM, K. H., SWEELEY, C. C., and TROST, B. M.: Die Strukter des Juvenilhormons. Angew. Chem., 79:190, 1967; The Structure of the Juvenile Hormone. Angew. Chem. Int. Ed., 6:179, 1967.

PART III
HORMONES AND PROTEIN
SYNTHESIS IN MAMMALS

HORMONES
and TRANSCRIPTIONAL
ACTIVITY of CHROMATIN

L. S. Hnilica, Y. H. Tsai and T. C. Spelsberg

INTRODUCTION

E ver since their discovery, hormones have been known to increase the rates of numerous metabolic processes *in vivo*. More recent research shows that the administration of hormones frequently induces or increases, in their target tissues, the activity of specific enzymes and initiates biosynthesis of new proteins as well as new RNA species. Many hormones, especially steroids, change the transcriptional activity of chromatin not only quantitatively, as demonstrated by its increased templating efficiency for RNA synthesis both *in vivo* and *in vitro*, but also modify the selectivity of genetic restriction as witnessed by compositional changes of the RNA biosynthesized under the influence of hormone. It can be assumed, therefore, that the interaction between certain hormones and their target tissues results in reprogramming of the DNA restriction in chromatin of the affected cells. The aim of this presentation is to discuss how such a genetic reprogramming can be effected at the molecular level.

DNA RESTRICTION IN CHROMATIN

Voluminous evidence in the literature, beginning with the discovery of histones by Kossel (1928), indicates that these basic proteins can form complexes with electronegative macromolecules. In the nucleus of the cell, histones are associated, mostly by electrostatic bonds, with the DNA in the form of chromatin. In addition to the DNA and histones, chromatin of most eucaryotic organisms also contains variable amounts of acidic or nonhistone proteins, RNA, and lipids. Although there is no doubt about the significance of DNA in the transfer and biochemical expression of heredity, the biological roles of histones and other chromatin components are uncertain. It has been suggested by Stedman and Stedman (1950, 1951) and perpetuated in the literature ever since, that histones may function as gene inhibitors. This hypothesis had no experimental basis until the reports by Huang and Bonner (1962) and Allfrey *et al.* (1963) who presented the first evidence that either the addition of histones to the DNA or their removal from isolated nuclei resulted in the inhibition of the ability of DNA to template for RNA synthesis *in vitro* and in the increase of RNA synthesis respectively. Experiments with isolated histone fractions demonstrated that lysine-rich histones inhibit RNA synthesis *in vitro* more efficiently than the arginine-rich fractions (Huang *et al.*, 1965; Barr and Butler, 1963; Liau *et al.*, 1965; Hnilica, 1967; Stellwagen and Cole, 1969; Johns and Hoare, 1970). However, in contrast to the results cited, Allfred *et al.* (1963), Hindley (1963), and others (Skalka *et al.*, 1966; Seligy and Neelin, 1970; Spelsberg and Hnilica, 1971) found that the arginine-rich and moderately lysine-rich histones are more potent inhibitors of RNA synthesis *in vitro* than the very lysine-rich ones in their hands. The amino-acid composition of the five main histones present in chromatin of most eucaryotic organisms as given in Table 1 stirred considerable controversy. Since the very lysine-rich F1 histones precipitate DNA much more efficiently than the other histone fractions, it was suggested (Hnilica and Billen, 1964; Johns and Forrester, 1970; Clark and Byvoet, 1970; Hoare and Johns, 1970) that their higher inhibitory activity may be due to the formation of insoluble nucleohistones during the reconstitution experiments, in which the DNA cannot function as a template. In accord with this suggestion, Sonnenberg and Zubay (1965) have demonstrated that RNA synthesis *in vitro* can be considerably increased by sonication of the chromatin.

Noticing that the high inhibitory activity of very lysine-rich F1 histones is reported for complexes made directly by interacting DNA with the histones, and that the controversy between the arginine-rich and lysine-rich histone inhibition affects on the RNA synthetic activity *in vitro* and not DNA replication *in vitro* (Hnilica and Billen, 1964; Gurley *et al.*, 1964; Wood *et al.*,

TABLE 1

AMINO–ACID COMPOSITION OF THE MAIN HISTONE FRACTIONS

Amino Acid	Calf Thymus F1*	Calf Thymus F2b	Calf Thymus F2a2	Calf Thymus F2a1	Calf Thymus F3
Lysine	*28.7*	*16.7*	*12.5*	9.8	10.1
Histidine	0.0	2.3	2.8	1.9	2.4
Arginine	1.7	6.4	9.3	*13.9*	*13.6*
ε-N-methyl-lysine	0.0	0.0	0.7	1.1	0.6
Aspartic Acid	2.0	4.9	5.5	5.0	4.4
Threonine	5.4	6.2	4.9	6.6	6.5
Serine	6.7	*10.9*	5.0	2.5	3.8
Glutamic Acid	3.4	7.6	8.7	6.2	10.2
Proline	*10.1*	4.8	4.1	1.3	4.4
Glycine	6.9	5.6	9.0	*15.9*	*5.8*
Alanine	*25.1*	10.2	*13.2*	*7.5*	*13.5*
Half Cystine	0.0	0.0	0.0	1.0	0.3
Valine	4.1	7.1	6.0	7.8	4.6
Methionine	0.0	1.6	0.3	1.0	1.5
Isoleucine	0.8	*4.9*	4.2	5.6	4.8
Leucine	4.1	*4.9*	10.1	8.0	9.0
Tyrosine	0.5	3.8	2.3	3.5	2.1
Phenylalanine	0.5	1.6	1.0	2.2	2.0

* Not Fractionated.

All values are expressed as percent of total moles of amino acids recovered.

The serine values were corrected (10) for hydrolytic losses.

The main features distinguishing each histone fraction are printed in italics.

1968). When Spelsberg and Hnilica investigated the inhibition of RNA polymerase by histones, arginine-rich histones were found to interact with both the bacterial and mammalian enzyme and inhibit the RNA synthesis *in vitro* to a much greater extent than when associated with the DNA. The inhibition is not proportional to the arginine content of the individual histone fractions (Spelsberg *et al.*, 1969). Whereas the very lysine-rich histones have a high affinity for the template DNA, their complexes with RNA polymerase are weak and dissociate at ionic strengths below the physiological value or in the presence of DNA (Spelsberg and Hnilica, 1969), releasing active enzyme. The arginine-rich histone-polymerase complexes are stable under these conditions, and the enzyme is inhibited. Although the biological meaning of these findings is not clear at the present time, they can explain some of the controversies reported in the literature. It can be concluded from the studies on DNA-histone complexes that the latter inhibit quantitatively the DNA as a template for the RNA synthesis *in vitro*.

Relatively recent work of several investigators (Zubay and Doty, 1959; Frenster *et al.*, 1963; Dingman and Sporn, 1964; Marushige and Bonner, 1966; Bonner *et al.*, 1968a; Bonner *et al.*, 1968b) showed the feasibility of preparing chromatin from the nuclei of numerous tissues without the loss of its structural and functional integrity. Isolated chromatin can template for the *in-vitro* RNA synthesis and the newly synthesized RNA can be analyzed for its base composition, nearest-neighbor frequencies, hybridization characteristics, *etc.* It has been demonstrated by Paul and Gilmour (1966a; 1966b; 1968; Gilmour and Paul, 1969; Paul, 1968; Paul, 1970), Bonner and associates (Bonner *et al.*, 1968; Bekhor *et al.*, 1969), and others (Smith *et al.*, 1969; Huang and Huang, 1969; Tan and Miyagi, 1970; Spelsberg and Hnilica, 1970; Spelsberg *et al.*, 1971) that the RNA templated by the isolated chromatin has hybridization properties almost identical to those of RNA made by intact cells.

Early experiments by Allfrey *et al.* (1963) demonstrated that the base composition of RNA made *in vitro* by nuclei devoid of histones (by exposure to trypsin) resembles the composition of DNA, indicating that the removal of histones resulted in the activation of new DNA segments, previously inhibited by histones. Similarly, Liau *et al.* (1965) working with isolated nucleoli and endogenous-RNA polymerase found the base composition of RNA synthesized by nucleoli stripped of histones by trypsin to change from the ribosomal GC-rich type to the DNA like AU-rich type. Reconstitution of histones to the trypsin-digested nucleoli restored the biosynthesis of GC-rich RNA (ribosomal) normally made by the intact nucleoli. These experiments, in addition to confirming the findings by Allfrey *et al.* (1963) that histones occupy sites on the DNA qualitatively different from those open for the transcription, also demonstrated that the sites designated to be transcribed are protected from the interaction with histones, since the reconstitution of histones to the trypsin-digested nucleoli did not result in the synthesis of RNA with a random base composition. It should be noted that less than 0.5 per cent of nucleolar DNA is active in genetic transcription.

As was already mentioned, selective dissociation of histones increases the transcriptional ability several fold (Hindley, 1963; Seligy and Neelin, 1970; Spelsberg and Hnilica, 1971; Marushige and Bonner, 1966; Bonner *et al.,* 1968; Paul and Gilmour, 1968; Tan and Miyagi, 1970; Spelsberg and Hnilica, 1971; O'Meara and Herrmann, 1970; and others). Whereas the removal of the very lysine-rich histones F1 affects the templating efficiency of chromatin only a little, removal of either the moderately lysine-rich fraction F1b or the arginine-rich histones F1a and F3 both results in a dramatic increase of the RNA synthesis *in vitro* templated by the dehistonized chromatin.

Analysis of the RNA species templated from isolated chromatin *in vitro* show that, as a consequence of cytodifferentiation, selected parts of the DNA genome are restricted and inactive in genetic transcription (Marushige and Bonner, 1966; Bonner *et al.,* 1968). As can be expected, this restriction is tissue specific (Bonner *et al.,* 1968; Paul and Gilmour, 1966b; Paul and Gilmour, 1968; Gilmour and Paul, 1969; Paul, 1968; Paul, 1970; Bekhor *et al.,* 1969; Smith *et al.,* 1969; Huang and Huang, 1969; Tan and Miyagi, 1970; Spelsberg and Hnilica, 1970; Spelsberg *et al.,* 1971) and a high degree of this specificity is retained in chromatin during its isolation. Complete removal of proteins from chromatin results in transcription of RNA very similar to that templated by pure DNA. Removal of only the histones produces chromatin which templates for a considerable number of new RNA species. This RNA is, however, not identical with the RNA made on pure (naked) DNA, indicating that nonhistone proteins contribute to the restriction of DNA (Spelsberg and Hnilica, 1971a, Spelsberg and Hnilica, 1971b; Paul and Gilmour, 1968). According to Paul and Gilmour (1968), reconstitution of histones to pure DNA produces a completely restricted nucleohistone. If such reconstitution is carried out with histones and dehistonized chromatin, instead of DNA, the reconstituted nucleohistone behaves similarly to the original sample. The dissociation and reconstitution of histones and nonhistone proteins from chromatin must be performed in the presence of concentrated urea in order to retain the transcriptional specificity of the reconstituted chromatin (Paul and Gilmour, 1968; Gilmour and Paul, 1969; Bekhor *et al.,* 1969; Huang and Huang, 1969; Spelsberg and Hnilica, 1970; Spelsberg *et al.,* 1971). The nonhistone proteins together with the histones appear, therefore, essential for the transcriptional function of chromatin.

The question whether, in chromatin, histones are associated with DNA segments different from those functioning in transcription was investigated by Spelsberg and Hnilica (1971a, 1971b). Studies on rates of the RNA synthesis *in vitro* and DNA-RNA hybridization revealed that the dissociation of any of the histones other than the F1 fraction causes partial loss of the specificity of RNA transcription. Selective removal of the lysine-rich histone F1 did not result in the biosynthesis of new species of RNA, indicating that this fraction either does not restrict the DNA qualitatively or that it is associated with DNA cistrons redundant to those that are transcriptionally active in un-

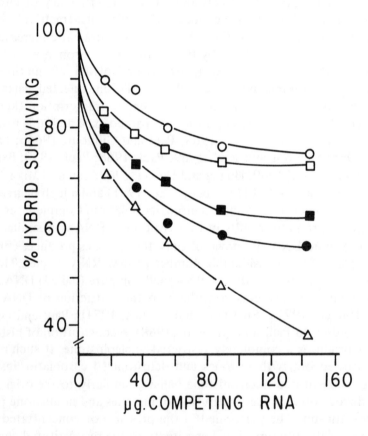

Figure 1

Competitive hybridization using RNA templated from rat-thymus chromatin which has been extracted with o——o = H_2O, □——□ = 0.2 M.$(NH_4)_2SO_4$, ■——■ = 0.3 M.$(NH_4)_2SO_4$, ●——● = 1.0 M.$(NH_4)_2SO_4$, and RNA templated from △——△ = pure rat DNA. ^{3}H-RNA templated from pure rat DNA was used at 50 μg. per reaction with 2 μg. DNA per filter.

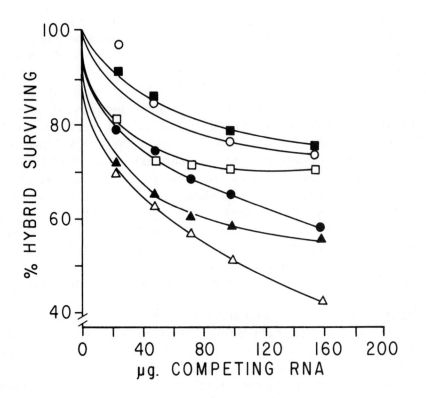

Figure 2

Competitive hybridization using RNA templated from rat-thymus chromatin which has been extracted with ○—○ = H$_2$O, ■—■ = 75 per cent ethanol, □—□ = 75 per cent ETOH + 2 per cent NaCl, ●—● = 75 per cent ETOH + 10 per cent Guan-HCl, ▲—▲ = 75 per cent ETOH - 0.25 N HCl, and RNA templated from △—△ = pure rat DNA. ^{3}H-RNA templated from pure rat DNA was used at 50 μg. per reaction with 2 μg. rat DNA per filter.

treated chromatin. If the F1 histones restricted relatively few unique DNA cistrons, the biosynthesis of such unique RNA species would remain undetected by the technique of competitive DNA-RNA hybridization employed by the authors. Dissociation of the moderately lysine-rich histone F2b substantially increased the number of different RNA species templated (Figure 1). Similarly, selective removal of the arginine-rich histone fractions F2a and F3 also resulted in the transcription of considerably more RNA species (Figure 2), indicating that, in intact chromatin, these two groups of histones inactivate transcriptional sites on the DNA which are qualitatively different from those originally accessible to the RNA-polymerase enzyme.

Realizing that the histones alone cannot restrict the DNA in chromatin specifically, several investigators initiated the search for substances necessary for tissue-specific restriction of chromatin. Bekhor *et al.* (1969) and Gilmour and Paul (1969) reported the necessity of using urea in the specific reconstitution of chromatin previously dissociated with 2.0 M. NaCl. Only chromatin dissociated by salt and reconstituted by slow dialysis in 5 M. urea produced templating patterns *in vitro* for RNA synthesis indistinguishable from the control samples. Based on the earlier discovery of chromosomal RNA (Huang and Bonner, 1965), Bekhor *et al.* (1969), and Huang and Huang (1969) proposed that this special chromosomal RNA (cRNA) is necessary for the specific reconstitution of dissociated chromatin. This cRNA is solubilized together with histones and nonhistone proteins during the dissociation of chromatin and appears to be firmly bound to a nonhistone-protein fraction (Huang and Huang, 1969; Bonner and Huang, 1966). The necessity for the urea to be included in reconstitution experiments to retain the tissue-specific restriction of chromatin indicated that the mechanism directing histones away from the DNA cistrons that are to remain active in transcription may involve hybridization of the chromosomal RNA to specific nucleotide sequences in the DNA.

On the other hand, Gilmour and Paul (1969) found that the nonhistone-chromatin proteins are essential for proper reconstitution of chromatin and that they confer specificity to the DNA restriction. These authors used serum albumin as a representative acidic protein not found in the nucleus to replace the nonhistone proteins in reconstituted chromatin. This produced a chromatin-like material which supported the RNA synthesis *in vitro* to an extent similar to the control sample, indicating that a nonspecific protein can protect quantitatively the DNA from total inhibition by histones. Analysis of the RNA templated by this artificial chromatin demonstrated, however, that the transcription of the DNA was completely random and nonspecific, indicating that albumin cannot confer the qualitative specificity of restriction to the DNA and histone complexes.

More recently, Gilmour and Paul (1970) and Spelsberg and Hnilica (1970; Spelsberg *et al.*, 1971) have found that the nonhistone proteins of chromatin are essential for the tissue-specific RNA transcription by reconstituted chromatin samples. Both groups found that the specificity of RNA synthesis *in vitro* detected by DNA-RNA hybridization can be changed from the pattern typical for one tissue to that of another by exchanging a fraction of nonhistone protein in isolated chromatin and reconstituting this fraction to the DNA and histones by slow dialysis in the presence of urea (Figure 3). Even the reconstitution of calf-thymus histones to dehistonized rat-liver chromatin complex of nonhistone proteins and DNA did not alter the RNA transcription specific for intact rat-liver chromatin (Figure 4). Since none of the investigators attempted to remove chromosomal RNA, the possibility that this RNA remained associated with the chromatin nonhistone proteins cannot be excluded. Curiously, the reconstitution experiments on chromatin resemble strongly the work on dissociation and reassembly of ribosomes (Nomura *et al.*, 1969). It would be interesting if both these mechanisms are governed by similar principles.

In conclusion, although it appears that histones alone do not possess sufficient molecular specificity to restrict the chromatin DNA qualitatively, it is evident that much of the quantitative restriction of DNA is due to its complexes with histones. Selective removal of histones results in the biosynthesis of new species of RNA indicating that DNA segments not previously trans-

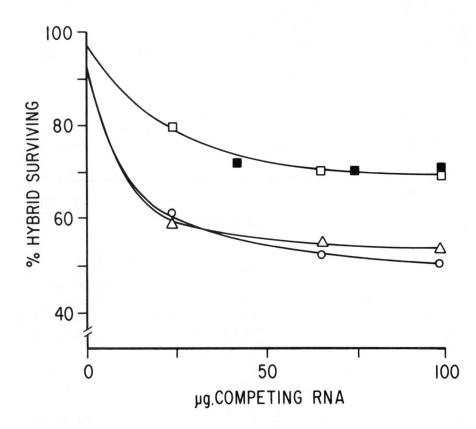

Figure 3

Competitive hybridization of unlabeled RNA templated *in vitro* from ○——○ native rat-liver chromatin, ■——■ hybrid chromatin composed of histones from rat liver and DNA with associated nonhistone proteins from rat-thymus chromatin, □——□ native rat-thymus chromatin, △——△ hybrid chromatin composed of histones from rat thymus and the DNA with associated nonhistone proteins from rat-liver chromatin. The reconstitution was performed by dialysis at pH 6.0. The unlabeled RNA was competed against ³H-RNA templated *in vitro* from native rat-liver chromatin. The 100 per cent hybridization represents 410 c.p.m. with 4 μg. of DNA per filter.

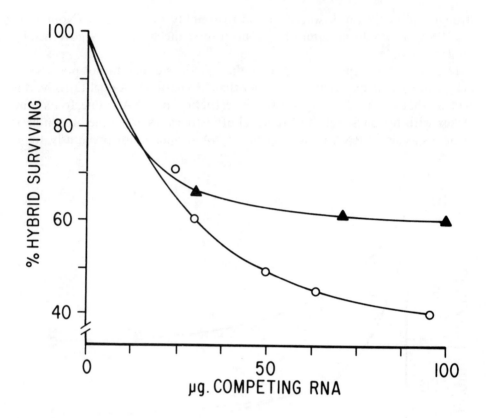

Figure 4

Competitive hybridization of unlabeled RNA templated *in vitro* from ●——● native rat-liver chromatin, ▲——▲ native rat-thymus chromatin, and ○——○ hybrid chromatin composed of whole calf-thymus histone and the DNA with associated nonhistone proteins from rat-liver chromatin. The unlabeled RNA was competed against ^{3}H-RNA templated *in vitro* from native rat-liver chromatin.

cribed became accessible to the RNA-polymerase enzyme. The presence of certain nonhistone proteins or RNA in chromatin is necessary for the DNA to be restricted specifically in individual tissues.

EFFECT OF HORMONES ON GENETIC TRANSCRIPTION.

One decade ago Zalokar (1961) and Karlson (1963) proposed that hormones affect the target tissues by regulating their gene activity. Evidence has been accumulated since then, suggesting that many plant and animal hormones regulate tissue metabolism by altering the pattern of RNA synthesis. These changes partially involve alterations in the qualitative restriction of chromatin. This has been demonstrated for the effect of hydrocortisone (Dahmus and Bonner, 1965) and cortisol (Stackhouse *et al.*, 1968) on the liver of the rat, estrogen on the uterus of the rat (Teng and Hamilton, 1968; Gorski *et al.*, 1965; Barker and Warren, 1967; Barker and Warren, 1966; Barker and Anderson, 1968), testosterone on skeletal muscle (Breuer and Florini, 1966) and prostatic nuclei (Liao *et al.*, 1966a; 1966b), thyroxine on liver of the tadpole (Kim and Cohen, 1966), progesterone on fowl oviduct (O'Malley *et al.*, 1969), and in other systems. The general pattern observed is that the chromatin samples of target tissues from animals treated with hormones are more effective templates for RNA synthesis *in vitro* than samples of chromatin from the same tissues of animals without treatment. When the histones and nonhistone proteins are removed from such chromatins, the differences in templating efficiency diminish substantially or disappear (Dahmus and Bonner, 1965; Breuer and Florini, 1966).

It was also reported that the addition of hormones to isolated nuclei causes an *in vivo*-like stimulation of RNA synthesis accompanied by changes of the templating capacity of their chromatin. In 1963, Roychoundhury and Sen (1963) found the endosperm nuclei of coconut milk enhance their RNA and DNA synthesis when treated with the plant hormone, indole-3-acetic acid. Other regulators of plant growth, kinetin and gibberellic acid, also enhance RNA synthesis and stimulate the RNA release from isolated nuclei (Roychoundhury *et al.*, 1965). Similar results were found with other botanical tissues (Cherry, 1967; Johri and Varner, 1968). However, recent studies (Matthysse, 1968 ; Matthysse and Phillips, 1969; Matthysse and Abrams, 1970; Matthysse, 1970) indicate the necessity for isolating the nuclei of plants in the presence of hormone, most likely to allow for the interactions between the cytosol receptor, hormone, and chromatin in the nucleus.

The effects of hormones were seen, with variable reproducibility, also in animal tissues. According to Sekeris *et al.* (1965; Dukes and Sekeris, 1965; Dukes *et al.*, 1966; Lukacs and Sekeris, 1967), addition of steroid hormones to isolated nuclei from tissues affected by the hormone (ecdysone and cortisol on epidermal-cell nuclei of insects and cortisol on hepatic nuclei in rats) enhances their RNA synthesis *in vitro*.

Barker and Warren (1967) reported that purified chromatin from uteri, but not lungs, of ovariectomized rats can be derepressed by estradiol *in vitro*. However, the 12-hour periods of incubation at 37° C. necessary for the effect of hormone to take place may produce artifacts as a result of chromatin degradation by nucleases or proteases. Other investigators have also reported increased RNA synthesis *in vitro* after addition of cortisol to hepatic chromatin in the rat (Beato *et al.*, 1970a; 1970b) or auxins to chromatin in plants (Matthysse and Phillips, 1969; Matthysse, 1970), but again critical measurements of proteolytic activity are essential. Other attempts to produce the derepression of RNA synthesis *in vitro* by cortisol in rat-liver chromatin (Dahmus and Bonner, 1965; Tsai and Hnilica, 1971), progesterone on chickoviduct chromatin (Spelsberg *et al.*, 1971), or estrogen on rat-uterine chromatin (Barker and Warren, 1967) were not successful.

As mentioned elsewhere in this volume, probably the best evidence supporting the concept of gene activation by hormones is the effect of ecdysone on locus-specific (puffs) activation of DNA transcription in polytene chromosomes in certain insect species. Although the hormone may act indirectly, *e. g.* through the activation of RNA-polymerase enzyme, by selective increase in the biosynthesis of certain nonhistone proteins, *etc.*, the first visible manifestation of the hormonal effect is the change in morphology of polytene chromosomes. Since individual puffs can be associated with the biosynthesis of specific salivary-gland proteins, the effect of ecdysone on polytene chromosomes is undoubtedly that of the derepression (activation) of specific genetic loci (Grossback, 1969).

In rat uteri, estrogen treatment of the animals results in an immediate synthesis of proteins, some of which are part of the chromatin nonhistone-protein complex (Teng and Hamilton, 1969; Notides and Gorski, 1966; Hamilton and Teng, 1969; Smith *et al.*, 1969; Teng and Hamilton, 1970). Some of these proteins are made within 30 minutes after the administration of hormone (Notides and Gorski, 1966). Recently, Shelton and Allfrey (1970) have discovered the synthesis of a specific protein of chromatin in livers of rats treated with cortisone. Although the biochemical identity of this protein is unknown, it may represent a hormone-induced increase of the synthesis of RNA polymerase or of a specific gene-activator protein. In uteri of the rat, the synthesis of a specific protein following treatment with estrogen is only secondary to the synthesis of RNA that was found by DeAngelo and Gorski (1970) to occur within 15 minutes after the injection of estrogen. The function of this rapidly-synthesized RNA is not known, but it represents the first detectable metabolic response of uterine cells to the hormone. It was reported by O'Malley *et al.* (1969) that the stimulation of fowl oviduct of the chicken by progesterone produces profound changes in the composition of RNA detectable by base analysis, nearest-neighbor frequency, and experiments of DNA-RNA hybridization. Consequently, changes in RNA transcription appear to be one of the first biochemical events brought about by hormonal action. This alteration of transcriptional activity and specificity, in many instances, has been preserved in isolated chromatin.

BINDING OF HORMONES TO CHROMATIN

Although direct binding of hormone to chromatin or to DNA is not a necessary prerequisite for its biological action, reports in the literature support the idea that such direct binding may be necessary for the biological activity of at least some hormones. Both histones and nonhistone proteins of chromatin have been implicated in mediating the change in genetic restriction produced by the administration of hormone. Since histones are known to inhibit the transcription of DNA and are associated with DNA segments not transcribed under normal circumstances, interaction of hormones with histones could provide a mechanism for selective removal of histone molecules from DNA or for specific changes in the conformation of chromatin allowing transcription from DNA sites previously inaccessible to RNA polymerase. On the other hand, if the chromatin nonhistone proteins play a decisive role in the tissue-specific restriction of DNA in chromatin, association of hormones with these proteins may change their locus-specific interactions with DNA, resulting in a modification of transcriptional specificity of chromatin.

Hormone Binding to Histones.

Since corticosteroid hormones were reported to cause an increase in the templating efficiency of rat-liver chromatin and biosynthesis of new RNA species in liver (Kidson and Kirby, 1964; Kidson, 1967), it has been suggested (Dahmus and Bonner, 1965; Sekeris and Lang, 1965; Sluyser, 1966a) that corticosteroid hormones may associate with histones, thereby stimulating RNA synthesis.

Sluyser (1966a) first reported that histones can form stable complexes with hydrocortisone when incubated together in NaCl solutions of low ionic strength. Arginine-rich histones were found to bind more hormone than the lysine-rich fractions (Sluyser, 1966a; 1966b). The binding *in vitro* of arginine-rich and other histones to cortisol, tetrahydrocortisol, cortisone, tetrahydrocortisone, progesterone, 17β-estradiol, and testosterone was confirmed by Sunaga and Koide (1967a; 1967b; 1967c). Labeled cortisone administered *in vivo* was detected in chromatin by Wilson and Loeb (1965), indicating that at least part of the injected hormone may accumulate at the site of its action. According to Sekeris and Lang (1965) the hormone was bound in a significant amount to the histones. The binding *in vivo* of hydrocortisone to histones was confirmed by Sluyser (1966a), who found the arginine-rich fraction F3 to accept the hormone most readily of all the histones. Similarly, injected testosterone was found associated with histones in prostate and in levator-ani muscle of rats and only to a much lesser extent in hepatic or splenic histones of the same animals. In contrast to hydrocortisone, labeled testosterone was bound preferentially to the very lysine-rich histone fraction F1. In spleen, the arginine-rich histone accepted more and retained labeled testosterone for a longer time than the other histone fractions.

Tsai and Hnilica (1971) investigated the binding of corticosteroid hormones to histones both *in vivo* and *in vitro*. They were able to confirm reports in the literature that administration of hormone to the rats or to hepatic slices *in vitro* produces approximately 20 per cent increase in the templating efficiency of chromatin isolated from treated tissues (Table 2). This ability

TABLE 2

TEMPLATE ACTIVITY OF CHROMATIN FROM MINCED LIVER INCUBATED
WITH CORTISOL

Chromatin Preparation	Time of Incubation in Minutes	$\mu\mu$Moles of Nucleotide Incorporated	Increase over Control
Control	15	76.6*	—
Cortisol	15	79.5*	3.8%
Control	30	50.1**	—
Cortisol	30	59.6**	18.9%
Control	60	36.8***	—
Cortisol	60	42.3***	14.9%

*   Based on 9 micrograms of DNA per assay.
**   Based on 14 micrograms of DNA per assay.
*** Based on 5 micrograms of DNA per assay.

The amount of RNA polymerase in each assay was capable of incorporating 1760 $\mu\mu$moles of H^3–CTP per 50 μg. of calf thymus DNA at 37C. in 10 minutes. The hepatic minces were incubated with 10 micrograms of cortisol per ml. of McCoy's medium.

of corticosteroid hormones to increase the rates of RNA synthesis templated by chromatin *in vitro* was lost, however, when isolated chromatin was used in a direct mixture with hormone. Occasional stimulation reported in the literature (Beato *et al.*, 1970a; 1970b) and also seen in our laboratory may be due to the contamination of isolated chromatin by cytoplasmic components. In search for the molecules capable of binding corticosteroid hormones *in vivo*, Tsai and Hnilica (1971) isolated nuclei from rats injected with labeled hydrocortisone or cortisone. Four different techniques for the isolation of nuclei were employed (Table 3). As can be seen, only nuclei contaminated by cytoplasmic particles [isotonic sucrose nuclei (Sekeris and Lang, 1965; Sluyser, 1966a; 1966b)] yielded histones associated with significant amounts of hormone. Hypertonic-sucrose procedure (Blobel and Potter, 1966; Chaveau *et al.*, 1956) produced hormone-labeled histones only if the isolated nuclei were extracted directly with diluted acid (without partial fractionation into the arginine-rich and lysine-rich histones), a technique known to result in considerable contamination of histones by ácid-soluble, nonhistone proteins. As can be seen in Table 3, the major part of radioactive hormone in the nucleus is associated with the acid-insoluble residue. It was concluded, from these experiments, that the labeling *in vivo* of histones with radioactive corticosteroid hormones in liver is due to their contamination by other proteins, most likely of cytoplasmic origin.

The interaction *in vitro* of corticosteroid hormones appeared, at first, less controversial. Isolated histone fractions, especially the arginine-rich F3, were found to bind labeled hormones readily, similar to the reports in the literature. As described by Sluyser (1969), the binding of labeled hydrocortisone to the F3 histones increased linearly with the time of incubation. The lysine-rich F1 histone accepted only small amounts of hormone *in vitro,* and F2a histones bound large amounts of hormone only when aggregated. Sluyser (1969) suggested that binding hydrocortisone to the arginine-rich histone is mainly through its hydrophobic amino-acid region which, due to a special folding of this fraction, is exposed on the outside of this molecule.

Monder and Walker (1970), who also studied the interactions of corticosteroid hormones with histones, concluded that, if cortisol is used for the interaction, the actual interacting molecule is 20-dehydrocortisol contaminating cortisol samples. This interaction involved terminal residues of basic amino acids, especially arginine. Electrophoretic analyses carried out in our laboratory on *in-vitro* complexes of unfractionated calf-thymus histone with hydrocortisone show the arginine-rich histones F3 are associated with over 65 per cent of the total hormonal radioactivity, although this fraction represents less than 20 per cent of the total histone protein. Approximately 33 per cent of the remaining radioactivity was associated with 1ysine-rich F1 his-

TABLE 3

INTERACTION OF CORTISTEROIDS WITH NUCLEAR PROTEINS *IN VIVO*

	1,2-³H-hydrocortisone		1,2-³H-Cortisone	
	A Hypertonic Sucrose (Chaveau *et al.*)	B Isotonic Sucrose (Sluyser)	C Hypertonic Sucrose (Blobel and Potter)	D Isotonic Sucrose (Sekeris and Lang)
Whole Nuclei	390**	—	3364*	16983*
Total Histones	—	—	841**	1759**
Histone Fractions			115***	159***
F1F2b	0	—		
F1		264***		
F2b	0	72***		
F2aF3	0	—		
F2a		173***		
F3		113***		

* DNA.

** Protein (based on serumalbumin standard).

*** Histone (based on histone standard).

Male rats (120—130/g.) were each injected with 0.97 mμmole of 1,2—³H-cortisone(50μCi., 51.6 mCi./μmole),or male rats (250—300/g.) were each injected with 1.14 mμmole of 1,2—³H-hydrocortisone (50μCi., 44mCi./μmole).The animals were sacrificed 30 minutes after the injection and nuclei isolated from their livers according to the procedures indicated.

tones (approximately another 20 per cent of the total histone protein). As determined by electrophoretic analysis, F3 histone contained less than 1 $\mu\mu$mole of hydrocortisone per mg. of protein; the F1 histone contained less than 0.2 $\mu\mu$mole of hydrocortisone per mg. of protein. The amount of hydrocortisone bound to the arginine-rich F3 histones represents approximately 15 $\mu\mu$moles of this hormone per mole of F3 histone, assuming the molecular weight of this fraction to be 15,000 daltons. This is about one molecule of hormone for every 6.6×10^4 molecules of F3 histone. Using data published by Sluyser (1969), similar combining ratios of the F3 histones can be calculated. Tsai and Hnilica (1971) interpreted this extremely low combining ratio to be due to actual association of the hormone with some other molecule, probably a nonhistone protein, contaminating the F3-histone fraction. This conclusion was supported by fingerprinting analysis of peptides resulting from tryptic digestion of F3-histone complexes with hydrocortisone. A considerable portion of the hormone remained at the origin, suggesting its binding to a trypsin-resistant, ninhydrin-positive substance. It is known that many acidic proteins are quite resistant to tryptic digestion. Since the arginine-rich hormones are known to contain significant amounts of contaminating nonhistone proteins that are difficult to remove (Hnilica and Bess, 1965; Stellwagen and Cole, 1968a; 1968b), part of this contamination may represent proteins that bind corticosteroid hormones. Although this conclusion cannot be generalized without additional experimental evidence, it appears that histones are not very likely candidates for the tissue-specific interactions of steroid hormones with chromatin.

Hormone Binding to Nonhistone Proteins in Chromatin.

Since histones most likely are not involved in the immediate interactions of steroid hormones with chromatin, there is a distinct possibility that chromatin nonhistone proteins may be involved in mediation of the metabolic effect of hormones. Recent studies have demonstrated that steroid hormone combines initially with a specific receptor protein in the cytoplasm of the target cells. The complexes are then transported to the nucleus and localized around the chromatin (O'Malley *et al.*, 1969; Jensen *et al.*, 1969; Rochefort and Baulieu, 1969; Shyamala and Gorski, 1967; Bruchovski and Wilson, 1968). A similar mechanism appears to operate in plants (Matthysse and Phillips, 1969; Matthysse, 1970; Liao and Hamilton, 1966; Spelsberg and Sarkissian, 1970). The nature of the hormone-receptor interaction and the transfer of the complexes into the nucleus is not completely understood.

Several investigators (Tsai and Hnilica, 1971; Shyamala and Gorski, 1967; Bruchovsky and Wilson, 1968; Fanestil and Edelman, 1966; Talwar *et al.,*

1964; King *et al.*, 1965; Beato *et al.*, 1969; King *et al.*, 1965; Maurer and Chalkley, 1967; King and Gordon, 1969; King *et al.*, 1969; Swaneck *et al.*, 1970) have reported that administered hormones *in vivo* accumulate preferentially in the fraction of nuclear nonhistone proteins that are frequently claimed to be part of the chromatin complex. The fact that steroid hormones can be released only from nuclei or chromatin by proteases, but not by nucleases, supports the conclusion that a proteinaceous component of nuclei or chromatin serves in the binding of the hormone (Fanestil and Edelman, 1966; Swaneck *et al.*, 1970; King and Gordon, 1967). The presence of specific receptor proteins in the cytoplasm poses the question whether the nuclear nonhistone protein complex with the hormone is a chromatin protein or whether it represents the complex of hormone with its cytosol receptor that became associated with chromatin in the nucleus of the cell. Brecher *et al.* (1967; Brecher and Wotiz, 1968; Brecher and Wotiz, 1969) found that the presence of uterine cytosol from the rat containing the receptor for estradiol was necessary for the binding of this hormone by isolated rat-uterus nuclei. Similar results were obtained in other laboratories with estradiol and rabbit hypothalmus (Chader and Villee, 1970) and progesterone with chick oviduct (O'Malley *et al.*, 1970). The binding of hormone required its biologically active form (inactive analogs failed), the cytosol of the target tissue containing the specific receptor protein for the hormone and nuclei from the target tissue. Recently O'Malley *et al.* (1971) have reported that progesterone, extracted from the oviduct nuclei labeled *in vitro*, is bound to a protein indistinguishable from the oviduct cytosol receptor-protein fraction. It appears, therefore, that the nonhistone proteins associated with various steroid hormones in nuclei or chromatin are actually the cytosol receptor-protein complexes with the hormone and probably not a specific fraction of the nonhistone protein in chromatin.

CYTOSOL RECEPTOR PROTEINS

It is known from the work of Jensen (Jensen *et al.*, 1969; DeSombre *et al.*, 1969), Gorski (Shyamala and Gorski, 1967), O'Malley (O'Malley *et al.*, 1964), their associates, and other investigators (Beato *et al.*, 1970a; Beato *et al.*, 1970b; Rochefort and Baulieu, 1969; Bruchovsky and Wilson, 1968; Beato *et al.*, 1969; *etc.*) that at least for steroid hormones such as estradiol, progesterone, cortisol, *etc.*, the hormone combines first with specific receptor proteins in the cytoplasm of target tissues. Partially purified receptor proteins appear relatively homogeneous with molecular weights lower than 100,000 daltons. The receptor protein for estradiol in calf uterine cytosol is present in the form of 8S complexes that can be dissociated reversibly into 4S subunits.

The approximate isoelectric points of the partially purified 8S and 4S receptor proteins are 5.8 and 6.4 respectively (DeSombre *et al.,* 1969).

The receptor protein for cortisol is different from the estradiol receptor. Although it has a similar molecular weight (50-60,000 daltons), it is more basic (Morey and Litwack, 1969; Litwack and Morey, 1970). There is a peculiar similarity in the properties of the receptor protein for cortisol and those of cytoplasmic proteins known to bind carcinogens *in vivo.* As shown by Litwack and Morey (1970) and by Ketterer *et al.* (1967), the cytoplasmic receptor proteins for cortisol and dimethylaminoazobenzene and perhaps for 3-methylcholanthrene may be identical in rat liver. This similarity suggests that the mechanisms of action of at least some carcinogens may be similar to those known for steroid hormones. It is also known that certain hormone analogs have both gonadotropic and carcinogenic activity.

Although the association of injected steroid hormones with cytoplasmic receptor proteins seems to be essential for its biological effect, it is not known whether the receptor protein serves only as a vehicle for the hormone to reach the nucleus or whether the entire complex becomes incorporated into the chromatin.

Using isolated chromatin and cytosol receptor-protein fractions from various chicken tissues including the oviduct, Spelsberg *et al.* (1971; Steggles *et al.,* 1971) found that the progesterone-cytosol complex is specific for the target tissue of this hormone (oviduct) and associates *in vitro* preferentially with oviduct chromatin. Therefore the cytosol proteins appear to furnish the specificity necessary for hormone binding to the chromatin of its target tissue only. Similar observations were reported for uterine chromatin of ovariectomized rats injected with estradiol or with chromatin of prostate in castrated male rats after the administration of dihydrotestosterone (Steggles *et al.,* 1971). This group demonstrated that the specificity of the interaction of the chicken oviduct cytoplasmic receptor protein-progesterone complex with chromatin of the same tissue depends on the origin of the nonhistone-chromatin proteins together with the DNA. Using interactions of specific cytoplasmic receptor protein-hormone complexes with chromatin of target and nontarget tissues, these authors demonstrated that the target-tissue chromatin is genetically programmed to receive the hormone-receptor protein complex. As in experiments on the tissue specificity of RNA synthesis on isolated chromatin templates discussed above, the selective binding of hormone-receptor protein complexes is directed by the macromolecules (most likely proteins) present in the nonhistone-protein fraction of chromatin. Histones play only the role of nonspecific repressors of the DNA and most likely do not participate directly in specific binding of steroid hormones to chromatin in their target tissues.

CONCLUSIONS

Reports from the literature briefly reviewed in this article suggest that chromatin proteins, both histones and the nonhistone proteins, are essential for the extent and specificity of DNA restriction in eucaryotic organisms. It is also known that many steroid hormones, in addition to increasing the rate of RNA synthesis in their target tissues considerably, also change the qualitative composition of newly synthesized RNA. This points to hormone-produced changes in the transcriptional specificity of chromatin. The exact mechanism of this tissue-specific activation is presently unknown. It appears to involve the interaction of hormone with a tissue-specific cytoplasmic receptor protein that facilitates its transfer into the nucleus. From the experimental data presented, the direct interaction of hormones with nuclear histones is unlikely. Possibly the entire cytoplasmic receptor-protein complex with the hormone interacts with specific loci in chromatin of the target tissue producing alterations manifested by changes in RNA synthesis. It was suggested by several investigators that the nonhistone chromatin proteins may serve as the actual interaction sites for either the hormone or more likely, the hormone-cytoplasmic receptor complex.

From the standpoint of the regulation of transcriptional specificity of chromatin, it is suggested that principally two kinds of restriction may exist in most eucaryotic organisms. A permanent restriction mediated by the histones is activated and determined during cytodifferentiation. At this time, histones are placed on DNA segments designated to remain inactive. This restriction is copied during each mitotic cycle and explains why DNA and histone biosynthesis coincide temporarily during the S phase of the cell cycle. Reprogramming of this histone-mediated permanent restriction of differentiated cells is rare, difficult, and most likely requires a cycle of DNA replication. The other type of restriction is variable and responds readily to various metabolic challenges. It probably involves numerous nonhistone proteins endowed with a sequence specificity of interaction with DNA. Existence of such proteins in chromatin was reported recently in the literature. It is possible that the cytosol receptor protein may represent one of these proteins capable of interacting with specific DNA cistrons previously protected by other nonhistone chromatin proteins. As was suggested by Allfrey and associates (Pogo *et al.*, 1969), a structural rearrangement of chromatin may be necessary to allow these highly specific nonhistone protein-DNA interactions to take place. Chemical modification of histones (acetylation, phosphorylation, thiolation, *etc.*) was suggested to be the necessary step in changing the conformation of chromatin and thereby opening the specific binding sites normally inaccessible to the interacting molecules.

Acknowledgement

This research was supported by grants from the USPHS (CA 07746 and HD 05803) and from the Robert A. Welch Foundation (G 138).

References

1. ALLFREY, V. G., LITTAU, V. C. and MIRSKY, A. E.: On the Role of Histones in Regulating Ribonucleic Acid Synthesis. Proc. Natl. Acad. Sci., U. S., *49:*414, 1963.

2. BARKER, K. L. and ANDERSON, J. M.: Displacement of Estradiol - 17β from the Uterus by Estradiol - 17α: Effect on Template Capacity of Uterine Chromatin. Endocrinology, *83:*585, 1968.

3. BARKER, K. L. and WARREN, J. C.: Effect of 17β - Estradiol *in Vitro* on the Template Capacity of Uterine Chromatin. Endocrinology, *80:*536, 1967.

4. BARKER, K. L. and WARREN, J. C.: Template Capacity of Uterine Chromatin: Control by Estradiol. Proc. Natl. Acad. Sci., U. S., *56:*1298, 1966.

5. BARR, G. C. and BUTLER, J. A. V.: Histones and Gene Function. Nature, *199:* 1170, 1963.

6. BEATO, M., BIESEWIG, D., BRAENDLE, W., and SEKERIS, C. E.: On the Mechanism of Hormone Action. XV. Subcellular Distribution and Binding of [1, 2-^{3}H] Cortisol in Rat Liver. Biochim. Biophys. Acta, *192:*494, 1969.

7. BEATO, M., SCHMID, W., BRAENDLE, W., and SEKERIS, C. E.: Partial Purification of a Cortisol Binding Protein from Rat Liver Cytosol. Steroids, *16:*207, 1970.

8. BEATO, M., SEIFART, K. H., and SEKERIS, C. E.: The Effect of Cortisol on the Binding of Actinomycin D to and on the Template Activity of Isolated Rat Liver Chromatin. Arch. Biochem. Biophys., *138:*272, 1970.

9. BEKHOR, I., KUNG, G. M., and BONNER, J.: Sequence-Specific Interaction of DNA and Chromosomal Protein. J. Molec. Biol., *39:*351, 1969.

10. BLOBEL, G. and POTTER, R. V.: Nuclei from Rat Liver: Isolation Method that Combines Purity with High Yield.Science, *154:*1662, 1966.

11. BONNER, J., CHALKLEY, G. R., DHAMUS, M. E., FAMBROUGH, D., FUJIMURA, F., HUANG, R. C. C., HUBERMAN, J., JENSEN, R., MARUSHIGE, K., OHLENBUSCH, H., OLIVERA, P., and WIDHOLM, J.: Isolation and Purification of Nuclear Proteins. *In*: L. Grossman and K. Moldave (ed.), Methods in Enzymology, *12B:*3. New York: Academic Press, 1968.

12. BONNER, J., DAHMUS, M. E., FAMBROUGH, D., HUANG, R. C. C., MARUSHIGE, K., and TUAN, D. Y. H.: The Biology of Isolated Chromatin. Science, *159:*47, 1968.

13. BONNER, J. and HUANG, R. C.: Histones as Specific Repressors of Chromosomal RNA Synthesis. *In*: A. V. S. DeReuck and J. Knight (ed.), Histones, p. 18, London, 1966.

14. BRECHER, P. I., VIGERSKY, R., WOTIZ, H. S., and WOTIZ, H. H.: An *in Vitro* System for the Binding of Estradiol to Rat Uterine Nuclei. Steroids, *10:*536, 1967.

15. BRECHER, P. I. and WOTIZ, H. H.: Dissociation of Estradiol from a Uterine Nuclear Receptor. Endocrinology, *84:*718, 1969.

16. BRECHER, P. I. and WOTIZ, H. H.: Stereospecificity of the Uterine Nuclear Hormone Receptors. Proc. Soc. Exptl. Biol. Med., *128:*470, 1968.

17. BREUER, C. B. and FLORINI, J. R.: Effects of Ammonium Sulfate, Growth Hormone and Testosterone Propionate on Ribonucleic Acid Polymerase and Chromatin Activities in Rat Skeletal Muscle. Biochemistry, *5:*3857, 1966.

18. BRUCHOVSKY, N. and WILSON, J. D.: The Intranuclear Binding of Testosterone and 5d-Androstan-17β-ol-3-one by Rat Prostate. J. Biol. Chem., *243:*5953, 1968.

19. CHADER, G. J. and VILLEE, C. A.: Uptake of Oestradiol by the Rabbit Hypothalamus. Specificity of Binding by Nucleic *in Vitro.* Biochem. J., *118:*93, 1970.

20. CHAVEAU, J. , MOULÉ, Y., and ROUILLER, C.: Isolation of Pure and Unaltered Liver Nuclei. Morphology and Biochemical Composition. Expt. Cell Res., *11:*317, 1956.

21. CHERRY, J. H.: Nucleic Acid Biosynthesis in Seed Germination: Influences of Auxin and Growth-regulating Substances. Ann. N. Y. Acad. Sci., *144:*154, 1967.

22. CLARK, P. R. and BYVOET, P.: Inhibition of RNA-Polymerase by Arginine-Rich Histone Fractions. Experientia, *26:*725, 1970.

23. DAHMUS, M. F. and BONNER, J.: Increase Template Activity of Liver Chromatin, a Result of Hydrocortisone Administration. Proc. Natl. Acad. Sci., U. S., *54:*1370, 1965.

24. DE ANGELO, A. B. and GROSKI, J.: Role of RNA Synthesis in the Estrogen Induction of a Specific Uterine Protein. Proc. Natl. Acad. Sci., U. S., *66:*693, 1970.

25. DE SOMBRE, E. R., PUCA, G. A., and JENSEN, E. V.: Purification of an Estrophilic Protein from Calf Uterus. Proc. Natl. Acad. Sci., U. S., *64:*148, 1969.

26. DINGMAN, C. W. and SPORN, M. B.: Studies on Chromatin. I. Isolation and Characterization of Nuclear Complexes of Deoxyribonucleic Acid, Ribonucleic Acid, and Protein from Embryonic and Adult Tissues of the Chicken. J. Biol. Chem., *239:*3483, 1964.

27. DUKES, P. P. and SEKERIS, C. E.: Stimulierung des Einbaus von (2-^{14}C) Uracil in Ribonucleinsaüre von Rattenleberkernen durch Cortisol *in Vitro.* J. Physiol. Chem., *341:*149, 1965.

28. DUKES, P. P., SEKERIS, C. E., and SCHMID. W.: On the Mechanism of Hormone Action. VI. Increase in Template Activity of Ribonucleic Acid from Isolated Nuclei Incubated in the Presence of Hormone. Biochim. Biophys. Acta, *123:*126, 1966.

29. FANESTIL, D. D. and EDELMAN, I. S.: Characteristics of the Renal Nuclear Receptors for Aldosterone. Proc. Natl. Acad. Sci., U. S., *56:*872, 1966.

30. FRENSTER, J. H., ALLFREY, V. G., and MIRSKY, A. E.: Repressed and Active Chromatin Isolated from Interphase Lymphocytes. Proc. Natl. Acad. Sci., U. S., *50:*1026, 1963.

31. GILMOUR, R. S. and PAUL, J.: Role of Nonhistone Components in Determining Organ Specificity of Rabbit Chromatins. FEBS Letters, *9:*242, 1970.

32. GILMOUR, R. S. and PAUL, J.: RNA Transcribed from Reconstituted Nucleo-proteins is Similar to Natural RNA. J. Molec. Biol., *40:*137, 1959.

33. GORSKI, J., NOTEBOOM, W. D., and NICOLETTE, J. A.: Estrogen Control of the Synthesis of RNA and Protein in the Uterus. J. Cell Comp. Physiol., *66:* 91, 1965.

34. GROSSBACH, U.: Chromosomen-Akitivität und Biochemische Zelldifferenzierung in den Speicheldrüsen von Camptochironomus. Chromosoma, *28:*136, 1969.

35. GURLEY, L. R., IRVIN, J. L., and HOLBROOK, D. J.: Inhibition of DNA Polymerase by Histones. Biochem. Biophys. Res. Comm., *14:*527, 1964.

36. HAMILTON, T. H. and TENG, C. S.: Regulation by Estrogen of Synthesis of Chromatin-directed RNA and of Nonhistone Chromatin Proteins. Genetics, Suppl., *61:*381, 1969.

37. HINDLEY, J.: The Relative Ability of Reconstituted Nucleohistones to Allow DNA-dependent RNA Synthesis. Biochem. Biophys. Res. Comm., *12:*175, 1963.

38. HNILICA, L. S.: Proteins of the Cell Nucleus. Prog. Nucl. Acid. Res. Molec. Biol., *7:*25, 1967.

39. HNILICA, L. S. and BESS, L. G.: The Heterogeneity of Arginine-rich Histones. Anal. Biochem., *12:*421, 1965.

40. HNILICA, L. S. and BILLEN, D.: The Effect of DNA-Histone Interactions on the Biosynthesis of DNA *in Vitro.* Biochim. Biophys. Acta, *91:*271, 1964.

41. HOARE, T. A. and JOHNS, E. W.: The Physical State of Deoxyribonucleo-Protein and its Ability to Direct Ribonucleic Acid Synthesis *in Vitro.* Biochem. J., *119:* 931, 1970.

42. HUANG, R. C. C. and BONNER, J.: Histone-bound RNA, A Component of Native Nucleohistone. Proc. Natl. Acad. Sci., *54:*960, 1965.

43. HUANG, R. C. C. and BONNER, J.: Histones, a Supressor of Chromosomal RNA Synthesis. Proc. Natl. Acad. Sci., U. S., *41:*1216, 1962.

44. HUANG, R. C. C., BONNER, J., and MURRAY, K.: Physical and Biological Properties of Soluble Nucleohistones. J. Molec. Biol., *8:*54, 1964.

45. HUANG, R. C. C. and HUANG, P. C.: Effect of Protein-bound RNA Associated with Chick Embryo Chromatin on Template Specificity of the Chromatin. J. Molec. Biol., *39:*365, 1969.

46. JENSEN, E. V., NUMATA, M., SMITH, S., SUZUKI, T., BRECHER, P. I., and DESOMBRE, E. R.: Estrogen-Receptor Interaction in Target Tissues. Develop. Biol. Suppl., *3:*151, 1969.

47. JOHNS, E. W. and FORRESTER, S.: Interactions between Histone Fractions and DNA. Biochim. Biophys. Acta, *209:*54, 1970.

48. JOHNS, E. W. and HOARE, T. A.: Histones and Gene Control. Nature, *226:*650, 1970.

49. JOHRI, M. M. and VARNER, J. E.: Enhancement of RNA Synthesis in Isolated Pea Nuclei by Gibberellic Acid. Proc. Natl. Acad. Sci., U. S., *59:*269, 1968.

50. KARLSON, P.: New Concepts on the Mode of Action of Hormones. Perspectives Biol. Med., *6:*203, 1963.

51. KETTERER, B., ROSS-MANSEL, P., and WHITEHEAD, J. K.: The Isolation of Carcinogen-binding Protein from Livers of Rats Given 4-Dimethylaminoazobenzene. Biochem. J., *103:*316, 1967.

52. KIDSON, C.: Cortisol in the Regulation of RNA and Protein Synthesis. Nature, *215:*779, 1967.

53. KIDSON, C. and KIRBY, K. S.: Selective Alterations of Mammalian m-RNA Synthesis: Evidence for Differential Action of Hormone on Gene Transcription. Nature, *203:*599, 1964.

54. KIM, K. H. and COHEN, P. P.: Modification of Tadpole Liver Chromatin by Thyroxine Treatment. Proc. Natl. Acad. Sci., U. S., *55:*1251, 1966.

55. KING, R. B. J. and GORDON, J.: Properties of a Purified Nuclear Acidic Protein Fraction. Biochem. J., *112:*32p, 1969.

56. KING, R. B. J. and GORDON, J.: The Assoication of [6, 7-^{3}H] Oestradiol with a Nuclear Protein. J. Endocrinology, *39:*533, 1967.

57. KING, R. B. J., GORDON, J., COWAN, D. M., and INMAN, D. R.: The Intra-nuclear Localization of [6, 7-^{3}H] Oestradiol - 17β in Dimethylbenzanthracene-induced Rat Mammary Adenocarcinoma and Other Tissues. J. Endocrinology, *36:* 139, 1966.

58. KING, R. B. J.. GORDON, J., and MARTIN, L.: The Association of [6, 7-^{3}H] Oestradiol with Nuclear Chromatin. Biochem. J., *97:*28p, 1965.

59. KING, R. B. J., GORDON, J., and STEGGLES, A. W.: The Properties of a Nuclear Acidic Protein Fraction that Binds [6, 7-^{3}H] Oestradiol - 17β. Biochem. J., *114:*649, 1969.

60. KOSSEL, A.: The Protamines and Histones. Longmans-Green, London, 1928.

61. LIAO, S., BARTON, R. W., and LIN, A. H.: Differential Synthesis of Ribonucleic Acid in Prostatic Nuclei: Evidence for Selective Gene Transcription Induced by Androgens. Proc. Natl. Acad. Sci., U. S., *55:*1593, 1966.

62. LIAO, S. and HAMILTON, R. H.: Intracellular Localization of Growth Hormones in Plants. Science, *151:*822, 1966.

63. LIAO, S., LIN, A. H., and BARTON, R. W.: Selective Stimulation Ribonucleic Acid Synthesis in Prostatic Nuclei by Testosterone. J. Biol. Chem., *241:*3869, 1966.

64. LIAU, M. C., HNILICA, L. S., and HURLBERT, R. B.: Regulation of RNA Synthesis in Isolated Nucleoli by Histones and Nucleolar Proteins. Proc. Natl. Acad. Sci., U. S., *53:*626, 1965.

65. LITWACK, G. and MOREY, K. S.: Cortisol Metabolite Binder. I. Identity with the Dimethylaminoazobenzene Binding Protein of Liver Cytosol. Biochem. Biophys. Res. Comm., *38:*1141, 1970.

66. LUKACS, I. and SEKERIS, C. E.: On the Mechanism of Hormone Action. IX. Stimulation of RNA Polymerase Activity of Rat Liver Nuclei by Cortisol *in Vitro.* Biochim. Biophys. Acta, *134:*85, 1967.

67. MARUSHIGE, K. and BONNER, J.: Template Properties of Liver Chromatin. J. Molec. Biol., *15:*160, 1966.

68. MATTHYSSE, A. G.: Organ Specificity of Hormone-Receptor-Chromatin Interaction. Biochim. Biophys. Acta, *199:*519, 1970.

69. MATTHYSSE, A. G.: The Effect of Auxin on RNA Synthesis. Plant. Physiol., *43:* S-42, 1968.

70. MATTHYSSE, A. G. and ABRAMS, M.: A Factor Mediating Interaction of Klinnis with Genetic Material. Biochim. Biophys. Acta, *199:*511, 1968.

71.   MATTHYSSE, A. G. and PHILLIPS, C.: A Protein Intermediary in the Interaction of a Hormone with the Genome. Proc. Natl. Acad. Sci., U. S., *63*:897, 1969.

72.   MAURER, R. and CHALKLEY, G. R.: Some Properties of a Nuclear Binding Site of Estradiol. J. Molec. Biol., *27:*431, 1967.

73.   MONDER, C. and WALKER, M. C.: Interaction between Corticosteroids and Histones. Biochem., *9:*2489, 1970.

74.   MOREY, K. S. and LITWACK, G.: Isolation and Properties of Cortisol Metabolite Binding Proteins of Rat Liver Cytosol. Biochemistry, *8:*4813, 1969.

75.   NOMURA, M., TRAUB, P., GUTHRIE, G., and NASHIMOTO, H.: The Assembly of Ribosomes. J. Cell Physiol., *74*:Suppl. 1 241, 1969.

76.   NOTIDES, A. and GORSKI, J.:Estrogen-induced Synthesis of a Specific Uterine Protein. Proc. Natl. Acad. Sci., U. S., *56*:230, 1966.

77.   O'MALLEY, B. W., McGUIRE, W. L., KOHLER, P. O., and KORENMAN, S. G.: Studies on the Mechanism of Steroid Hormone Regulation of Synthesis of Specific Proteins. Rec. Prog. Horm. Res., *25*:105, 1969.

78.   O'MALLEY, B. W., SHERMAN, M. R., and TOFT, D. O.: Progesterone 'Receptors' in the Cytoplasm and Nucleus of Chick Oviduct Target Tissue. Proc. Natl. Acad. Sci., U. S., *67*:501, 1970.

79.   O'MALLEY, B. W., TOFT, D. O., and SHERMAN, M. R.: Progesterone-binding Components of Chick Oviduct. J. Biol. Chem., *246:*117, 1971.

80.   O'MEARA, A. R. and HERRMANN, R. L.: A Biphase Activation of Template by Removal of Protein from Liver Chromatin., Federation Proc., *29:*913a, 1970.

81.   PAUL, J.: DNA Masking in Mammalian Chromatin: A Molecular Mechanism for Determination of Cell Type. Current Topics in Develop. Biol., *5:*317, 1970.

82.   PAUL, J.: Molecular Aspects of Cytodifferentiation. Adv. Comp. Physiol. Biochem., *3:*115, 1968.

83.   PAUL, J. and GILMOUR, R. S.: Organ-specific Restriction of Transcription in Mammalian Chromatin. J. Molec. Biol., *34:*305, 1968.

84.   PAUL, J. and GILMOUR, R. S.:Template Activity of DNA is Restricted in Chromatin. J. Molec. Biol., *16:*242, 1966.

85.   PAUL, J. and GILMOUR, R. S.: Restriction of Deoxyribonucleic Acid Template Activity in Chromatin is Organ Specific. Nature, *210:*992, 1966.

86.   POGO, B. G. T., POGO, A. O. and ALLFREY, V. G.: Histone Acetylation and RNA Synthesis in Rat Liver Regeneration. Genetics, *61*:Suppl. 1,373, 1969.

87;   ROCHEFORT, H. and BAULIEU, E.: New *in-Vitro* Studies of Estradiol Binding in Castrated Rat Uterus. Endocrinology, *84*:108, 1969.

88.   ROYCHOUNDHURY, R. DATTA, A., and SEN, S. P.: The Mechanism of Action of Plant Growth Substances: The Role of Nuclear RNA in Growth Substance Action. Biochim. Biophys, Acta, *107:*346, 1965.

89.   ROYCHOUNDHURY, R. and SEN, S. P.: Metabolic Conversion of Thymine-2-C^{14} and Its Incorporation into Nuclear RNA of Endosperm Nuclei of *Cocos nucifera*, Linn. Biochem. Biophys. Res. Comm., *14:*7, 1963.

90. SEKERIS, C. E., DUKES, P. P., and SCHMID, W.: Wirkung von Ecdyson auf Epidermiszellkerne von Calliphora-Larven *in Vitro.* J. Physiol. Chem., *341:*152, 1965.

91. SEKERIS, C. E. and LANG, N.: Binding von (^{3}H)Cortison an Histone aus Rattenleber. Hoppe-Seyler's Z. Physiol. Chem., *340:*92, 1965.

92. SELIGY, V. L. and NEELIN, J. M.: Transcription Properties of Stepwise Acid-Extracted Chicken Erythrocyte Chromatin. Biochim. Biophys. Acta, *213:*380, 1970.

93. SHELTON, K. R. and ALLFREY, V. G.: Selective Synthesis of a Nuclear Acidic Protein in Liver Cells Stimulated by Cortisol. Nature, *228:*132, 1970.

94. SHYAMALA, G. and GORSKI, J.: Estrogen Receptors in the Rat Uterus. J. Biol. Chem., *244:*1097, 1967.

95. SKALKA, A., FOWLER, A. V., and HURWITZ, J.: The Effect of Histones on the Enzymatic Synthesis of Ribonucleic Acid. J. Biol. Chem., *241:*588, 1966.

96. SLUYSER, M.: Interaction of Steroid Hormones with Histones *in Vitro.* Biochim. Biophys. Acta, *182:*235, 1969.

97. SLUYSER, M.: Binding of Hydrocortisone to Rat Liver Histones. J. Molec. Biol., *19:*591, 1966.

98. SLUYSER, M.: Binding of Testosterone and Hydrocortisone to Rat-Tissue Histones. J. Molec. Biol., *22:*411, 1966.

99. SMITH, J. A., MARTIN, L., and KING, R. J. B.: Effect of Oestradiol-17β and Progesterone on Nuclear-Protein Synthesis in the Mouse Uterus. Biochem. J., *114:*59p, 1969.

100. SMITH, K. D., CHURCH, R. B., and McCARTHY, B. J.: Template Specificity of Isolated Chromatin. Biochemistry, *8:*4271, 1969.

101. SONNENBERG, B. P. and ZUBAY, G.: Nucleohistone as a Primer for RNA Synthesis. Proc. Natl. Acad. Sci., U. S., *54:*415, 1965.

102. SPELSBERG, T. C. and HNILICA, L. S.: Proteins of Chromatin in Template Restriction. I. RNA Synthesis *in Vitro.* Biochim. Biophys. Acta, *228:*202, 1971a.

103. SPELSBERG, T. C. and HNILICA, L. S.: Proteins of Chromatin in Template Restriction. II. Specificity of RNA Synthesis. Biochim. Biophys. Acta, *228:*212, 1971b.

104. SPELSBERG, T. C. and HNILICA, L. S.: Deoxyribonucleoproteins and Tissue-Specific Restriction of the Deoxyribonucleic Acid in Chromatin. Biochem. J., *120:* 435, 1970.

105. SPELSBERG, T. C. and HNILICA, L. S.: Studies on the RNA Polymerase-Histone Complexes. Biochim. Biophys. Acta, *195:*55, 1969.

106. SPELSBERG, T. C., HNILICA, L. S., and ANSEVIN, A. T.: Proteins of Chromatin in Template Restriction. III. The Macromolecules in Specific Restriction of the Chromatin DNA. Biochim. Biophys. Acta, *228:*550, 1970.

107. SPELSBERG, T. C. and SARKISSIAN, I. V.: Isolation and Analysis of the Proteins of Plant Nuclei: Interaction of Hormones with Nuclear Proteins in Isolated Nuclei of *Phaseolus vulgaris.* Phytochemistry, *9:*1203, 1970.

108. SPELSBERG, T. C. and STEGGLES, A. W., and O'MALLEY, B. W.: Progesterone-binding Components of Chick Oviduct. III. Chromatin Acceptor Sites. J. Biol. Chem., *246:*4188, 1971.

109. SPELSBERG, T. C., TANKERSLEY, S., and HNILICA, L. S.: Inhibition of RNA Poly-
     merase Enzyme by Arginine-rich Histones. Experientia, *25:*129, 1969.

110. STACKHOUSE, H. L., CHETSANGA, C. J., and TAN, C. H.: The Effect of Cortisol on
     Genetic Transcription in Rat Liver Chromatin. Biochim. Biophys. Acta,
     *155:*159, 1968.

111. STEDMAN, E. and STEDMAN, E.: The Basic Proteins of Cell Nuclei. Phil. Trans.
     Royal Soc., London, B*235:*565, 1951.

112. STEDMAN, E. and STEDMAN, E.: Cell Specificity of Histones. Nature, *166:*780, 1950.

113. STEGGLES, A. W., SPELSBERG, T. C., GLASSER, S. R., and O'MALLEY, B. W.: Sol-
     uble Complexes between Steroid Hormones and Target-tissue Receptors Bind
     Specifically to Target-tissue Chromatin. Proc. Natl. Acad. Sci., U. S., *68:*1479,
     1971.

114. STEGGLES, A. W., SPELSBERG, T. C., and O'MALLEY, B. W.: Tissue Specific Bind-
     ing *in Vitro* of Progesterone-Receptor to the Chromatin of Chick Tissue. Biochem.
     Biophys. Res. Comm., *43:*20, 1971.

115. STELLWAGEN, R. H. and COLE, R. D.: Chromosomal Proteins. Ann. Rev. Biochem.
     *38:*951, 1969.

116. STELLWAGEN, R. H. and COLE, R. D.: Danger of Contamination in Chromatograph-
     ically Prepared Arginine-rich Histone. J. Biol. Chem., *243:*4452, 1968.

117. STELLWAGEN, R. H. and COLE, R. D.: Comparison of Histones Obtained from
     Mammary Gland at Different Stages of Development and Lacation. J . Biol. Chem..
     *243:*4456, 1968.

118. SUNAGA, K. and KOIDE, S. S.: Interaction of Calf Thymus Histones and DNA with
     Steroids. Steroids, *9:*451, 1967.

119. SUNAGA, K. and KOIDE, S. S.: Factors Influencing the Interaction of Steroids with
     Calf Thymus Histones. Arch. Biochem. Biophys., *122:*670, 1967.

120. SUNAGA, K. and KOIDE, S. S.: Structural Specificity of the Steroids Interacting
     with Calf Thymus Histones. Biochem. Biophys. Res. Comm., *26:*342, 1967.

121. SWANECK, G. E., CHU, L. L. H., and EDELMAN, I. S.: Sterospecific Binding of Aldo-
     sterone to Renal Chromatin. J. Biol. Chem., *245:*5382, 1970.

122. TALWAR, G. P., SEGAL, S. J., EVANS, A., and DAVIDSON, O. W.: The Binding of
     Estradiol in the Uterus: A Mechanism for Derepression of RNA Synthesis.
     Proc. Natl. Acad. Sci., U. S., *52:*1059, 1964.

123. TAN, C. H. and MIYAGI, M.: Specificity of Transcription of Chromatin *in Vitro*.
     J. Molec. Biol., *50:*641, 1970.

124. TATA, J. R.: Hormone and the Synthesis and Utilization of Ribonucleic Acid. Prog.
     Nucl. Acid. Res. Molec. Biol., *5:*191, 1966.

125. TENG, C. S. and HAMILTON, T. H.: Regulation by Estrogen of Organ-specific
     Synthesis of a Nuclear Acidic Protein. Biochem. Biophys. Res. Comm., *40:*
     1231, 1970.

126. TENG, C. S. and HAMILTON, T. H.: Role of Chromatin in Estrogen Action in the
     Uterus. II. Hormone-induced Synthesis of Nonhistone Acidic Proteins which
     Restore Histone-inhibited DNA-dependent RNA Synthesis. Proc. Natl. Acad.
     Sci., U. S., *63:*465, 1969.

127. TENG, C. S. and HAMILTON, T. H.: The Role of Chromatin in Estrogen Action in the Uterus. I. The Control of Template Capacity and Chemical Composition and and the Binding of H^3-Estradiol-17β. Proc. Natl. Acad. Sci., U. S., *60:*1410, 1968.

128. TREWAVAS, A. J.Effect of IAA on RNA and Protein Synthesis. Effect of 3-Indolylacetic Acid on the Metabolism of Ribonucleic Acid and Protein in Etiolated Subapical Sections of *Pisum sativum.* Atch. Biochem. Biophys., *123:*324, 1968.

129. TSAI, Y. H. and HNILICA, L. S.: Interaction of Histones with Corticosteroid Hormones. Biochim. Biophys. Acta, *238:*277, 1971.

130. WILSON, J. D. and LOEB, P. M.: Estrogen and Androgen Control of Cell Biosynthesis in Target Organs. *In*: Developmental and Metabolic Control Mechanism and Neoplasia, p. 375. Baltimore: Williams and Wilkins, 1965.

131. WOOD, W. G., IRVIN, J. L., and HOLBROOK, D. J.: Inhibition of Calf Thymus Deoxyribonucleic Acid Polymerase by Histones. Biochemistry, *7:*2256, 1968.

132. ZALOKAR, M.: *In:* D. M. Bonner (ed.), Control Mechanisms in Cellular Processes. p. 87. New York: Ronald Press, 1961.

133. ZUBAY, G. and DOTY, P.: The Isolation and Properties of Deoxyribonucleoprotein Particles Containing Single Nucleic Acid Molecules. J. Molec. Biol., *1:*1, 1959.

MECHANISMS of RNA SYNTHESIS and POSSIBLE SITES for INTERACTION with HORMONES

R. B. Hurlbert

HORMONAL EFFECTS ON RNA SYNTHESIS

The request to discuss some of the aspects of mammalian RNA synthesis and metabolism which might be the most susceptible to regulation by hormones will be met by mentioning some of our own work which may be the most pertinent to mechanism of action of steroid hormones with only a very limited review of the literature. Several excellent reviews are cited below (Grant, 1969; Hamilton, 1971; Tata, 1970). Although none of our own work on RNA syntheses in nuclei and nucleoli has specifically utilized hormone-dependent systems, we have sought to study regulatory steps in these processes which might, with equal likelihood, be involved in carcinogenic transformation or hormone responses.

It is clear that, whatever the initial sites of action of these steroid hormones are (whether on DNA, RNA, enzymes, carrier proteins, regulatory proteins, membrane components, or other agents), the stimulation of RNA synthesis is the first major effect to be consistently observed thus far, and that this change in RNA synthesis is necessary for expression of the hormonal action *via* an altered balance of enzymatic activities of the target organ. First the possibilities of a direct effect of a hormone on the transcription of RNA will be considered in a general way, and then the various species of RNA will be considered separately.

Messenger RNA

Much of current thinking rests upon Jacob and Monod's theory of regulation of genetic activity in microorganisms, and according to Professor Karlson's concepts (Karlson, 1968) it is believed that the hormone derepresses the transcription of the mRNAs for certain enzymes. Since a number of coordinated cellular activities are stimulated by this class of hormones, it would appear either that a common repressor (capable of binding the hormone to cause a transition between repressive activity and inactivity) exists for this group of mRNAs, that an appropriate number of different repressors (each capable of binding the hormone) exists, or that some mechanism for amplifying the action of the hormone exists. Professor Karlson has already discussed those possibilities, including the theory of Britten and Davidson (1969), which might provide the necessary amplification (Chapter 3).

Transfer RNA

It is not, however, essential to consider that these hormones act exclusively on transcription of mRNA. Any alteration in the rate of synthesis of selected transfer RNAs could well exert definite effects on the synthesis of specific proteins. Redundancy of the genetic code and the existence of iso-accepting tRNAs both permit the possibility that expression of a certain critical mRNA can be controlled by the availability of a tRNA unique to that mRNA. Changes in the amount and proportion of the different components of the tRNA population have been correlated with differences in species, state of differentiation, malignancy, and other metabolic states, including response to hormones (Novelli, 1969).

Ribosomal RNA

The growth-and-development types of hormones cause a generalized increase in many diverse enzymatic activities. It appears logical that a stimulation of synthesis of rRNA and ribosomes could readily account for such an effect. Because the rRNA molecules are transcribed from a relatively small number of (presumably) identical cistrons, the control by a small number of active ribosomes should accentuate the phenotypic characteristics of the cell by permitting greater utilization of the available genetic messages. (One must however assume here that the production of mRNAs is in excess, or is controlled by availability of ribosomes, and that the proportions of the critical mRNAs are such that they would be selected in significantly different amounts upon alteration in the flux of new ribosomes.) Much of the evidence regarding the stimulation by these hormones points to increased formation of ribosomal RNA (Tata, 1970), although this interpretation is by no means unequivocal (Church and McCarthy, 1970).

Regulation of Transcription

Dr. Hnilica has discussed in another chapter the role of histone and non-histone proteins in modifying the template ability of chromatin by binding to the DNA and acting as general repressors or specific repressors, which could in turn be modulated by the binding of hormones.

The possibility of a regulatory action of hormones on RNA polymerase itself must also be considered. Microbial RNA polymerases have been shown to consist of cooperative subunits plus initiation (Travers and Burgess, 1969) and termination (Roberts, 1969) factors. The sigma factor aids the polymerase molecule in recognizing and binding to the correct site for initiation of a genetic message (phage), whereas the rho factor aids the polymerase in recognizing the correct termination point with the release of the mRNA. Whether animal cells possess similar factors or a multiplicity of them has not been established; it is, however, apparent that interaction of such factors with regulatory chemical signals (whether representing feedback from cellular processes or consisting of hormonal agents) is an attractive possibility.

The existence of several forms of RNA polymerase in animal cells has however been demonstrated, and more importantly some of these forms have been localized in either nucleolus or nucleoplasm, with a strong indication that they possess specificity for synthesis of rRNA or mRNA, respectively (Roeder and Rutter, 1970). Dr. Sekeris has just discussed his own work with these multiple forms of the enzyme. It is quite apparent that many interesting mechanisms of the regulation of RNA polymerase activity remain to be discovered, and the question is whether intervention of hormones will be among them.

Possible Action of Hormones on RNA Synthetic Processes Other than Transcription

It is assumed that these hormones act by binding to specific receptor sites on appropriate proteins, thereby changing the conformation of the protein and its ability to carry out yet another binding or catalytic action. (Other possibilities may exist, but direct binding of steroids to DNA or RNA now seems unlikely to be effective at physiological concentrations.) Within this assumption, several other sites of action of hormones could quite conceivably exert a dramatic effect on the rate of production of metabolically effective RNA molecules or transportation of these molecules from nucleus to cytoplasm. Examples of such sites are:

1.   Alteration of the activity or specificity of the enzyme that methylates preribosomal RNA in the nucleolus (Muramatsu and Fujisawa, 1968). It is believed that the location of methyl groups on the 45 S preribosomal RNA controls the sites of action of the nucleases that process the molecule to the smaller 28 and 18 S ribosomal RNA subunits.

2.   The rate or specificity of the enzymes that methylate transfer tRNAs could be altered, which might have rather subtle effects initially but result later in a considerable change in the metabolic balance.

3.   The rate and selectivity of the transport of mRNA molecules to the cytoplasm could be altered, perhaps by modification of the carrier protein or by modulation of a mechanism for destruction of surplus mRNA molecules.

These three examples are by no means the only conceivable ones; they are selected mainly because some of our work provides systems by which these examples could be tested.

It should also be considered that hormones might have their primary effect on systems that we do not yet know how to test. It seems almost certain (more or less intuitively) that feedback regulatory systems must exist in the cell whereby the rate of formation of specific mRNAs is governed in some way by the net activity of the enzymes for which they code. Small-molecule chemical signals, possibly substrates or products or components of the enzymes involved, could conceivably interact specifically with the mechanisms for synthesis, transport, or translation of these corresponding messenger RNAs. By alteration of the production of these chemical signals, hormones could even act on such regulatory systems without themselves entering the nucleus or participating directly.

STUDIES ON SYNTHESIS OF RNA AND PROTEIN
IN ISOLATED NUCLEI AND NUCLEOLI

Since we tend to the view that some of the mechanisms of action of hormones will have to be resolved at the nuclear or subnuclear level, some of our own work has a bearing on the subject of this volume. First some of our recent findings on the synthesis and processing of ribosomal RNA and synthesis of protein in isolated nucleoli will be mentioned, and then recent work on the mechanism of turnover of rapidly labeled or heterogeneous nuclear RNA will be discussed.

The nucleolus of the Novikoff tumor cell is a surprisingly complex organelle. Its previously known components include RNA polymerase (Liau *et al.*, 1965) and the cistrons for ribosomal RNA (Hurlbert *et al.*, 1969) in addition to other components common to nucleoli; condensed DNA nucleoprotein, preribosomal RNA in the form of ribonucleoprotein particles, and the enzymes, DPN pyrophosphorylase, ribonuclease, and ATPase. A number of low-molecular-weight RNAs have also been observed (Nakamura *et al.*, 1968). Our recent work shows that this organelle also contains one or more ribosomal RNA methylases and several tRNA methylases (Liau *et al.*, 1970), a large number of tRNAs, and a corresponding number of amino-acid-activating enzymes. It has been found that these nucleoli contain a complete protein-synthesizing system that is tightly integrated and does not require an exogenous source of energy.

Synthesis of Preribosomal RNA

Dr. Ming C. Liau has developed techniques for following some of the steps in biosynthesis of ribosomal RNA in nucleoli isolated from the Novikoff tumor. He can observe *in vitro* the initial formation of labeled 45 S preribosomal RNA and the shift of label into intermediates in the degradative conversion of this RNA into 18 and 28 S RNA molecules. He can measure the action of rRNA methylase, which utilizes S-adenosyl methionine to methylate the 2'-OH position of the ribose group of a few of the RNA nucleotides and has demonstrated that it acts on the nascent rRNA. Isolated nucleoli have thereby been shown to offer practical subjects for further studies on initiation of the polymerase action, transcription of the ribosomal cistrons, and the relationships between the action of specific methylases and the processing by nucleases. Study of the action of other agents, such as histones and nonhistone proteins on these steps is now needed. It is also apparent that action of regulatory agents, such as hormones, on one or more of these steps could exert definite effects on rate of synthesis of ribosomes.

Dr. Liau has also found and described in these nucleoli another class of methylases, which methylate some of the purine and pyrimidine bases of exogenous transfer RNAs (Liau *et al.*, 1970). The nucleolar tRNA methylases represent about 5 per cent of the total cellular tRNA methylase activity and have a unique pattern of specificity for the purine and pyrimidine bases. We suggest that they function as part of the system for synthesizing nucleolar protein.

Protein Synthesis in Isolated Nucleoli

Lamkin (Lamkin and Hurlbert, 1972) has shown conclusively that Novikoff nucleoli do contain a complete, tightly-integrated, protein-synthesizing system. Labeled amino acids, singly or in full complement, are incorporated into nucleolar protein without addition of any of the factors known to be necessary for the cytoplasmic system (ATP, tRNA, activating and transfer enzymes, *etc.*) She has found that these nucleoli contain activating enzymes for each of the amino acids and that each amino acid is transferred to low-molecular-weight RNA as an aminoacyl substituent. Presumably, other components of protein synthesis are also present; it will be of interest to characterize the types of protein synthesized and determine whether they have roles in synthesis of ribosomal nucleoprotein or regulation thereof.

Turnover and Nature of Heterogeneous Nuclear RNA

HnRNA is synthesized in the extranucleolar regions of the nucleus; the term is derived from the wide distribution of molecular weights of the newly synthesized RNA, as analyzed by sucrose-gradient centrifugation. This type of RNA represents a large (up to 80 per cent) portion of the newly synthesized, nonribosomal RNA and has most of the properties expected of messenger RNA. That is, it is rapidly synthesized, turns over rapidly, is heterogeneous in size, is complementary to many sites on the genome, and has a DNA-like composition. Yet, the anomalous situation exists that this RNA is apparently degraded within the nucleus and is never utilized as the messenger strand of the polysomes. Further knowledge of the function and process of degradation of this type of RNA is needed. It is not known whether heterogeneous nuclear RNA is truly messenger RNA. If it is, mechanisms must exist for selection of those messages needed for actual translation and selection of those to be destroyed. The choice between utilized and nonutilized RNA may be a vital part of the mechanism for control of genetic expression. Even if the heterogeneous nuclear RNA is nonmessage RNA, the questions of its function remain pertinent; Bonner (Mayfield *et al.*, 1971) has recently postulated that HnRNA is the source of chromosomal RNA which he believes to be a regulator of genic transcription.

Knowledge of the degradative mechanism is a necessary part of studies on the origin, function, and selection of these RNA species and is also interesting from the viewpoint of energy metabolism. The biosynthesis of nucleotides and polynucleotides consumes a large amount of metabolic energy (in terms of ATP utilized). Much of this energy would be wasted if the degraded RNA species were hydrolyzed to the 2'-(3')-nucleotides, nucleosides, and bases by the usual action of nucleases, phosphatases, and nucleosidases. It is more reasonable to postulate that the RNA is degraded by mechanisms that permit re-utilization of the components at some higher level of energy, such as the 5'-nucleotides, that would be in close equilbrium with RNA. That this mechanism of turnover indeed exists has been indicated by the work of H. Harris and J. Watts in 1961 (Watts, 1969), who showed that some 5'-adenosine nucleotides were released from nuclear RNA, although the quantitative yield was low. Lazarus and Sporn (1967) have also identified an exonuclease in ascites nuclei that cleaves RNA to 5'-nucleotides.

We have recently examined several aspects of this turnover of RNA by use of nuclei first labeled *in vivo* then incubated *in vitro*. These nuclei were isolated in isotonic sucrose from the livers of rats 2 hours after injection of ^{14}C-orotic acid, a procedure that labels hepatic RNA uracil preferentially. The nuclei then were incubated in media containing ATP, UTP, CTP, and GTP under conditions known from previous work (Hurlbert *et al.*, 1969; Takahashi *et al.*, 1963) to permit optimal incorporation of these precursors into RNA. The loss of the labeled RNA to acid-soluble materials was studied. It was found that a 60 per cent loss of ^{14}C-RNA to acid-soluble materials occurred in 30-40 minutes, whereas only 10-15 per cent of the total (unlabeled) nuclear RNA was degraded. During this same period of incubation, a normal incorporation of ^{3}H-CTP *in vitro* into nuclear RNA was measured showing that both synthesis and degradation can occur simultaneously (Figure 1).

The ^{14}C-labeled, acid-soluble material was found by electrophoretic analysis to contain about 40 per cent uridine and 30 per cent uridine phosphate. The question was whether the uridine phosphate was the 2'-(3')- or the 5'-isomer, and whether the uridine was split off directly or arose from hydrolysis of the uridine nucleotides. Both of the nucleotide isomers can be attacked by phosphatases to give uridine, but only the 5'-isomer can be phosphorylated enzymatically to UTP. Therefore, an ATP-generating system and a nucleotide phosphokinase (present in an extract of rat liver) were included in the incubation; these permitted the recovery of 70-75 per cent of the label as UTP, 7 per cent as UDP, 5 per cent as UMP, and 12-16 per cent as uridine. This proved with reasonable certainty that the degradation of the rapidly labeled RNA results in conversion of most of the uracil moiety to 5'-UMP, which is then readily available by normal cellular mechanisms for phosphorylation to UTP and re-incorporation into RNA. A cycle for turnover of the heterogeneous nuclear RNA therefore exists and is practical from the stand-

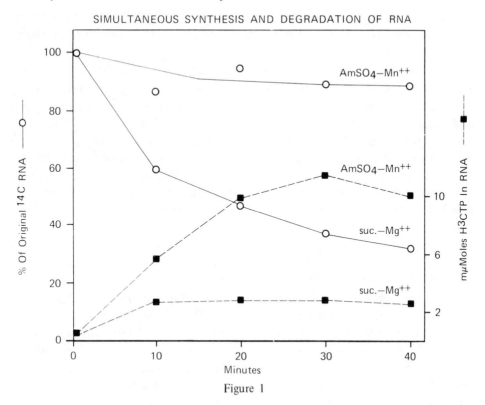

Figure 1

Turnover of RNA in Hepatic Nuclei *in Vitro*

Nuclei were prepared by isotonic procedures (Hurlbert *et al.*, 1969) from the liver of a 150-G. rat that had received 3.3 μCi. (3.3 μmoles) of orotic acid-6-^{14}C two hours previously. The nuclei were incubated at $37°$ C. in isotonic sucrose-Mg[++] or 0.4 M. ammonium sulfate-Mn[++] medium containing ^{3}H-CTP for the times indicated, then were precipitated and washed with cold perchloric acid. The nucleic acids (only RNA was labeled under these conditions) were extracted by hot perchloric acid ($100°$ C., 15 minutes) and the amounts of ^{14}C and ^{3}H in the extracts were determined by direct counting of 0.5 ml. aliquots in 10 ml. of Aquasol scintillation solution (New England Nuclear Corp.). Amounts of RNA and DNA were also determined. The solid lines represent loss of ^{14}C-uracil from prelabeled RNA, and the dashed lines represent incorporation into RNA of ^{3}H-CMP from CTP, both during the incubation.

The Suc-Mg[++] medium contained in a final volume of 2.0 ml.: 100 mM. tris-HCl, pH 8.5; 150 mM. sucrose; 7.5 mM. MgCl$_2$; 1.0 mM. each of UTP, CTP, GTP, and ATP; 5 mM. phosphoenol pyruvate and 20 μG./ml. of PEP kinase; and 20 mM. cysteine. The AmSO$_4$-Mn[++] medium contained 1.2 mM. MnCl$_2$ and 2.5 mM. MgCl$_2$ instead of the above Mg[++] concentration and, in addition to the above components, 400 mM. ammonium sulfate. Each tube also contained 20 x 10[6] d.p.m. of ^{3}H-CTP and an amount of nuclei containing 0.35–0.40 mg. of DNA.

lation to UTP and re-incorporation into RNA. A cycle for turnover of the heterogeneous nuclear RNA therefore exists and is practical from the standpoint of energy metabolism.

Inhibition of the presumed exonuclease activity was studied. The activity was the same whether or not RNA synthesis was occurring (*i.e.*, actinomycin or omission of nucleotides had no effect.) Phosphate ions had no effect; this and other evidence rule out formation of UDP by polynucleotide phosphorylase as the degradative mechanism. Fluoride, pyrophosphate, uridine-3'-phosphate, and cytidine-3'-phosphate were inhibitory, as reported for the exonuclease purified by Lazarus and Sporn (1967). Ammonium sulfate, 0.2-0.4 M., inhibited almost completely the degradation of both labeled and unlabeled RNA while at the same time stimulating the incorporation of ^{3}H-CMP from CTP (Figure 1).

The inhibition by ammonium sulfate of the degradation of heterogeneous nuclear RNA is of some interest by itself. Following the observations of Widnell and Tata (Tata, 1970), it has been observed frequently that addition of 0.4 M. ammonium sulfate (or other salts of comparable ionic strength) to a suspension of nuclei engaged in RNA synthesis will stimulate both the rate and extent of RNA synthesis. As we (Hurlbert *et al.*, 1969) and others have described, the composition of the RNA formed is shifted from ribosomal RNA-like in the isotonic medium (with Mg^{++}) to DNA-like in the high-ionic-strength medium (with Mn^{++}). It appears that the high-ionic-strength medium permits the partial activity of any previously formed complex of template DNA with RNA polymerase and initiated RNA strands while inhibiting completely the formation of any new complexes.

When nuclei from target tissues of animals treated with steroid hormones are incubated under the isotonic conditions (with Mn^{++}), the rRNA-like RNA synthesizing activity is significantly increased in comparison with control nuclei (Grant, 1969; Hamilton, 1971; Tata, 1970). When, however, the comparison is made under conditions of high ionic strength, both treated and control nuclei are stimulated, but the difference is no longer observed, at least for short-term hormonal effects. The inference is that the effect of the hormone is on actual, or net, template activity (isotonic sucrose-Mg^{++}), whereas potential activity of RNA polymerase and DNA template (ammonium sulfate-Mn^{++}) remains unaffected for the first few hours of hormonal action. We have previously favored the viewpoint (Hurlbert *et al.*, 1969) that the effect of ammonium sulfate was primarily to dissociate histones (and perhaps other proteins) from the DNA template to permit unrestricted transcription and regarded the observed inhibition of ribonuclease as a secondary benefit.

It now seems more likely that the main effect of the ammonium sulfate is to inhibit the exonuclease responsible for degradation of heterogeneous nuto inhibit the exonuclease responsible for degradation of heterogeneous nuclear RNA, and that HnRNA is the primary product being measured under isotonic conditions; heterogeneous nuclear RNA is formed but is immediately degraded, leaving the nucleolar rRNA precursor as the main product measured.

In conclusion then, we postulate the following:

Heterogeneous nuclear RNA represents the products of transcription of the chromosomal genes and much of it is potentially messenger RNA. These potential messenger RNAs are, however, susceptible to stepwise hydrolysis by an exoribonuclease that clips off 5′-nucleotides. These nucleotides are readily rephosphorylated to the nucleoside-5′-triphosphates and re-incorported into new RNA strands. We believe that a mechanism must exist for selection of certain HnRNA molecules to be translated. This mechanism would involve protection of an RNA molecule from the exonuclease (and an endonuclease that is also observed to be present) plus association with a carrier protein during transport to the cytoplasm and combination with ribosomes into a functional polysome. While some of this is conjecture, it is apparent that some means must exist to protect a true messenger RNA from the nuclease action and that selection between those RNA molecules to be expressed and those to be destroyed is a critical process which is a potential site for the hormonal action.

Acknowledgement

This work was supported by Grants CA 10244 from USPHS and E-609 from the American Cancer Society. Institutional Grants from the John Q. Gaines Foundation and from the American Cancer Society (IN-43-K) specifically for the work on HnRNA are also gratefully acknowledged. The major participation of Miss Dorothy Norlin and Miss Marian Stankovitch in the HnRNA work is also greatly appreciated.

References

1. BRITTEN, R. J. and DAVIDSON, E.: Gene Regulation for Higher Cells: A Theory. Science, *165:*349, 1969.

2. CHURCH, R. B. and McCARTHY, B. J.: Unstable Nuclear RNA Synthesis Following Estrogen Stimulation. Biochim. Biophys. Acta, *199:*103, 1970.

3. GRANT, J. K.: Actions of Steroid Hormones at Cellular and Molecular Levels. *In:* P. N. Campbell and G. D. Greville (ed.), Essays in Biochemistry, *5:*1. New York: Academic Press, 1969.

4. HAMILTON, T. H.: Effects of Sexual Steroid Hormones on Genetic Transcription and Translation. In; *Basic Actions of Sex Steroids in Target Organs*, pp. 56-92,

5. HURLBERT, R. B., MILLER, E. G. and VAUGHAN, C. L.: Control of RNA Poly-merase Reactions in Isolated Nuclei and Nucleoli. In: *Advances in Enzyme Regulation,* 7, p. 219, Ed., G. Weber; Pergamon Press, 1969.

6. KARLSON, P.: Regulation of Gene Activity by Hormones. Humangenetik, *6:*99. 1968.

7. LAMKIN, A. F., and HURLBERT, R. B.: Amino Acid Activation by Nucleoli Isolated from the Novikoff Asciter Tumor. Biochem. Biophys. Acta, *272:*321, 1972.

8. LAZARUS, H. M. and SPORN, M. B.: Purification and Properties of a Nuclear Exoribonuclease from Ehrlich Ascites Tumor Cells. Proc. Natl. Acad. Sci. (U. S.), *57:*1386, 1967.

9. LIAU, M. C., FLATT, N. C., and HURLBERT, R. B.: Methylation of Preribosomal and Transfer RNA's by Isolated Nucleoli of the Novikoff Rat Tumor. Biochem. Biophys. Acta, *224:*282, 1970.

10. LIAU, M. C., HNILICA, L. S., and HURLBERT, R. B.: Regulation of RNA Synthe-sis in Isolated Nucleoli by Histones and Nucleolar Proteins. Proc. Natl. Acad. Sci. (U. S.), *53:*626, 1965.

11. MAYFIELD, J. E., HOLMES, D. S., and BONNER, J.: Rapidly-labeled Nuclear RNA is the Precursor of Chromosomal RNA. Biophysical Society Abstracts, *11:*150a, 1971.

12. MURAMATSU, M. and FUJISAWA, T.: Methylation of Ribosomal RNA Precursor and tRNA in Rat Liver, Biochem. Biophys. Acta, *157:*476, 1968.

13: NAKAMURA, T., PRESTAYKO, A. W., and BUSCH, H.: Studies on Nucleolar 4-6 S RNA of Novikoff Hepatoma Cells. J. Biol. Chem., *243:*1368, 1968.

14. NOVELLI, G. D.: The Separation of Isoaccepting Transfer RNA's and the Possible Role of tRNA in Regulation. J. Cell Physiol., *74*(1):121-148, 1969.

15: ROBERTS, J. W.: Termination Factor for RNA Synthesis. Nature, *224:*1168, 1969.

16: ROEDER, R. G. and RUTTER, W. J.: Specific Nucleolar and Nucleoplasmic RNA Pojymerases. Proc. Natl. Acad. Sci. (U. S.), *65:*675, 1970.

17. TAKAHASHI, T., SWINT, R. B., and HURLBERT, R. B.:Synthesis of RNA in Isolat-ed Nuclei of the Novikoff Ascites Tumor. Exptl. Cell Res., Suppl. *9:*330, 1963.

18. TATA, J. R.: Regulation of Protein Synthesis by Growth and Developmental Hormones. In: *Biochemical Actions of Hormones,* 1, 89, Ed., G. Litwack, Academic Press, 1970.

19. TRAVERS, A. A. and BURGESS, R. R.: Cyclic Reuse of the RNA Polymerase Sig-ma Factor. Nature, *222:*537, 1969.

20. WATTS, J.: The Loss of Rapidly-labeled RNA from Isolated HeLa Cell Nuclei. Biochem. J., *112:*71, 1969.

ROLE OF HORMONES
in the BIOSYNTHESIS
of POLYPEPTIDES

A. Clark Griffin and Dianne D. Black

The cytoplasmic-polysomal system accounts for a high proportion of all proteins, including many of the hormones, that are synthesized in mammalian cells. However, protein or polypeptide synthesis does occur in the mitochondria and the nucleus. Mention should also be made of the fact that other mechanisms for the biosynthesis of peptides exist, such as the nucleic acid-independent formation of gramicidin S from the interaction of an enzyme-phenylalanine complex with a polyenzyme system charged with the four addition amino acids (Kleinkauf *et al.,* 1969). Most studied of these is the cytoplasmic-polysomal system, and a rather universal mechanistic pattern is beginning to emerge. *In-vitro* systems for incorporating amino acids now have been isolated from a large number of mammalian tissues including rabbit reticulocytes, liver, tumor cells, pancreas, brain, human tissues, etc. From these investigations, it is quite evident that the basic mechanism of protein biosynthesis is similar in all mammalian cells. In fact, the elaborate studies *in vitro* involving components isolated from plant and from microbial sources suggest that this basic mechanism operates in all living cells.

Although it is obvious that hormones may play a major role in affecting the rate and types of proteins or polypeptides that are synthesized, including their own kind(s), there is a paucity of information as to the specific manner in which the hormones exert their effects. The possibility that most of the hormonal influences may be directed to transcriptional events rather than subsequent translational steps must be given serious consideration. Dr. Karlson reaffirms in this volume his long-standing view that ecdysone and hormones in general act directly at the chromosomal level, presumably in the transcription of mRNA. However, there is also some indication that hormones may be involved in one or more of the stages of the assembly of amino acids into polypeptide structures.

Initially, the components and individual reactions involved in protein synthesis will be considered and then the complete mechanism as it now exists. An attempt will be made to review at least a portion of the rather voluminous literature presenting evidence that hormones may affect polypeptide synthesis at the various stages indicated above. There are some obvious difficulties in studying the regulation of protein synthesis employing approaches utilizing *in-vitro* systems. The process has been removed from the organized environment in the cell and also removed from the host of regulatory and modulatory influences, including those exerted by hormones that are present *in vivo*. However, the complexity of the intact organism does require some degree of resolution if individual events are to be studied.

MECHANISM OF PROTEIN BIOSYNTHESIS

The model proposed by Drs. Crick and Lipmann (Lipmann, 1969) (and presented in modified forms by several other authors in other chapters) illustrates the major events in the translational stages of protein biosynthesis. This overall mechanism may be broken down into four stages:

1. **Amino-acid activation**
   Amino acid + ATP, Mg^{++}

   $\longrightarrow$ Amino acid-enzyme-ATP + PPi
   Aminoacyl synthetase

   Amino acid-enzyme-AMP + tRNA $\longrightarrow$ Aminoacyl tRNA + enzyme + AMP + PPi

2. **Initiation of polypeptide chain**
   Initiating tRNA (f-methionyl tRNA in bacteria)
   mRNA
   GTP

Mg^{++}

Initiating factors

30S and 50S ribosomal subunits

3. **Peptide-chain elongation**

Aminoacyl tRNAs

Mg^{++}

Factors T_1. T_2 (T and G)

GTP

SH, K^+ or NH^+_4. Peptidyl synthetase

4. **Termination**

Codon, m RNA

Factor R

During amino-acid activation, the aminoacyl synthetases, each specific for an amino acid, and tRNA are involved in the formation of amino-acid adenylates. These intermediates are then esterified to corresponding tRNAs by the same enzyme through an ester linkage between the carboxyl group of the amino acid and the hydroxyl group of ribose in the terminal adenosine of the tRNA. The final products are aminoacyl tRNAs, AMP, and Ppi (Zachau *et al.*, 1958; Berg, 1961).

Initiation of a peptidyl chain requires the native or free 30S and 50S ribosomal subunits, initiator codon AUG or GUG, factors F_1, F_2, and F_3 and GTP. Essential for microbial or yeast cell-free systems is the specific chain initiator, formylmethionyl tRNA (f-Met tRNA). In general, the initiation factors F_1, F_2, and F_3, mRNA, and f-Met tRNA interact with the 30S ribosomal unit to form an initiation complex, and concomitantly to attach to the 50S particle, thereby assembling an active 70S ribosome. To occur, this process is stimulated by GTP, the codon AUG or GUG and a Mg^{++} concentration of 5 mM. (Lipmann, 1969; Mukundan *et al.*, 1968; Ohta *et al.*, 1967; Rudland *et al.*, 1969).

Although f-Met tRNA has been identified in cellular extracts from HeLa cells (Galper and Darnell, 1969), Ehrlich ascites cells (Li and Yu, 1969) and hepatic mitochondria of the rat (Smith and Marcker, 1968), the function of this tRNA in mammalian systems is still uncertain. Using cellular extracts from murine ascites-tumor cells, Smith and Marcker (1970) have demonstrated the interaction of an f-Met tRNA species with an initiation complex, and with the ribosomal dependent initiator codon AUG. Likewise, Kerwar *et al.* (1970) reported similar findings for hepatic homogenates from rabbits. Hardesty and coworkers, employing extracts from reticulocytes in rabbits (Culp *et al.*, 1969a; Culp *et al.*, 1969b; Culp *et al.*, 1970; Mosteller *et al.*, 1968), are of the opinion that a specific species of deacylated tRNA serves as a chain initiator.

Chain elongation by mammalian or microbial ribosomes entails soluble transfer enzymes T_1 and T_2 (see Griffin and Black, 1971 for literature designation of the transfer enzymes) and inherent ribosomal peptidyl transferase GTP. NH_4^+, Mg^{++}, and a sulfhydryl compound. Each functional ribosome has two sites that are necessary for location or alignment of the aminoacyl tRNAs. An initiator or peptidyl tRNA must be in the peptidyl or donor site before another tRNA can hydrogen bond to its codon in the vacant aminoacyl or acceptor sites. Factor T_1, in the presence of Mg^{++} and NH_4^+ or K^+, attaches to GTP and an acyl tRNA, with subsequent binding of the ternary complex to the ribosomal-acceptor slot and messenger codon (Lipmann, 1969; McKeehan and Hardesty, 1969; Miller and Weissbach, 1969; Shorey *et al.*, 1969; Skoultchi *et al.*, 1970).

Thus far, mammalian T_1 has not been separated into two components as reported for *Escherichia coli* (Lucas-Lenard and Haenni, 1968; Ravel *et al.*, 1968) or *Bacillus stearothermophilus* (Skoultchi *et al.*, 1970). Mammalian enzymatic binding occurs at concentrations of 1.5-6.7 mM. Mg^{++}, 67-120 mM. KCl or 80 mM. NH_4^+, and 1 x 10^{-4} M. GTP, and interacts mainly with the 40S ribosomal subunit (Arlinghaus *et al.*, 1968; Shaeffer *et al.*, 1968; Skogerson and Moldave, 1968a). Hydrolysis of GTP occurs prior to or concurrently with peptide-bond formation (Lipmann, 1969; Ono *et al.*, 1969; Skogerson and Moldave, 1968a).

Peptidyl transferase is an integral part of the 50S or 60S ribosomal component, but its successful detachment from the larger subunit has not been achieved. Even so, this enzymatic factor is responsible for catalyzing peptide-bond formation between the carboxy group of the amino acid in the peptidyl site and the α-amino group of the amino acid in the acceptor site and for transfer of the nascent peptidyl moiety from the peptidyl site to the amino acceptor on the aminoacyl site (Fahnestock *et al.*, 1970; Monro, 1967; Skogerson and Moldave, 1968a; Skogerson and Moldave, 1969b; Skogerson and Moldave, 1969c). Both NH_4^+ and K^+ stimulate activation of this ribosomal protein (Ravel *et al.*, 1970; Skogerson and Moldave, 1968a), and inhibition can be induced with antibiotics such as chloramphenicol, lincomycin, hydroxypuromycin, N-acetylpuromycin, and sparsomycin (Vogel *et al.*, 1969).

At this stage of protein synthesis, the aminoacyl site now holds the peptidyl moiety, and the deacylated tRNA occupies the peptidyl site. Another factor T_2 then complexes with GTP and both ribosomal subunits to translocate peptidyl tRNA from the acceptor to the peptidyl socket with concurrent clearance of the deacylated tRNA in the peptidyl site. Simultaneously, GTP is hydrolyzed to GDP and Pi, and mRNA moves three nucleotides so that a new codon will be at the unoccupied acceptor site (Brot *et al.*, 1969; Parmeggiani and Gottschalk, 1969; Siler and Moldave, 1969; Skogerson and

Moldave, 1968a; Skogerson and Moldave, 1968b; Skogerson and Moldave, 1968c). Sulfhydryl compounds aid in activation and protection of the T_2 enzyme (Felicetti and Lipmann, 1968; Siler and Moldave, 1969). Shifting of the peptidyl tRNA, now one amino acid longer, provides a free aminoacyl site for the oncoming aminoacyl tRNA. A mechanism for removal of the donor tRNA from the peptidyl site for translocation to be completed has not been established. However, a soluble factor and GTP facilitate release of the deacylated tRNA (Kuriki and Kaji, 1968; Lucas-Lenard and Haenni, 1969). Aminoacyl tRNA binding and translocation continues on the same ribosome, each time resulting in the addition of an amino acid to a growing peptidyl chain.

Messenger termination triplets UAA, UAG, or UGA at the ribosomal acceptor site and supernatant factors S and R signal termination of the peptidyl chain (Goldstein *et al.,* 1970; Scolnick *et al.,* 1968). The R factor can be separated into two components, R_1 specific for codons UAA and UAG and R_2 specific for codons UAA and UGA. Release or hydrolysis of the completed peptide from tRNA in the peptidyl site is not completely understood (Tompkins *et al.,* 1970; Vogel *et al.,* 1969).

Numerous references related to systems for incorporating amino acids *in vitro* and to methodology employed for isolation of the components synthesizing protein appear in the literature for mammalian tissues (Bermek and Matthaei, 1970a; Bermek and Matthaei, 1970b; Culp *et al.,* 1969; Goodwin *et al.,* 1969; Grau and Favelukes, 1968; Hardesty *et al.,* 1963; Hoagland *et al.,* 1964; Hradeĉ, 1970; Ibuki and Moldave, 1968; Mahler and Brown, 1968; Means and Hall, 1969; Means *et al.,* 1969; Rosen *et al.,* 1967), Novikoff ascites-tumor cells (Black and Griffin, 1970; Krisko *et al.,* 1969), microbial systems (Lucas-Lenard and Lipmann, 1966; Nishizuka and Lipmann, 1966a; Nishizuka and Lipmann, 1966b; Parmeggiani, 1968; Ravel *et al.,* 1968), and yeast systems (Ayuso and Heredia, 1967; Richter and Lipmann, 1970). Methods for the preparation and study of systems incorporating amino acids in mammalian tissues were reviewed by Griffin and Black (1971) covering the literature to 1969. The reader's attention is directed also to Volume 34, *Cold Spring Harbor Symposia on Quantatitive Biology,* 1969: *The Mechanism of Protein Synthesis.*

EFFECT OF HORMONES UPON THE BIOSYNTHESIS OF POLYPEPTIDES

The consensus still prevails that the effect of hormones upon protein synthesis is mediated through the formation of mRNA at the transcriptional level (Karlson, this volume; Florini and Breuer, 1966; Korner, 1965; Means and Hall, 1969; Means *et al.,* 1969). Turkington and Riddle (1970), in studying the hormone-dependent initiation of casein synthesis in mammary cells, have demonstrated the coupling of the increase in transcriptional activity with greatly enhanced polysome formation. Palmiter *et al.* (1970) have arrived at similar conclusions from studies of the administration of estrogen to the immature chick.

There is increasing indication that hormones, in addition to their established effects at the genetic or transcriptional level, may also influence one or more of the translational stages that are involved in peptide synthesis. This is mentioned briefly since complete coverage of the many investigations that are emerging in this area is not feasible.

Hormones may alter the transfer RNA patterns and also the aminoacyl synthetase activities of target tissues. This could be associated with the regulation of protein synthesis. Altered tRNA patterns, as measured by various chromatographic procedures, have been observed during sporulation, embryogenesis, differentiation, carcinogenesis, viral infection, *etc.* (Griffin, 1971; Griffin and Black, 1971). Recently, Gefter and Russell (1969) have observed that infection of *E. coli* with defective transducing bacteriophage leads to the synthesis of three forms of suppressor tRNAs that differ in the base adjacent to the anticodon. The cytokinins that promote cell division and morphogenesis in plants have been found as integral components of tRNAs from different species (Armstrong *et al.,* 1969). The complete nucleotide sequence of approximately twenty different tRNAs has been reported in the literature (Griffin and Black, 1971). With the increasing knowledge of the structural aspects of tRNAs from tissues in varying states of physiologic or pathologic activities, it will be possible to assess the role of these nucleic acids as regulatory factors.

Studies carried out in this laboratory have been concerned largely with the interaction of chemical carcinogens with essential components of the cells or tissues (Goldman and Griffin, 1970). The tRNAs were selected since they could possibly reflect the changes induced by the carcinogens, or metabolites thereof, upon DNA; or, alternatively, it is quite possible that the carcinogens may react directly with the tRNAs to modify their structures. In a typical study, albino rats were fed diets containing the hepatocarcinogen, 3 -methyl-4-dimethylaminoazobenzene, for 3 to 4 weeks. Livers were removed from these animals and from comparable control rats, and the tRNA was isolated by the usual phenol procedure. The tRNA from the precancerous livers was charged with a labeled amino acid (*i. e.,* ^{14}C-phenylalanine) and the normal hepatic tRNA with the same amino acid labeled with another isotope (^{3}H-phenylalanine). The two aminoacylated preparations were then co-chromatographed employing reversed-phase column chromatography (Weiss and Kelmers, 1967) and the elution patterns established. The tRNA-elution patterns

Figure 1

Reversed Phase Chromatography Elution Profile of Phenylalanyl Transfer Ribonucleic Acids from Normal Rat Livers and from Livers of Rats Fed Diets Containing a Carcinogenic Azo Compound

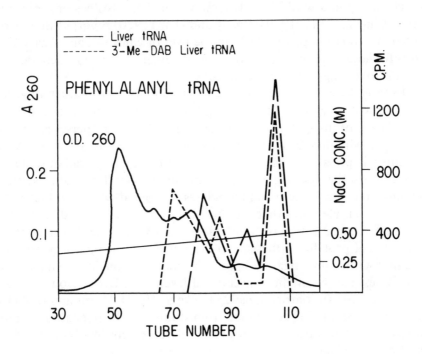

for tRNA^{Phe} are given in Figure 1. It was observed previously that the patterns for arginine are very close for the normal and the precancerous livers. In contrast, the tRNA^{Phe} profiles differ in two tissues. Two of the three tRNA^{Phe} peaks of the carcinogen-fed rats emerged earlier than the corresponding peaks from livers of the normal animals. Studies are in progress to ascertain the structural changes that caused this shift in the chromatographic behavior. Several investigators, employing this same general procedure, have observed alterations in the transfer-RNA patterns of target organs following the administration of hormones.

Ilan and Ilan (1970) have presented evidence that control of genic expression in *Tenebrio molitor* mediated by juvenile hormone is at the translational level and involves the appearance of a new transfer RNA and probably the corresponding synthetase. Correspondingly, major quantitative variations in tRNA^{Ser} were observed by Mäenpää and Bernfield (1969) during the hepatic synthesis of the yolk phosphoprotein, phosphovitin, in roosters treated with estrogen. This protein contains over 50 per cent serine. Alterations in tRNA methylases and a change in the $tRNA^{Ser}$ pattern in the uterus in ovariectomized rats were reported by Sharma and Borek (1970). These effects were reversed by physiological doses of estradiol.

A large increase in nuclear and cytoplasmic tRNA was noted in oviducts from chicks treated with diethylstibesterol or diethylstilbesterol plus progesterone (Dingman *et al.,* 1969). Busby and Hele (1970) reported that estrogen resulted in a variation of $tRNA^{Lys}$ in the liver of chickens, and Agarwal *et al.* (1969) found an approximate 20 per cent general increase in hepatic tRNAs of the rat following cortisone administration.

Jackson *et al.* (1970), employing reversed-phase chromatography, noted two additional species of $tRNA^{Asp}$ in livers of rats treated with growth hormone. This is of interest in view of the findings of Gallo (personal communication) that viral-induced tumors have an additional aspartyl tRNA peak.

Palmiter (in press) has observed that administration of estradiol to newborn chicks triggers the cytodifferentiation of tubular-gland cells that synthesize ovalbumin and conalbumin and modulates the rate at which oviduct proteins are synthesized. He notes that the three major effects of estradiol are: (1) increase in the concentration of translatable mRNA, (2) stimulation of the rate of initiation of protein synthesis, and (3) increase in the rate of peptide-chain elongation. Other investigators have concluded that one of the major effects of hormones may be at the translational level, *i. e.,* GH at elongation steps, Stage 3, and FSH (initiator, Stage 2) (Korner, 1969). Means and Hall (1969) and Morgan *et al.* (1971) concluded from studies on the regulation of protein synthesis in cardiac muscle that insulin accelerates steps involved in the initiation of peptide chains.

The information reported above are only indicative of the many investigations now in progress to determine more precisely the mechanism of action of the hormones. Many of the findings are suggestive that the hormonal effects may be mediated at one or more of the translational steps of protein biosynthesis. The major progress that has been made in recent years in elucidating the mechanism of protein synthesis, as well as the observations relating to the structure and formation of the tRNAs, should provide more stimulus and opportunity for the study of the effects of hormones at the various translational stages.

Acknowledgement

Studies reported in this chapter were supported by grants from the Robert A. Welch Foundation and The American Cancer Society.

References

1. AGARWAL, M. K., HANOUNE, J., YU, F. L., WEINSTEIN, I. B., and FEIGELSON, P.: Studies on the Effect of Cortisone on Rat Liver Transfer Ribonucleic Acid. Biochemistry, *8*:4806-4812, 1969.

2. ARLINGHAUS, R., SHAEFFER, S., BISHOP, J., and SCHWEET, R.: Purification of the Transfer Enzymes from Reticulocytes and Properties of the Transfer Reaction. Arch. Biochim. Biophys, *125*:604-613, 1968.

3. ARMSTRONG, D. J., BURROWS, W. J., SKOOF, F., ROY, K. L., and SÖLL, D. CY-TOKININS: Distribution in Transfer RNA Species of *Escherichia coli.* Proc. Natl. Acad. Sci. U. S., *63*:834-841, 1969.

4. AYUSO, M. and HEREDIA, C. F.: Simple Resolution of the Yeast Amino Acid Transfer System into Two Complementary Factors. Biochim. Biophys. Acta, *145*:199-201, 1967.

5. BERG, P.: Annual Reviews Biochemistry. *In*: Annual Review, California, *30*:293-374, 1961.

6. BERMEK, E. and MATTHAEI, H.: Elongation Factors From Human Lymphatic Tissue: Isolation and Some Properties. FEBS Letters *10*:121-124, 1970a.

7. BERMEK, E. and MATTHAEI, H.: The Effect of Antibiotics on an Optimized Poly-phenylalanine Synthesizing Cell-free System from Human Lymphatic Tissue. Hoppe-Seyler's Z. Physiol. Chem., *351*:1377-1383, 1970.

8. BLACK, D. D. and GRIFFIN, A. C.: Similarity of the Transfer Factors in Novikoff Ascites Tumor and Other Amino-acid Incorporating Systems. Cancer Res., *30*:1281-1286, 1970.

9. BROT, N., SPEARS, C. and WEISSBACH, H.: The Formation of a Complex Containing Ribosomes, Transfer Factor G and A and A Guanosine Nucleotide. Biochem. Biophys. Res. Comm., *34*:843-848, 1969.

10. BUSBY, W. F. and HELE, P.: Estrogen-induced Variation of Lysine Transfer Ribonucleic Acid Isoacceptors in Chicken Livers. Biochim. Biophys. Acta, *224*:413-422, 1970.

11. CULP, W. J., MCKEEHAN, W. L., and HARDESTY, B.: Deacylated tRNA[Phe] Binding to a Reticulocyte Ribosomal Site for the Initiation of Polyphyenlalanine Synthesis. Proc. Natl. Acad. Sci. U. S., *63*:1431-1438, 1969.

12. CULP, W., MCKEEHAN, W., and HARDESTY, B.: The Mechanism of Messenger RNA Translocation through Ribosomes. Proc. Natl. Acad. Sci. U. S., *64*:388-395, 1969.

13. CULP, W., MORRISEY, J., and HARDESTY, B.: Initiator tRNA for the Synthesis of Globin Peptides. Biochem. Biophys. Res. Comm., *40*:777-785, 1970.

14. DINGMAN, C. W., ARONOW, A., BUNTING, S. L., PEACOCK, A. C ., and O'MAL-LEY, B. W.: Changes in Chick Oviduct Ribonucleic Acid Following Hormonal Stimulation. Biochemistry, *8*:489-495, 1969.

15. FAHNESTOCK, S., NEUMANN, H., SHASHOUA, V., and RICH, A .: Ribosome-Catalyzed Ester Formation. Biochemistry, *9*:2477-2483, 1970.

16. FELICETTI, L. and LIPMANN, F.:   Comparison of Amino Acid Polymerization Factors Isolated from Rat Liver and Rabbit Reticulocytes. Arch. Biochim. Biophys., *125:*548-557, 1968.

17. FLORINI, J. R. and BREUER, C. B.:   Amino Acid Incorporation into Protein by Cell-free Systems from Rat Skeletal Muscle. V. Effects of Pituitary Growth Hormone on Activity of Ribosomes and Ribonucleic Acid Polymerase in Hypophysectomized Rats. Biochemistry, *5:*1870-1876, 1966.

18. GALPER, J. B. and RUSSELL, R. L.: The Presence of N-Formyl-Methionyl-tRNA in HeLa Cell Mitochondria. Biochem. Biophys. Res. Comm., *34:*205-214, 1969.

19. GEFTER, M. L. and RUSSELL, R. L.: Role of Modifications in Tyrosine Transfer RNA: A Modified Base Affecting Ribosome Binding. J. Mol. Biol., *39:* 145-157, 1969.

20. GOLDMAN, M. and GRIFFIN, A. C.:   Transfer RNA Patterns in Livers of Rats Fed Diets Containing 3'-Methyl-4-dimethylaminoazobenzene. Cancer Res., *30:*1677 – 1680, 1970.

21. GOLDSTEIN, J., MILMAN, G., SCOLNICK, E., and CASKEY, T.:   Peptide Chain Termination. VI. Purification and Site of Action of S. Proc. Natl. Acad. Sci. U. S., *65:*430-437, 1970.

22. GOODWIN, F., SHAFRITZ, D., and WEISSBACH, H.: *In Vitro* Polypeptide Synthesis in Brain. Arch. Biochem. Biophys., *130:*183-190, 1969.

23. GRAU, O. and FAVELUKES, G.:   Polyribosomes in Extracts of Hepatic Bone Marrow Erythroid Cells and Their Preservation by Hepatic Ribonuclease Inhibitor. Arch. Biochem. Biophys., *125:*647-657, 1968.

24. GRIFFIN, A. C.: Molecular Translational Factors in Carcinogenesis. Role of the Transfer Ribonucleic Acids. The U. of Texas M. D. Anderson Hospital and Tumor Institute 24th Annual Symposia on Basic Cancer Research, in press.

25. GRIFFIN, A. and BLACK, D. D.: Protein Biosynthesis. *In*: H. Busch (ed.), Methods in Cancer Research, *VI*:189-251. New York: Academic Press, 1971.

26. HARDESTY, B., ARLINGHAUS, R., SHAEFFER, J., and SCHWEET, R.: Hemoglobin and Polyphenylalanine Synthesis with Reticulocyte Ribosomes. *Cold Spring Harbor Symp. on Quant. Biol, 28:*215-222, 1963.

27. HOAGLAND, M. B., SCORNIK, O. A., and PFEFFERKORN, L. C.: Aspects of Control of Protein Synthesis in Normal and Regenerated Rat Liver, II. A Microsomal Inhibitor of Amino Acid Incorporation Whose Action is Antagonized by Guanosine Triphosphate. Proc. Natl. Acad. Sci. U. S., *51:*1184-1191, 1964.

28. HRADEC, J.: Separation of Two Different Peptidyl Transfer RNA Translocases from Mammalian Tissues. FEBS Letters, *10:*159-162, 1970.

29. IBUKI, F. and MOLDAVE, K.:   Evidence for the Enzymatic Binding of Aminoacyl Transfer Ribonucleic Acid to Rat Liver Ribosomes. J. Biol. Chem., *243:* 791-798, 1968.

30. ILAN, J. and ILAN J.: Mechanism of Gene Expression in *Tenebrio molitor*. J. Biol. Chem., *245:*1275-1281, 1970.

31. JACKSON, C. D., IRVING, C. C., and SELLS, B. H.: Changes in Rat Liver Transfer RNA Following Growth Hormone Administration and in Regenerating Liver. Biochim. Biophys. Acta, *217:*64-71, 1970.

32. KERWAR, S. S., SPEARS, C., and WEISSBACH, H.: Studies on the Initiation of Protein Synthesis in Animal Tissues. Biochem. Biophys. Res. Comm., *41:*78-84, 1970.

33. KLEINKAUF, H., GEVERS, W., and LIPMANN, F.: Interrelation between Activation and Polymerization in Gramicidian S Biosynthesis. Proc. Natl. Acad. Sci. U. S. *62:*226-233, 1969.

34. KORNER, A.: Growth Hormone Control of Biosynthesis of Protein and Ribonucleic Acid. *In*: G. Pincus (ed.), Recent Progress in Hormone Research, *1:*205-240. New York: Academic Press, 1965.

35. KORNER, A.: The Effect of Growth Hormone on Protein Synthesis in the Absence of Peptide Chain Initiation. Biochim. Biophys. Acta, *174:*351-358, 1969.

36. KRISKO, I., GORDON, J., and LIPMANN, F.: Studies on the Interchange Ability of One of the Mammalian and Bacterial Supernatant Factors in Protein Biosynthesis. J. Biol. Chem., *244:*6117-2123, 1969.

37. KURIKI, Y. and KAJI, A.: Factor and Guanosine 5'-Triphosphate-Dependent Release of Deacylated Transfer RNA from 70S Ribosomes. Proc. Natl. Acad. Sci. U. S., *61:*1399-1405, 1968.

38. LI, C. and YU. C.: Formylation of Methionyl Transfer RNA in a Mammalian System. Biochim. Biophys. Acta, *182:*440-443, 1969.

39. LIPMANN, F.: Polypeptide Chain Elongation in Protein Biosynthesis. Science, *164:*1024-1031, 1969.

40. LUCAS-LENARD, J. and HAENNI, A. L.: Requirement of Guanosine 5'-Triphosphate for Ribosomal Binding of Aminoacyl-sRNA. Proc. Natl. Acad. Sci. U. S., *59:* 554-560, 1968.

41. LUCAS-LENARD, J. and HAENNI, A. L.: Release of Transfer RNA During Peptide Chain Elongation. Proc. Natl. Acad. Sci. U. S., *63:*93-97, 1969.

42. LUCAS-LENARD, J. and LIPMANN, F.: Separation of Three Microbial Amino Acid Polymerization Factors. Proc. Natl. Acad. Sci. U. S., *55:*1562-1566, 1966.

43; MÄENPÄÄ, P. H. and BERNFIELD, M. R.: Quantitative Variation in Serine Transfer Ribonucleic Acid During Estrogen-induced Phosphoprotein Synthesis in Rooster Liver. Biochemistry, *8:*4926-4934, 1969.

44. MAHLER, H. R. and BROWN, B. J.: Protein Synthesis by Cerebral Cortex Polysomes: Characterization of the System. Arch. Biochem. Biophys., *125:* 387-400, 1968.

45. McKEEHAN, W. L. and HARDESTY, B.: Purification and Partial Characterization of the Aminoacyl Transfer Ribonucleic Acid Binding Enzyme from Rabbit Reticulocytes. J. Biol. Chem., *244:*4330-4339, 1969.

46. MEANS, A. R., ABRASS, I. B., and O'MALLEY, B. W.: Protein Biosynthesis on Chick Oviduct Polyribosomes. I. Changes During Estrogen-mediated Tissue Differentiation. Biochemistry, *10:*1561-1569, 1971.

47. MEANS, A. R. and HALL, P. F.:   Protein Biosynthesis in the Testis. V. Concerning the Mechanism of Stimulation by Follicle Stimulating Hormone. Biochemistry, *8:*4293-4298, 1969.

48. MEANS, A. R., HALL, P. F., NICOL, L. W., SAWYER, W. H., and BAKER, C. A.: Protein Biosynthesis in the Testis. IV. Isolation and Properties of Polyribosomes. Biochemistry, *8:*1488-1495, 1969.

49. MILLER, D. E; and WEISSBACH, H.:   An Interaction Between the Transfer Factors Required for Protein Synthesis. Arch. Biochem. Biophys., *132:*146-150, 1969.

50. MONRO, R. E.:   Catalysis of Peptide Bond Formation by 50S Ribosomal Subunits from *Escherichia coli.* J. Molec. Biol, *26:*147-151, 1967.

51. MORGAN, H. E., JEFFERSON, L. S., WOLPERT, E. B., and RANNELS, D. E.:   Regulation of Protein Synthesis in Heart Muscle, II. Effect of Amino Acid Levels and Insulin on Ribosomal Aggregation. J. Biol. Chem., *243:*6343-6352, 1968.

52. MOSTELLER, R. D., CULP, W. J., and HARDESTY, B.:   Deacylated Transfer Ribonucleic Acid as a Factor for Peptide Chain Initiation in Rabbits Reticulocyte Systems. J. Biol. Chem., *243:*6343-6352, 1968.

53. MUKUNDAN, M. A., HERSHEY, J. W. B., DEWEY, K. F., and THACH, R. E.:   Binding of Formylmethionyl-tRNA to 30S Ribosomal Subunits. Nature, *217:* 1013-1016, 1968.

54. NISHIZUKA, Y. and LIPMANN, F.: Comparison of Guanosine Triphosphate Split and Polypeptide Synthesis with a Purified *E. coli* System. Proc. Natl. Acad. Sci. U. S., *55:*212-219, 1966.

55. NISHIZUKA, Y. and LIPMANN, F.: The Interrelationship Between Guanosine Triphosphate and Amino Acid Polymerization. Arch. Biochem. Biophys., *116:* 344-351, 1966.

56. OHTA, T., SARKAR, S. and THACH, R. E.: The Role of Guanosine 5'-Triphosphate in the Initiation of Peptide Synthesis, III. Binding of Formylmethionyl-tRNA to Ribosomes. Proc. Natl. Acad. Sci. U. S., *58:*1638-1644, 1967.

57. ONO, Y., SKOULTCHI, A., WATERSON, J., and LENGYEL, P.: Peptide Chain Elongation: GTP Cleavage Catalyzed by Factors Binding Amino-acyl-Transfer-RNA to the Ribosome. Nature, *222:*645-648, 1969.

58. PALMITER, R. D.:   Regulation of Protein Synthesis in Chick Oviducts. J. Molec. Biol., in press.

59. PALMITER, R. D., CHRISTENSEN, A. K., and SCHIMKE, R. T.:   Organization of Polysomes from Pre-existing Ribosomes in Chick Oviduct by a Secondary Administration of Either Estradiol or Progesterone. J. Biol. Chem., *245:* 833-845, 1970.

60. PARMEGGIANI, A.: Crystalline Transfer Factors from *Escherichia coli.* Biochem. Biophys. Res. Comm., *30:*613-619, 1968.

61. PARMEGGIANI, A. and GOTTSCHALK, E. M.:   Properties of the Crystalline Amino Acid Polymerization Factors from *Escherichia coli.* Binding of G to Ribosomes. Biochem. Biophys. Res. Commun., *35:*861-867, 1969.

62. RAVEL, J. M., SHOREY, R. L., FROEHNER, S., and SHIVE, W.: A Study of the Enzymic Transfer of Aminoacyl-RNA to *Escherichia coli* Ribosomes. Arch. Biochem. Biophys., *125:*514-526, 1968.

63. RAVEL, J. M., SHOREY, R. A. L., and SHIVE, W.: Relationship between Peptidyl Transferase Activity and Interaction of Ribosomes with Phenylalanyl Transfer Ribonucleic Acid-Guanosine 5'-Triphosphate-TI$_u$ Complex. Biochemistry, *9:* 5028-5033, 1970.

64. RIEHTER, D. and LIPMANN, F.: Separation of Mitochondrial and Cytoplasmic Peptide Chain Elongation Factors from Yeast. Biochemistry, *9:*5065-5070, 1970.

65. ROSEN, L., MURRAY, E. L., and NOVELLI, G. D.: Cell-free Incorporation of Amino Acids by a Trout-Liver System. Heat-labile Aminoacyl Transferase Activity. Canad. J. Biochem., *45:*2005-2014, 1967.

66. RUDLAND, P. S., WHYBROW, W. A., MARCHER, K. A., and CLARK, B. F. C.: Recognition of Bacterial Initiator tRNA by Initiation Factors. Nature,*222:* 750-753, 1969.

67. SCOLNICK, R., TOMPKINS, R., CASKEY, T., and NIRENBERG, M.: Release Factors Differing in Specificity for Terminator Codons. Proc. Natl. Acad. Sci. U. S., *61:*768-774, 1968.

68. SHAEFFER, J., ARLINGHAUS, R., and SCHWEET, R.: Effect of Varying the KCl and MgCl$_2$ Concentration on the Enzymic and Nonenzymic Binding of Phenylalanyl-RNA to Reticulocyte Ribosomes. Arch. Biochem. Biophys., *125:*614-622, 1968.

69. SHARMA, O. K. and BOREK, E.: Hormonal Effect on Transfer Ribonucleic Acid Methylases and on Serine Transfer Ribonucleic Acid. Biochemistry,*9:*2507-2513, 1970.

70. SHOREY, R. L., RAVEL, J. M., GARNER, C. W., and SHIVE, W.: Formation and Properties of the Aminoacyl Transfer Ribonucleic Acid-Guanosine Triphosphate-protein Complex. J. Biol. Chem. *244:*4555-4564, 1969.

71. SILER, J. and MOLDAVE, K.: Studies on the Kinetics of Peptidyl Transfer RNA Translocase from Rat Liver. Biochim. Biophys. Acta., *195:*138-144, 1969.

72. SKOGERSON, L. and MOLDAVE, K.: Evidence for Aminoacyl-tRNA Binding, Peptide Bond Synthesis, and Translocase Activities in the Aminoacyl Transfer Reaction. Arch. Biochem. Biophys., *125:*497-505, 1968.

73. SKOGERSON, L. and MOLDAVE, K.: Characterization of the Interaction of Aminoacyltransferase II with Ribosomes. J. Biol. Chem., *243:*5354-5360, 1968.

74. SKOGERSON, L. and MOLDAVE, K.: Evidence for the Role of Aminoacyltransferase II in Peptidyl Transfer Ribonucleic Acid Translocation. J. Biol. Chem., *243:* 5361-5367, 1968.

75. SKOULTCHI, A., ONO, Y., WATERSON, J., and LENGYEL, P.: Peptide Chain Elongation: Indications for the Binding of an Amino Acid Polymerization Factor, Guanosine 5'-Triphosphate-Aminoacyl Transfer Ribonucleic Acid Complex to the Messenger-Ribosome Complex. Biochemistry, *9:*508-514, 1970.

76. SMITH, A. E. and MARCKER, K. A.: N-Formylmethionyl Transfer RNA in Mitochondria from Yeast and Rat Liver. J. Mol. Biol., *38:*241-243, 1968.

77. SMITH, A. and MARCKER, K.: Cytoplasmic Methionine Transfer RNAs from Eukaryotes. Nature, *226:*607-610, 1970.

78. TOMPKINS, R. K., SCOLNICK, E. M., and CASKEY, C. T.: Peptide Chain Termination, VII. The Ribosomal and Release Factor Requirements for Peptide Release. Proc. Natl. Acad. Sci., U. S., *65*:702-208, 1970.

79. TURKINGTON, R. W. and RIDDLE, M.: Hormone-dependent Formation of Polysomes in Mammary Cells *In Vitro*. J. Biol. Chem., *245*:5145-5152, 1970.

80. VOGEL, Z., ZAMIR, A., and ELSON, D.: The Possible Involvement of Peptidyl Transferase in the Termination Step of Protein Biosynthesis. Biochemistry, *8:* 5161-5168, 1969.

81. WEISS, J. F. and KELMERS, A. D.: A New Chromatographic System for Increased Resolution of Transfer Ribonucleic Acids. Biochemistry, *6:*2507-2513, 1967.

82. ZACHAU, H. G., ACS, G., and LIPMANN, F.: Isolation of Adenosine Amino Acid Esters from a Ribonuclease Digest of Soluble, Liver Ribonucleic Acid. Proc. Natl. Acad. Sci., U. S., *44*:885-889, 1958.

REGULATION of ENZYMATIC ACTIVITY by HORMONES

Antonio Orengo

This discussion will be limited to a few pertinent correlations between hormones and molecular properties of enzymes, and no attempt will be made to furnish a catalogue of the numerous biochemical effects produced by hormones in higher organisms. In order to avoid diffusiveness, the term, hormone, is here restricted to any substance produced by a distinct set of cells and able to modulate the metabolism of target cells for the benefit of the whole organism (Huxley, 1935).

At the present time several lines of evidence support the view that hormonal action consists primarily in a modulation effect of the metabolic coordination of target cells. As a consequence, the mechanism of hormonal action can only be understood when detailed descriptions at the molecular level of coordinating mechanisms operating in the metabolism of the target cells is available. However, it should be clear that the function of a hormone cannot be deduced from the chemical description of its molecule, the hormones that we extract and study today are the consequence of a purposeful selection. The teleology is illusory, since only what was selected by the criterion of survival of the fittest is available for perusal. Hormonal function as well as controls in regulation of metabolism are grasped better from the point of view of semiology; that is, recognition that a code mechanism is underlying these phenomena.

From the point of view of chemistry, the plethora of effects mediated by a single hormone is disturbing. In recent years the problem of regulating metabolism has been understood much better by virtue of the description of controls. In particular an exploitable molecular basis for such a description has been furnished by studies of the macromolecular properties of enzymes. The biological meaning of protein conformation has begun to be more fully appreciated and a more dynamic picture of enzyme molecules has been disseminated extensively.

The restrictive model of the substrate as a key and of the enzyme as a lock furnishes a gratuitous degree of rigidity to the enzyme molecule. The acceptance of such a model pictorially describing enzyme specificity in the past has compelled one to handle certain kinetic findings with models that consider the enzyme as a rigid surface. Since this is such a coarse approximation, first it is desirable to review the chemical basis of protein conformation in order that the proteiform character of proteins will become more evident.

Proteins are sequences of amino acids arranged in a linear array by a peptide bond. In a linked sequence of amino acids only three types of covalent bonds are represented: the peptide bond (a), the a-carbon-carbonyl bond (b), and the a-carbon-nitrogen bond (c) (Figure 1). The modality of biosynthesis of these macromolecules is unique. The biopolymer is arranged under the guidance of DNA templates through a mechanism of transcription to RNA templates and a mechanism of translation by which ribosomes and transfer RNAs play their role. This synthetic modality has an immediate consequence: identicalness. The molecules produced will have a very narrow range of molecular distribution and identical amino-acid sequence. However, since there is no apparent limitation in the rotation around the axis of a-carbon-carbonyl bonds, the atoms of a polypeptide chain may arrange themselves in space in an almost infinite number of ways. However, only few of the many possible conformations actually occur and of these few even fewer have any biological meaning.

What then are the constraints? The main constraints of protein conformation are related to the nature of the peptide bond and to the chemical diversity of the side chains on amino-acid residues. Analysis by x-rays indicates that the four atoms of the peptide linkage, -NH-CO-, lie on a quasiplanar configuration and that the interatomic distance between carbon and the nitrogen atoms is shorter when compared to average values.

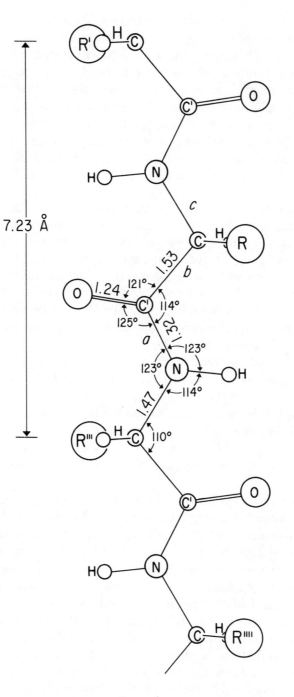

Figure 1

From R. B. Corey and L. Pauling, Proc. Roy. Soc. B141, 10 (1953).

This suggests an overlapping of electron shells with an induced electron deficiency in the imino group and an electron excess on the oxygen of the carbonyl group. These are proper conditions for strong hydrogen bonding. Therefore, the carbonyl of one peptide bond is able to form linkage with the imino group of another peptide bond present in its own chain or in a neighboring chain. Such hydrogen bonding can freeze segments of the polypeptide chain in a more or less stable conformation. Pauling and Corey proposed a periodic structure in which the hydrogen bonds are directed along the axis of the chain linking peptide bond 1 to peptide bond 5, bond 2 to 6, and so on (Pauling *et al.*, 1951; Corey and Pauling, 1953) (Figure 2).

Native proteins have various degrees of a helicity. For example the hormone, insulin, has 51 per cent of its amino-acid residues in an a-helix conformation whereas the enzyme, ribonuclease, exhibits only 17 per cent. Although there are other hydrogen-bonded structures such as the β-structure, discussion of them will not be pertinent and would far exceed the limit of the present context. If the nature of the peptide bond is responsible for these segments of chain in a periodical structure, the amino-acid side chains, as a result of their chemical diversity, appear to be the determinants of the overall folding of the protein molecule.

Among the weak interactions in a protein molecule that can be listed are:

(1)   hydrogen bonds between the -OH and $-NH_2$ group such as the -OH group of serine and the $-NH_2$ group of lysine;

(2)   ionic bonds between COO^- and NH_3^+ groups, such as the COO^- of glutamic and the $-NH_3^+$ of arginine; and

(3)   the disulfide bonds among the -SH groups of cystine residues The hydrophobic interactions (Kauzmann, 1959), however, are of particular significance.

Of the twenty amino acids that may occur in a polypeptide chain, ten are classified as nonpolar, having a very limited solubility in water. As a result of the hydrogen-bonded structure of water (Nemethy and Scheraga, 1962), the nonpolar side chains tend to interact with themselves through Van-der-Waals forces and hydrogen bonding. As consequence of such interaction, the polypeptide chain may assume a more or less globular shape with the hydrophobic side chains of the amino-acid residues arranged in the core of the protein globule whereas the hydrophilic residues are displayed on the surface. The picture of a globular protein that is derived from these considerations is constituted by segments of periodical structures interrupted by amino-acid sequences in a nonperiodical conformation. Therefore, the degree of conformational stability of the entire molecule is based on weak interactions, and the emerging character of a globular protein in solution appears to be its conformational ductility.

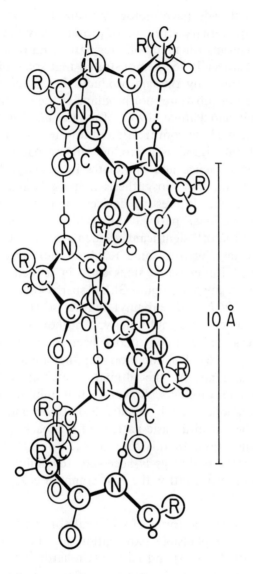

Figure 2

Diagrammatic drawing of the α-helix after Pauling and Corey

Only in the last decade have biologists realized the possibility that allosteric linkage and quaternary struction of proteins may function as elements in molecular mechanisms for metabolic regulation. Early studies (Umbarger, 1956; Yates and Pardee, 1956) demonstrated that some biosynthetic pathways could be controlled by the end products. Later, the existence of sites for ligands that are not substrates nor products of the reaction catalyzed was suggested (Gerhardt and Pardee, 1962; Monod *et al.*, 1963). This property of some enzymes may allow coordination of different sequences of chemical transformations if the ligand is a product of one pathway but binds the catalyst of another sequence and modulates its activity. Alternatively, the ligand may regulate its own biosynthesis if it binds and inhibits the first catalyst of the sequence. Interesting devices for regulation have been described for multifunctional pathways in which control by the ultimate metabolite could turn off significant segments of metabolism (Figure 3). Enzymic species catalyzing the same reactions but structurally dissimilar have been described for enzymic steps early in sequences branching into different metabolic segments (Figure 3b). Asparto-kinase (Stadtman *et al.*, 1961; Patte *et al.*, 1967) and carbamyl synthetase (Lacroute *et al.*, 1965) are two examples of enzyme multiplicity. Another type of feedback inhibition, the sequential feedback control, has been found by Nester and Jensen (Nester and Jensen, 1966). The common step, here, is inhibited by the last common product and not by the ultimate metabolites of the sequence. Each of the ultimate products, however, will inhibit the first enzyme unique to the metabolic branch (Figure 3c). Datta and Gest (Datta and Gest, 1964) described a third basic pattern of feedback inhibition: the concerted feedback inhibition. In this case an excess of all the ultimate products of the branching pathways is necessary to inhibit; none of the ultimate products alone can control the first common enzymatic step (Figure 3d).

The existence of isomeric forms of self regulatory enzymes in equilibrium has been invoked as a plausible explanation for such findings. Koshland (Koshland, 1963; 1964; 1966) and Pardee (Gerhardt and Pardee, 1962) suggested that the conformational transition of the enzymic molecule takes place as a consequence of the binding of ligands. The induced conformation, in turn, enhances or reduces the affinity for the substrate or alters the $K_{catalytic}$ of the enzyme. Monod (Monod *et al.*, 1965) proposed a more general model in which it is assumed that the regulatory protein can exist in two or more conformations that differ in their affinity for substrate or modifier. Wyman (Wyman, 1967) extended this model, introducing the concept of allosteric linkage. The concept is based on the assumption that

Figure 3

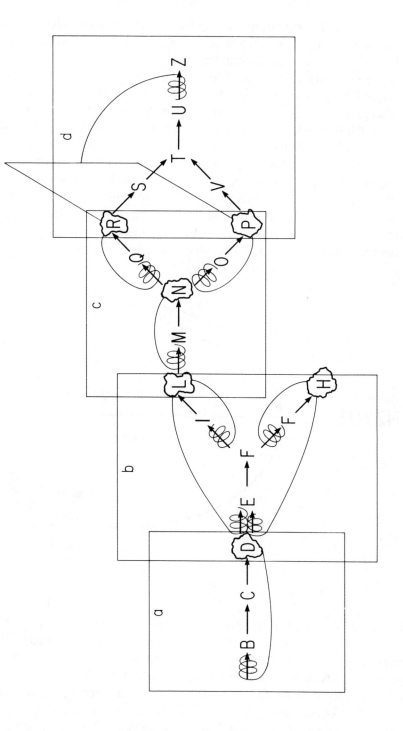

the binding of the substrate or regulatory ligand takes place exclusively because of the prevalence of one of the many conformations among which a polypeptide chain may fluctuate. Neither of these conformations may necessarily have any affinity at all for the ligands.

It should be clear indeed that the term, enzyme, denotes the association of a polypeptide chain in a defined sequence and a set of conformations among which the molecule fluctuates. The term is reduced to a mere abstraction if one of the elements of the association is neglected (Figure 4). To equate enzymic activities to protein molecules may turn out to be very unrewarding and perhaps DNA intervention has been invoked too often in molecular biology. The supposition that enzymic activities exist before polypeptide chains is erroneous because it suggests a simple relationship between a primary structure and the meaningful folding of the chain. Perhaps there are far more activities than polypeptide chains.

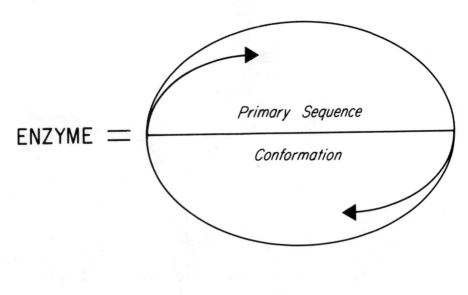

Figure 4

In a recent review, Klotz (Klotz *et al.*, 1970) has listed 108 proteins that may dissociate into subunits under mild treatments. Such aggregation of polymers has been described among identical polypeptide chains or among chains with different amino-acid sequences. The finding known for some time has never been viewed from the angle of metabolic regulation until recently. It is conceivable, in fact, that modulation in the degree of freedom in the folding of the chain may be achieved through a mechanism of dissociation-association of subunits. The freedom in folding could be viewed as an unavoidable consequence of the length of chain necessary to perform the basic function. Two examples of hormonal modulation of metabolisms have been chosen to conclude this discussion because they represent two types of mechanisms for molecular control.

GLUTAMATE DEHYDROGENASE

Some steroid hormones, diethylstilbestrol in particular, inhibit glutamate-*a*-ketoglutarate conversion (Yielding and Tomkins, 1960). Under identical conditions the hormone stimulates a monocarboxylic amino-acid dehydrogenase reaction with alanine and several other amino acids (Tomkins *et al.*, 1961). Moreover, ADP was found to stimulate the glutamic-dehydrogenase reaction (Frieden, 1959), to prevent its inhibition by diethylstilbestrol, Yielding and Tomkins, 1960) and finally to inhibit the alanine-dehydro – genase reaction (Tomkins *et al.*, 1961). Crystalline, bovine, L glutamate dehydrogenase exists in solution in two states of aggregation: a high molecular weight form of about 1,000,000 and species with molecular weight of about 250,000 (Olson and Anftinsen, 1951; Frieden, 1958; Kubo *et al.*, 1959). The forms are in equilibrium with a prevalence of heavier species at high concentration of protein, and both catalyze the glutamate-*a*-ketoglutarate conversion. Since the factors enhancing the glutamate reaction prevent the alanine reaction and *vice versa*, the findings have been rationalized with the hypothesis that two conformations of the enzyme were in

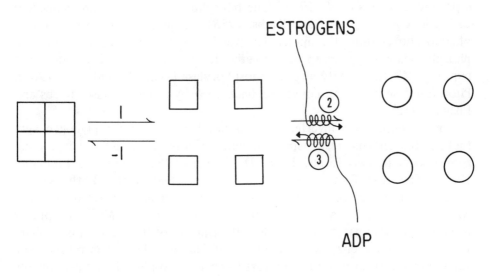

Figure 5

equilibrium and ADP or estrogens shift the equilibrium in opposite directions, generating the prevalence of one enzymatic activity over the other. Also it has been necessary to assume that the conformation prevalent in the presence of ADP is in equilibrium with the tetrameric form of the enzyme, since both the monomeric and tetrameric forms catalyze the glutamate reaction (Tomkins *et al.*, 1965) (Figure 5). The model is supported by the finding that estrogens dissociate the polymeric forms (Yielding and Tomkins, 1962). In fact, the estrogen would shift the first equilibrium to the right in stabilizing a monomeric conformation. In this case, the hormone appears to affect enzymatic physics with a concomitant alteration of the quaternary structure and substrate specificity.

THE GLYCOGEN SYNTHETASE-GLYCOGEN PHOSPHORYLASE SYSTEM

The glycogen synthetase-glycogen phosphorylase system offers an example of the cascade mechanism and introduces the concept of a second messenger in hormonal action. The appearance of a metabolite (cyclic AMP) or its increase above a threshold level initiates a series of phosphorylations of enzymes involved in the storage and production of energy with pleomorphic metabolic effects. Glycogen phosphorylase, the enzyme responsible for glycogen depolymerization, exists as a dimer, phosphorylase *b*, and as a tetramer, phosphorylase *a* (Keller and Cori, 1953; Krebs *et al.*, 1958). The *b* form can be converted to *a* form by a protein kinase, phosphorylase *b* kinase, with a transfer of 4 moles of phosphate per mole of phosphorylase *a* produced (Krebs *et al.*, 1958). The phospho donor is ATP, and a divalent cation is required (Fisher and Krebs, 1955) for the reaction. In the process of phosphorylation, the molecular weight of the enzyme doubles, and phosphorylase *a* appears to be the active form of the enzyme and does not require AMP for activity as does phosphorylase *b* (Brown and Cori, 1961). Phosphorylase *a* can be converted back to *b* by a phosphatase (Krebs and Fisher, 1962).

An analogous but inverted pattern has been found for glycogen synthetase, the enzyme responsible for glucose polymerization. Again the enzyme exists in two forms, I and D (Larner, 1966; Trout and Lipmann, 1963). The first form is glucose 6-P independent (I form), the second depends on the presence of hexosephosphate for activity (D form). The conversion of the I form to the D form requires ATP and Mg^{++}; it appears to be of enzymic nature and involves the transfer of the terminal phosphate from ATP to the enzyme (Friedman and Larner, 1963). The reverse conversion of the D form to the I appears to be a dephosphorylation presumably catalyzed by a phosphatase (Friedman and Larner, 1963).

The evidence therefore indicates that the interconversion of the synthetase enzymic species, as in the case of interconversion of the phosphorylase forms, is produced through a phosphorylation-dephosphorylation reaction. The difference lies in the fact that the phosphorylated form is active in the case of the phosphorylase; whereas the inverse is true for the synthetase.

The intrinsic elegance of the two symmetrical and inverted cycles had no meaning in the regulation of the main route of energy until it was found that another system of phosphorylation and dephosphorylation, dependent now on $3,5'$-AMP, could connect degradation and synthesis of glycogen. The enzyme, responsible for the phosphorylation and activation of glycogen phosphorylase b, appears to exist in two forms also. The inactive form in the presence of $3,5'$-AMP is phosphorylated by ATP and converted to an active phosphorylated form by another protein kinase (Walsh *et al.*, 1968). This protein kinase appears to be the same enzyme that catalyzes the phosphorylation of glycogen synthetase, *i. e.*, the inactivating enzyme of the glycogen synthetase system (Soderbing *et al.*, 1970). The finding, therefore, suggests that a single enzyme, a cyclic $3,5'$-AMP-stimulated protein kinase, inactivates glycogen synthetase and conversely activates phosphorylase b kinase and therefore glycogen phosphorylase (Figure 6).

It has been known for a long time that epinephrine increases the rate of release of glucose from the liver. Hepatic slices were found suitable for the study of the hormonal effect. The effect was lost, however, when hepatic homogenate was centrifuged and the supernatant used for the study; it was found later that epinephrine interacts with the particulate fractions of the homogenate, producing a factor which was identified as cyclic AMP (Rall *et al.*, 1957; Sutherland and Rall, 1957). Studies on the distribution of adenylate cyclase (Davoren and Sutherland, 1963; Sutherland *et al.*, 1962; Rabinowitz *et al.*, 1965), the enzyme that catalyzes the conversion of ATP to cyclic AMP, revealed its wide distribution in membranes of cells suggesting the idea that this protein could be considered a cellular chemical receptor. It is then apparent that the interaction of the hormone, epinephrine, with the adenylate cyclase of cellular membranes can start a significant series of events in the main route supplying energy to tissues (Figure 6).

This is an example of how hormone, through chemical modifications of preformed polypeptide chains, may control important segments of metabolism.

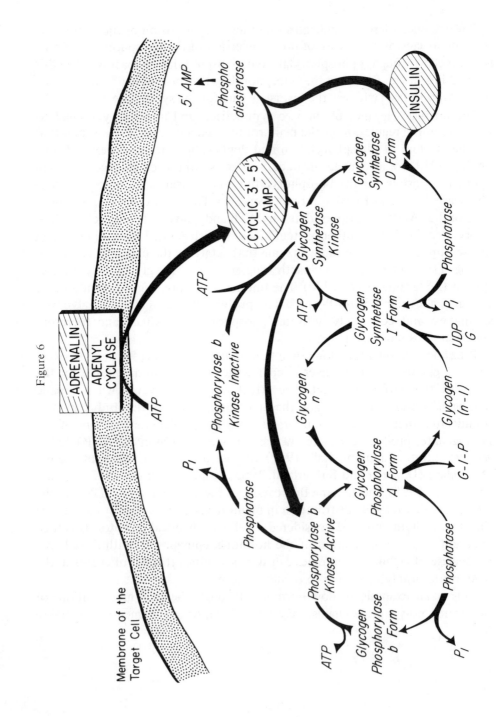

Figure 6

References

1. BROWN, D. and CORI, C. F.: Animai and Plant Polysaccharide Phosphorylases. The Enzymes, *5:*207, 1961.

2. COREY, R. B. and PAULING, L.: Fundamental Dimensions of Polypeptide Chains. Proc. Roy. Soc. (London), *141:*10, 1953.

3. DATTA, P. and GEST, H.: Alternative Patterns of End-Product Control in Biosynthesis of Amino Acids of the Aspartic Family. Nature, *203:*1259, 1964.

4. DAVOREN, P. R. and SUTHERLAND, E. W.: The Cellular Location of Adenyl Cyclase in the Pigeon Erythrocyte. J. Biol. Chem., *238:*3016, 1963.

5. FISHER, E. H. and KREBS, E. H.: Conversion of Phosphorylase b to Phosphorylase a in Muscle Extracts. J. Biol. Chem., *216:*121, 1955.

6. FRIEDEN, C.: Glutamic Dehydrogenase II. The Effect of Various Nucleotides on on the Association-Dissociation and Kinetic Properties. J. Biol. Chem., *234:* 815, 1959.

7. FRIEDEN, C.: The Dissociation of Glutamic Dehydrogenase by Reduced Disphosphopyridine Nucleotide (DPNH). Biochim. Biophys. Acta, *27:*431, 1958.

8. FRIEDMAN, D. L. and LARNER, J.: Studies on UDGP-Glucan Transglucosylase. III. Interconversion of two Forms of Muscle UDPG-Glucan Transglucosylase by a Phosphorylation-Dephosphorylation Reaction Sequence. Biochemistry, *2:* 669, 1963.

9. GERHARDT, J. C. and PARDEE, A. B.: The Enzymology of Control by Feedback Inhibition. J. Biol. Chem., *237:*891, 1962.

10. HUXLEY, J. S.: Chemical Regulation and the Hormone Concept. Biol. Rev., *10:*427, 1935.

11. KAUZMANN, W.: Some Factors in the Interpretations of Protein Denaturation. Advances in Protein Chem., *14:*1, 1959.

12. KELLER, P. J. and GORI, G. T.: Enzymic Conversion of Phosphorylase a to Phosphorylase b. Biochim. Biophys. Acta, *12:*235, 1953.

13. KLOTZ, I. M., LANGERMAN, N. R., and DARNALL, D. W.: Quanternary Structure of Proteins. Ann. Rev. of Biochem., *39:*25, 1970.

14. KOSHLAND, D. E.: Enzyme Conformation in Relation to Controlled Activity Conformation Changes at the Active Site during Enzyme Action. Federation Proc., *23:*719, 1964.

15. KOSHLAND, D. E.: The Role of Flexibility in Enzyme Action. *Cold Spring Harbor Symp. Quant. Biol.,* 28:473, 1963.

16. KOSHLAND, D. E., NEMETHY, G., and FILMER, D.: Comparison of Experimental Binding Data and Theoretical Models in Proteins Containing Subunits. Biochem., *5:*365, 1966.

17. KREBS, E. G. and FISHER, E. H.: Molecular Properties and Transformation of Glycogen Phosphorylase in Animal Tissues. Advan. Enzym., *24:*263, 1962.

18. KREBS, E. G. and FISHER, E. H.: The Phosphorylase b to a Converting Enzyme of Rabbit Skeletal Muscle. Biochim. Biophys., Acta, *20:*150, 1956.

19. KREBS, E. G., KENT, A. B., and FISHER, E. H.: The Muscle Phosphorylase b Kinase Reaction. J. Biol. Chem., *231:*73, 1958.

20. KUBO, H., IWATSUBO, M., WATARI, H., and SOYAMA, T.: Sur la Polymerisation et la Forme Moleculaire de la Glutamico–Deshydrogenase. J. Biochem. (Tokyo), *46:*1171, 1959.

21. LACROUTE, F., PICRARD, A., GRENSON, M., and WIAME, S. M.: The Biosynthesis of Carbamyl Phosphate in *Saccharomyces cerevisiae.* J. Gen. Microbiol., *40:*127, 1965.

22. LARNER, J.: Hormonal and Nonhormonal Control of Glycogen Metabolism. N. Y. Acad. Sci., Ser. II, *29:*192, 1966.

23. MONOD, J., WYMAN, J., and CHANGEUX, J. P.: Allosteric Proteins and Cellular Control Systems. J. Mol. Biol., *6:*306, 1963.

24. MONOD, J. WYMAN, J., and CHANGEUX, J. P.: On the Nature of Allosteric Transitions: A Plausible Model. J. Mol. Biol., *12:*88, 1965.

25. NEMETHY, G. and SCHERAGA, H.: Structure of Water and Hydrophobic Bonding in Proteins I. A Model for the Thermodynamic Properties of Liquid Water J. Chem. Phys., *36:*3382, 1962.

26. NESTER, E. W. and JENSEN, R. A.: Control of Aromatic Acid Biosynthesis in *Bacillus subtilis*: Sequential Feedback Inhibition. J. Bacteriol., *91*:1594, 1966.

27. OLSON, J. A. and ANFINSEN, C. B.: The Crystallization and Characterization of L-Glutamic Acid Dehydrogenase. J. Biol. Chem., *197*:67, 1952.

28. PATTEN, J. C., LEBRAS, G., and COHEN, G. N.: Regulation by Methionine of the Synthesis of a Third Aspartokinase and of a Second Homoserine Dehydrogenase in *Escherichia coli* K_{12}. Biochim. Biophys. Acta, *136:*245, 1967.

29. PAULING, L., COREY, R. B., and BRANSON, H. R.: The Structure of Proteins: Two Hydrogen-bonded Helical Configurations of the Polypeptide Chains. Proc. Natl. Acad. Sci., U. S., *37*:205, 1951.

30. RABINOWITZ, M., DESALLES, L., MEISLER, J., and LORAND, L.: Distribution of Adenyl-cylase Activity in Rabbit Skeletal Muscle Fractions. Biochim. Biophys. Acta, *97:*29, 1965.

31. RALL, T. W., SUTHERLAND, E. W., and BERTHET, J.: The Relationship of Epinephrine and Glucagon to Liver Phosphorylase. IV. Effect of Epinephrine and Glucagon on the Reactivation of Phosphorylase in Liver Homogenates. J. Biol. Chem., *224:*463, 1957.

32. SODERBING, T. R., HICKENBOTTOM, J. P., REIMANN, E. M., HUNKELER, F. L., WALSH, D. A., and KREBS, E. G.: Inactivation of Glycogen Synthetase and Activation of Phosphorylase Kinase by Muscle Adenosine 3′, 5′-Monophosphate - dependent Protein Kinases. J. Biol. Chem., *245*:6317, 1970.

33. STADTMAN, E. R., COHEN, G. N., LEBRAS, G., and DE ROBICHON-SZULMAJSTER, H.: Feedback Inhibition and Repression of Aspartokinase Activity in *Escherichia coli* and *Saccharomyces cerevisiae.* J. Biol. Chem., *236:*2033, 1961.

34. SUTHERLAND, E. W. and RALL, T. W.: The Properties of an Adenine Ribonucleotide Produced with Cellular Particles, ATP Mg^{++} and Epinephrine or Glucagon. J. Amer. Chem. Soc., *79:*3608, 1957.

35. SUTHERLAND, E. W., RALL, T. W., and MENON, T.: Adenyl Cyclase-Distribution, Preparation, and Properties. J. Biol. Chem., *237:*1220, 1962.

36. TOMKINS, G. M., YIELDING, K. L., and CURRAN, J. F.: Steroid Hormone Activation of L-Alanine Oxidation Catalyzed by a Subunit of Crystalline Glutamic Dehydrogenase. Proc. Natl. Acad. Sci., U. S., *47:*270, 1961.

37. TOMKINS, G. M., YIELDING, K. L., CURRAN, J. F., SUMMERS, M. R., and BITENSKY, M. W.: The Dependence of the Substrate Specificity on the Conformation of Crystalline Glutamate Dehydrogenase. J. Biol. Chem., *240:*3793, 1965.

38. TROUT, R. R. and LIPMANN, F.: Activation of Glycogen Synthetase by Glucose 6-Phosphate. J. Biol. Chem., *238:*1213, 1963.

39. UMBARGER, H. E.: Evidence for a Negative-feedback Mechanism in the Biosynthesis of Isoleucine. Science, *123:*848, 1956.

40. WALSH, D. A., PERKINS, S. P., and KREBS, E. G.: An Adenosine 3 ,5′-Monophosphate-dependent Protein Kinase from Rabbit Skeletal Muscle. J. Biol. Chem., *243:*3763, 1968.

41. WYMAN, J.: Allosteric Linkage. J. Amer. Chem. Soc., *89:*2202, 1967.

42. YATES, R. A. and PARDEE, A. B.: Control of Pyrimidine Biosynthesis in *Escherichia coli* by a Feedback Mechanism. J. Biol. Chem., *221:*757, 1956.

43. YIELDING, K. L. and TOMKINS, G. M.: Studies on the Interaction of Steroid Hormones with Glutamic Dehydrogenase. Recent Prog. on Hormone Res., XVIII, 467, 1962.

44. YIELDING, K. L. and TOMKINS, G. M.: Structural Alterations in Crystalline Glutamic Dehydrogenase Induced by Steroid Hormones. Proc. Natl. Acad. Sci., U. S., *46:*1483, 1960.

CELLULAR
MEMBRANES as AMPLIFIERS
of HORMONAL ACTION

Earl F. Walborg, Jr. and N. Burr Furlong

CELLULAR MEMBRANES AS SITES OF HORMONAL ACTION

Hormonal regulation of cellular processes can be described in terms of molecule-mediated information transfer, initiated by the interaction of hormone and a cellular receptor. The basic elements of such a system have been described by Hechter (1966):

"... two complementary aspects are involved in the primary reaction of hormone with its receptor—one cybernetic, the other energetic. The cybernetic component involves (a) the environmental informational message brought to the cell by hormone which is selectively received by a macromolecule coded to recognize and discriminate between closely related molecular structures and (b) the translation of the message into intracellular language of information signals, which then flow through the cell to diverse effector sites. The energetic component involves amplification of the message so that it may be transmitted with an energy content sufficient to 'trigger' the underlying effector mechanisms. ..."

During the last decade the activity of adenyl cyclase was found to be controlled by a variety of polypeptide hormones and catechol amines (Robison *et al.*, 1968). As a result of these investigations, the two-messenger concept of hormonal action was proposed (Robison *et al.*, 1968). The adenyl-cyclase complex was postulated to function both as the discriminator of environmental messengers and as a generator of intracellular messengers. Sutherland and his associates consider adenyl cyclase to be composed of a regulatory and catalytic subunit, with hormonal specificity being ascribed to the regulatory subunit (Robison, 1967). Hechter and his colleagues designate the hormonal receptors as discriminators and do not specify the mode of coupling between discriminator and adenyl cyclase (Schwartz and Hechter, 1966).

Figure 1 illustrates the basic components of the two-messenger hypothesis. The nomenclature adopted for the various components of the system is consistent with the concept of molecule-mediated information transfer, formulated by Hechter (1966; Robison *et al.*, 1966). Figure 1 should not be construed to espouse either the Sutherland or Hechter models for the association of hormonal receptor and adenyl cyclase, since available experimental evidence cannot distinguish between these mechanistic alternatives. The role of cyclic adenosine-3′, 5′-monophosphate (C-AMP) in amplification of the signal of the extracellular messenger has been discussed by Bowness (1966).

Adenyl cyclase has been demonstrated to be membrane bound (Davoren and Sutherland, 1963), a fact that has served to focus attention on cellular membranes as sites of hormonal action. Fat cell ghosts (Braun and

Figure 1

The Two-messenger Concept of Hormonal Action.

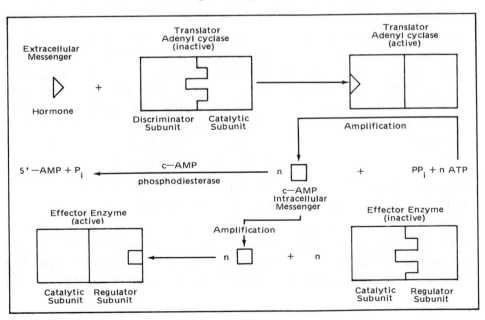

Hechter, 1970) and hepatic cell plasma membranes (Pohl *et al.,* 1969) have been utilized to investigate the effect of hormones on membrane-bound adenyl cyclase. The recent evidence of Turkington (1970) that sepharose-bound insulin and prolactin stimulate the synthesis of rapidly labeled RNA in epithelial cells of the mammary gland in mice indicates that these hormones regulate transcription through an initial interaction with the plasma membrane.

Recent investigations by Rodbell and associates (Pohl *et al.,* 1971; Birnbaumer *et al.,* 1971; Rodbell *et al.,* 1971) on the glucagon-sensitive adenyl cyclase present in hepatic cell plasma membranes of rats will serve to illustrate the recent focus on membranes as sites of hormonal action; they also will provide a basis for further exploration into the role of cellular membranes in molecule-mediated information transfer. Rodbell has summarized the results of these investigations very succinctly:

> "Glucagon binds to liver membranes at sites which are specific for glucagon, finite in number, and which display characteristics of a lipoprotein. Specificity of binding, similarity in range of concentrations over which the hormone binds and activates adenyl cyclase, and the correlations observed between loss of binding and loss of activation of adenyl cyclase by the hormone suggest that the binding sites are components of the glucagon-sensitive adenyl cyclase system in rat-liver membranes .
>
> "An understanding in molecular terms, of the mechanism or mechanisms by which polypeptide hormones control these systems depends upon identification, characterization and resolution of the components of which such a system are made (Pohl *et al.,* 1971)."

Clearly, the future elucidation of the macromolecular nature of hormone-sensitive adenyl cyclase systems will require a clearer understanding of the molecular intricacies of membrane structure. The exemplary progress in unraveling the molecular components of the electron-transfer chain, present in the membrane of mitochondrial cristae (Yamashita and Racker, 1969) demonstrates that complex, membrane-bound, enzymatic systems are amenable to the disruptive experimental approach of the biochemist and finally to reconstitution from its separate components.

MEMBRANE MODELS – IMPLICATIONS OF LIPOPROTEIN SUBUNIT MODELS OF MEMBRANE STRUCTURE

Since cellular membranes are indeed sites of hormonal action, it is reasonable to assume that progress in research on membranes will contribute to clarifying the molecular mechanism of the propagation of information contained in an extracellular messenger into activation of membrane-bound effector enzymes. The conceptual framework for the structure of membranes has undergone evolution from an emphasis on universality and structure to an emphasis on diversity and function. The Davson-Danielli paucimolecular model (lipid bilayer model) of membrane structure (Danielli and Davson, 1935) dominated biological thought for some thirty years. This theory was originally proposed to explain certain biological, chemical, and physical properties of the erythrocyte ghost. It later received support from x-ray diffraction investigation of myelin and from electron-microscopic examination of fixed and stained biological material; and it was finally incorporated into the unit membrane (Robertson, 1959) proposed by J. D. Robertson. The central feature of the paucimolecular model was the arrangement of the lipids in a continuous bimolecular lipid layer in which the polar portions of the lipids were directed outward and the nonpolar portions inward. Proteins were associated with the polar portion of the lipid bilayer by ionic bonds to form a complex in which the structure was primarily determined by the lipid bilayer.

The investigation of the metabolically active mitochondrial membranes prompted Green to question the validity of the lipid-bilayer model and to propose instead that membranes are expressions of repeating lipoprotein units (Green and Pardue, 1966; Green *et al.,* 1967). This model was based on a number of observations, including the following:

(1)   Under appropriate staining conditions, the trilaminar unit membrane generally seen in electron micrographs was replaced by a repeating globular structure.

(2)   Mitochondria extracted with lipid solvents, prior to fixation, continued to show the trilaminar structure when stained sections were observed in the electron microscope, indicating that protein was the determinant of structure.

(3)   Membranes were dissociated by agents that interrupted hydrophobic bonds, indicating that the primary type of bonding between lipid and protein in the membrane was hydrophobic, not electrostatic, in nature.

(4)   Membranes, dissociated into their monomeric subunits, were shown to reassemble by hydrophobic recombination to form membranes. On the basis of these considerations Green and Pardue (1966) proposed that biological membranes were two dimensional continua of nesting lipoprotein repeating units. This model and other variations of the lipoprotein-subunit model (Green *et al.,* 1967; Lucy, 1964; Lenard and Singer, 1966; Benson, 1966; Korn, 1968) have served to emphasize the role of protein as the determinant of membrane structure.

It now seems evident that it will not be possible to explain the widely different properties of widely different membranes (*e.g.,* the myelin sheath and the membrane of mitochondrial cristae) using some universal membrane model. A more reasonable solution would appear to be the existence of a spectrum of structures similar to that proposed by Vanderkooi (Vanderkooi and Green; Vanderkooi and Sundaralingam, 1970). This model envisions two layers of loosely packed globular proteins with crevices or inter-stices between the protein molecules being filled with the nonpolar tail of lipid molecules, so that the polar heads of the lipids lie at the two membrane-water interfaces. The proteins are assumed to have more or less hydrophobic regions on their surfaces, permitting hydrophobic bonding with the lipid molecules. The protein molecules have limited regions of con-tact with each other, meaning that protein interactions will be involved in giving structural stability to the membrane. In the spectrum of membrane structures, the size of the interstitial space would vary, thereby allowing varying amounts of lipid bilayer. The central feature of all subunit models would still be applicable to such a spectrum of membranes; *i.e.,* the protein-to-protein interactions would remain a dominant feature. It is therefore pos-sible to view membranes as lattices of interacting lipoproteins, an arrange-ment that has considerable significance for molecule-mediated information transfer and amplification of the hormone-receptor interaction.

Changeux and colleagues (1967) have considered this aspect of mem-brane structure in developing their theory of cooperativity in biological membranes. The concept of cooperativity is based on several assumptions:

(1) Biological membranes exist as "an ordered collection of globular lipoprotein units organized into a two-dimensional crystalline lattice."

(2) Several conformational states are reversibly accessible to each lipoprotein unit.

(3) The conformation of the lipoprotein depends upon its association with neighboring lipoproteins in the lattice and thus is submitted to a lattice constraint.

The information contained in the extracellular messenger may be propagated through conformational changes of the lipoproteins in the membrane lat-tice. The energetic component necessary to trigger cooperative effects with-in membranes may reside in the membrane-bound, adenyl-cyclase system.

CURRENT MODELS OF COOPERATIVITY

Much of the chemistry upon which life processes depend involves very specific associations between molecular species; for example, substrate for enzyme or hormone for receptor. Mathematical formulations relating to enzymatic associations were developed by Henri (1903), Michaelis and Menton (1913), Briggs and Haldane (1925), and others in this period which served as suitable models for certain simple enzymatically-catalyzed reactions. However as early as 1910, A.V. Hill (1910), proposed a model for oxygen binding to hemoglobin in which interaction occurred among successively bound oxygen molecules, thus altering the binding properties of the hemoglobin-oxygen complex at each stage. The phenomenon whereby the binding of a ligand to a molecule alters the binding of ligands to the same or neighboring molecules is called cooperativity. Cooperativity has been found to provide a much more suitable model for many enzymatic reactions than the simple Michaelis theory and, in addition, is able to provide a formulation encompassing a variety of other biological phenomena. In the case where a ligand binds singly to a molecule and no interaction with other binding sites occurs, the extent of the binding, under the usual assumptions, will vary with ligand concentration in the form of an hyperbola and a double reciprocal plot will be linear. However, if the binding of successive ligands is promoted by those previously bound, the basic relationship becomes sigmoid, *i.e.,* a double reciprocal plot is no longer linear. The importance of sigmoid behavior is that, for certain ligand concentrations, a relatively small change in concentration is capable of producing a profound difference in the amount of ligand bound. Changeux and co-workers (1967) have developed a formulation for cooperativity in which the interdependence of ligand binding is summarized in a convenient manner. Their model applies whether or not the interaction occurs between units that are arrayed linearly on a surface or distributed in three dimensions. In the simplest form, their model assumes that ligand, f, can bind to one or both interconvertible forms of a molecule, R or S, according to the following reactions:

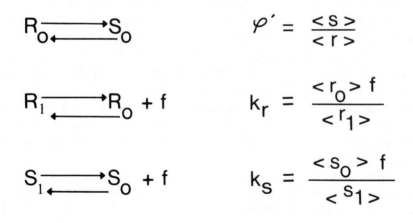

$$R_0 \rightleftarrows S_0 \qquad \varphi' = \frac{<S>}{<r>}$$

$$R_1 \rightleftarrows R_0 + f \qquad k_r = \frac{<r_0> f}{<r_1>}$$

$$S_1 \rightleftarrows S_0 + f \qquad k_s = \frac{<s_0> f}{<s_1>}$$

In each case, the triangular brackets "$<>$" signify the fraction of molecules in the given form, R or S. The equilibrium constant φ' is related to the free energy of conversion from S to R by the usual relationship:

$$\varphi n\, \varphi' = \frac{\Lambda F}{RT}$$

The binding of f to R at a mean energy, η, affects the basal free energy of interconversion ϵ, so that

$$\Delta F = \epsilon - <r>\eta.$$

The contributions to the equilibrium constant, then, can be analyzed into two factors:

$$\varphi n\, \varphi' = \varphi n\, \varphi + <r>\varphi n\, \Lambda$$

where

$$\varphi = \, _e N_0 \epsilon / RT$$

and

$$\Lambda = e^{-N_0 \eta} / RT.$$

Thus, the energy alteration due to ligand binding conveniently appears in the Λ term. Equations are developed giving $<r>$ (the fraction of sites on R occupied by f) as a function of $a = f/k_r = \frac{<r_1>}{<r_0>}$, (the ratio of bound to free sites) in terms of φ, Λ, and , c where $c = K_r/k_s$:

$$r = (1 + a) / [1 + a + \varphi \Lambda^{<r_1>}(1 + ca)].$$

Under certain reasonable assumptions for a ligand that binds only to R, it can be demonstrated that a nearest neighbor interaction value, η, of about 2.4 Kcal./mole will be sufficient to bring about an all-or-none shift in ligand bound: that is, for certain concentrations of f and R, a sudden transition in the ability to bind f occurs. (If f binds to both R and S, the interaction energy, in general, must be greater to achieve this bistable condition). Thus an amplification in the ability of R to bind f occurs in this region. This type of cooperativity provides one means whereby a very slight increase in the concentration of a given substance may be greatly amplified in altering some other metabolite or process.

The problem of amplification has also been approached by Gilbert Ling cooperativity. The recent Changeux (*op. cit.*) model described above is developed on assumptions similar to those used by Ling except that Ling proposes that the binding of ligand occurs simultaneously with the change in form of the molecule responsible for the binding, since he conceives that the ligands compete for sites that determine the conformational state of the proteins. Ling hypothesizes certain specific cardinal absorption sites that determine protein conformational alternatives in an all-or-none fashion. If ions or other ligands are bound differently by the various conformations of the protein, the ligand responsible for altering the conformation will be able to produce profound effects on all the other ligands bound. In the more extended treatments, Changeux has focused attention on the theoretical formulation of the process-as-a-whole, whereas Ling has attempted to provide a reasonable microscopic mechanism for an essentially similar phenomenon. In both of these models of cooperativity, proposals are made whereby single molecular events can be amplified to multimolecular effects, and it is this aspect of cooperativity which probably has the greatest implications for molecular mechanisms of hormonal action.

Acknowledgement

The considerations proposed in this paper were developed in connection with research supported in part by the following grants: G-120 (N. B. F) and G-354 (E. F. W.) from the Robert A. Welch Foundation and a research grant from the Paul and Mary Haas Foundation (E. F. W.).

One of us (E. F. W.) is indebted to Dr. George N. Holcomb, Ferris State College, Big Rapids, Michigan, and Dr. D. N. Ward, Biochemistry Department, University of Texas M. D. Anderson Hospital & Tumor Institute at Houston, for assistance in searching the literature concerned with the role of adenyl cyclase in hormonal action.

References

1. BENSON, A.: On the Orientation of Lipids in Chloroplast and Cell Membranes. J. Am. Oil. Chem. Soc., *43*:265, 1966.

2. BIRNBAUMER, L., POHL, S. L., and RODBELL, M.: The Glucagon-sensitive Adenyl Cyclase System in Plasma Membranes of Rat Liver II. Comparison between Glucagon and Fluoride Stimulated Activities. J. Biol. Chem., *246*:1857-1860, 1971.

3. BOWNESS, J. M.: Epinephrine: Cascade Reactions and Glycogenolytic Effects. Science, *152*:1370-1371, 1966.

4. BRAUN, T. and HECHTER, O.: Glucocorticoid Regulation of ACTH Sensitivity of Adenyl Cyclase in Rat Fat Cell Membranes. Proc. Natl. Acad. Sci., U. S., *66*:995-1001, 1970.

5. BRIGGS, C. E. and HALDANE, J. B. S.: A Note on the Kinetics of Enzyme Action. Biochem. J., *19*:338-343, 1925.

6. CHANGEUX, J. P., THIERY, J., TUNG, Y., and KITTEL, C.: On the Cooperativity of Biological Membranes. Proc. Natl. Acad. Sci., U. S., *57*:335-341, 1967.

7. DANIELLI, J. F. and DAVSON, H.: A Contribution to the Theory of Permeability of Thin Films. J. Cell. Comp. Physiol., *5*:495-508, 1935.

8. DAVOREN, P. R. and SUTHERLAND, E. W.: The Cellular Location of Adenyl Cyclase in the Pigeon Erythrocyte. J. Biol. Chem., *238*:3016-3023, 1963.

9. GREEN, D. E., ALLMANN, D. W., BACHMANN, E., BAUM, H., KOPACZYK, K., KORMAN, E. F., LIPTON, S., MACLENNAN, D. H., McCONNELL, D. G., PERDUE, J. F., RIESKE, J. S., and TZAGOLOFF, A.: Formation of Membranes by Repeating Units. Arch. Biochem. Biophys., *119*:312-335, 1967.

10. GREEN, D. E. and PARDUE, J. F.: Correlation of Mitochondrial Structure and Function. Ann. N. Y. Acad. Sci., *137*:667-684, 1966.

11. HECHTER, O.: Hormone Action at the Cell Membrane. *In*: P. Karlson (ed.), Mechanisms of Hormone Action - A NATO Advanced Study Institute, pp. 61-82. New York: Academic Press, 1966.

12. HENRI, V.: Lois Generales de l'Action des Diastases. Hermann, Paris, 1903.

13. HILL, A. V.: The Possible Effects of the Aggregation of the Molecules of Haemoglobin on Its Dissociation Curves. J. Physiol. (London), *40*:iv, 1910.

14. KORN, E. D.: Structure and Function of the Plasma Membrane. A Biochemical Perspective. J. Gen. Physiol., *52*:257-278, 1968.

15. LENARD, J. and SINGER, S. J.: Protein Conformation in Cell Membrane Preparations as Studied by Optical Rotary Dispersion and Circular Dichroism. Proc. Natl. Acad. Sci., U. S., *56*:1828-1835, 1966.

16. LING, G. N.: A New Model for the Living Cell: A Summary of the Theory and Recent Experimental Evidence in Its Support. *In*: G. H. Bourne and J. F. Danielli (ed.), Review of Cytology, pp. 42-68. New York: Academic Press, 1969.

17. LUCY, J. A.: Globular Lipid Micelles and Cell Membranes. J. Theoret. Biol., *7*:360-373, 1964.

18. MICHAELIS, L. and MENTEN, M. L.: Die Kinetik der Invertinwirkung. Biochem. Z., *49*:333-353, 1913.

19. POHL, S. L., BIRNBAUMER, L., and RODBELL, M.: The Glucagon-sensitive Adenyl Cyclase System in Plasma Membranes of Rat Liver I. Properties. J. Biol. Chem., *246*:1849-1856, 1971.

20. POHL, S. L., BIRNBAUMER, L. and RODBELL, M.: Glucagon-sensitive Adenyl Cyclase in Plasma Membrane of Hepatic Parenchyme Cells. Science, *164*:566, 1969.

21. ROBERTSON, J. D.: The Ultrastructure of Cell Membranes and Their Derivatives. Biochem. Soc. Symp., *16*:1-43, 1959.

22. ROBISON, G. A., BUTCHER, R. W., and SUTHERLAND, E. W.: Cyclic AMP. Ann. Rev. Biochem., *37*:149, 1968.

23. ROBISON, G. A., BUTCHER, R. W. and SUTHERLAND, E. W.: Adenyl Cyclase as an Adrenergic Receptor. Science, *139*:703-723, 1967.

24. RODBELL, M., KRANS, H. M. J., POHL, S. L., and BIRNBAUMER, L.: The Glucagon-sensitive Adenyl Cyclase System in Plasma Membranes of Rat Liver III. Binding of Glucagon: Methods of Assay and Specificity. J. Biol. Chem., *246*:1861-1871, 1971.

25. RODBELL, M., KRANS, H. M. J., POHL, S. L., and BIRNBAUMER, L.: The Glucagon-sensitive Adenyl Cyclase System in Plasma Membranes of Rat Liver IV. Effects of Guanyl Nucleotides on Binding of ^{125}I-Glucagon. J. Biol. Chem., *246*:1872-1876, 1971.

26. RODBELL, M., BIRNBAUMER, L., POHL, S. L., and KRANS, H. M. J.: The Glucagon-sensitive Adenyl Cyclase System in Plasma Membranes of Rat Liver V. An Obligatory Role of Guanyl Nucleotides in Glucagon Action. J. Biol. Chem., *246*:1877-1882, 1971.

27. SCHWARTZ, I. L. and HECHTER, O.: Insulin Structure and Function. Am. J. Med., *40*:765-772, 1966.

28. TURKINGTON, R. W.: Stimulation of RNA Synthesis in Isolated Mammary Cells by Insulin and Prolactin Bound to Sephrarose. Biochem. Biophys. Res. Commun., *41*:1362, 1970.

29. VANDERKOOI, G. and GREEN, D. E.: Biological Membrane Structure, I. The Protein Crystal Model for Membranes. Proc. Natl. Acad. Sci., U. S., *66*:615-621, 1970.

30. VANDERKOOI, G. and SUNDARALINGAM, M.: Biological Membrane Structure, II. A Detailed Model for the Retinal Rod Outer Segment Membrane. Proc. Natl. Acad. Sci., U. S., *67*:233-238, 1970.

31. YAMASHITA, S. and RACKER, E.: Resolution and Reconstitution of the Mitochondrial Electron Transport System. II. Reconstitution of Succinoxidase from Individual Components. J. Biol. Chem., *244*:1220-1227, 1969.

CORRELATION of HORMONAL STRUCTURE with HORMONAL FUNCTION in MAMMALIAN TISSUES

Darrell N. Ward

The hope is often expressed that knowledge of the structure of protein hormones will lend new insight into their mechanism of action. This is true only to the same extent that knowledge of the structure of a steroid or a hormone derived from amino acid, such as thyroxin, has given new insight. Karlson comments on the mode of action of hormones, saying: "As a chemical substance, a hormone can have only chemical effects; it must influence some chemical processes. The observed 'physiological effects' usually appear much later, as a consequence of the primary chemical effect" (Karlson, 1965). This is acceptable if chemical effects include physico-chemical effects. Attention should be directed particularly to the latter part of the statement, ". . . the primary chemical effect." Conceptually, the idea is very simple. A hormone sent to initiate some action in a tissue must have a place to start: a primary chemical effect. In practice, however, the identification of this primary chemical effect has proved very elusive indeed.

A simple diagram is useful to illustrate why the primary chemical effect has been so difficult to identify (Figure 1) The term, primary chemical effect, implies an effect for any specific hormone, not a single primary chemical effect common to all hormones. In Figure 1 the primary chemical event is depicted at A, whereas 1,2,3, *etc.* indicate levels of reaction removed from A but which are initiated by it. To the extent that a hormone may invoke a reaction in more than one tissue or type of cell other primary chemical events may occur, e.g., B, C, etc. The net effect (illustrated here as the fourth level) may represent in summation the so-called physiological effect which could be growth of an organ, growth of the whole animal, or production of biochemical compounds. These usually represent the first observation of the endocrinologist. The usual approach is to trace backward from such an observation through the maze making up the triangles in this series to the more proximal levels leading to A. The difficulty comes in the decision whether the reaction is located at level 2, level 1, or actually at the primary chemical effect. Unfortunately, despite thousands of papers and hundreds of conferences on the mechanism of action of hormones, the detailed mechanism of action of any hormone specifying a mechanism at the molecular level cannot be written at present.

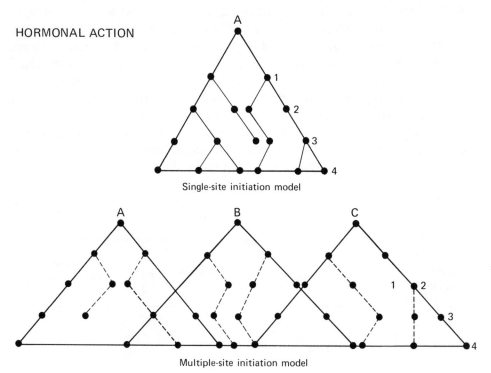

HORMONAL ACTION

Single-site initiation model

Multiple-site initiation model

Figure 1.

Model for hormonal mechanism of action sequelae. The letters designate the primary chemical effect and levels 1, 2, 3, and 4 the subsequent biochemical processes affected.

The studies of mechanisms of action of hormones that would approach the level of 1 or 2 in our diagram would undoubtedly be:

a.   stimulation of m-RNA synthesis.

b.   stimulation of an adenyl cyclase system, and

c.   alteration of cell-membrane permeability
      or transport.

By definition, the primary chemical effect may have been reached in the last instance for those hormones reacting in this fashion, and all that remains is to describe the details of molecular events.

In a recent series of papers, Rodbell and his associates have made impressive progress in their studies of the mechanism of action of glucagon on the cellular membrane of adipose tissue (Birnbaumer *et al.*, 1969 a and 1969 b) and on the membrane of hepatic cells (Pohl *et al.*, 1971; Birnbaumer *et al.*, 1971; Rodbell *et al.*, 1971 a, b, and c). The model on which their studies are based (Figure 2.) is a refinement of one proposed by Hechter and colleagues (Bar *et al.*, 1969 and Hechter *et al.*, 1964). The model of Hechter *et al.*, (1964) is in turn an alternative statement to the unitized receptor subunit model of Sutherland and colleagues (Robison *et al.*, 1968 and Sutherland *et al.*, 1966). The model of Rodbell and colleagues consists of a hormone as the "signal," a "discriminator" to detect the signal, a "transducer" of unspecified nature to transmit the signal to the "amplifier." In the systems they were studying the amplifier represents the adenyl-cyclase system. The amplifier response or output must then continue to affect an enzyme system, etc. in order to obtain the desired end-point.

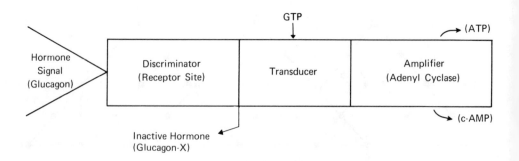

Figure 2.

Schematic representation of the studies of Birnbaumer, Rodbell, Pohl, and Krans (1971) on the mechanism of action of glucagon on hepatic cellular membranes.

In the system for the membrane of hepatic cells studied by Rodbell and coworkers, the reaction *in vitro* was very slow unless GTP was added (Rodbell *et al.*, 1971 a and b). Apparently GTP is involved in an allosteric effect which facilitates the interaction of the discriminator and the transducer. In their particular system, GTP stimulated the rate and degree of dissociation of the bound hormone. Since systems *in vitro* have long been notorious for their lack of sensitivity to hormone, perhaps this will provide a clue to the improvement of such systems for tools in studies on mechanisms of hormonal action.

One more characteristic of the system studied by Rodbell *et al.*, (1971a) that deserves mention is their finding that glucagon was inactivated in proportion to the quantity of membrane present. Although this has not been studied in detail, it would appear that some provision for removal of the input signal is an important part of this model.

The elegant series of papers by Rodbell and coworkers forms an excellent model on which to design structural studies for glucagon analogues, etc. as they may relate to the correlation of hormonal structure with hormonal function in mammalian tissues.

There are now many protein hormones whose amino-acid sequence is known. Obviously, with suitable systems for testing, this knowledge can be put to good use, and luteinizing hormone (LH) will be used to illustrate specific points in relating structure to hormonal function. In 1964, Li and Starman showed LH underwent a monomer-dimer type subunit dissociation. In 1966 we (Ward *et al.*, 1966) were able to show that the subunits were dissimilar and shortly thereafter began our studies on sequence which now have been completed for both subunits (Liu *et al.*, 1970; Liu *et al.*, 1971; and Ward *et al.*, 1972). One of the interesting things that has developed has been that the sequence of the LH-*a* subunit (Liu *et al.*, 1971) from ovine pituitaries is identical to the TSH-*a* subunit from bovine pituitaries as determined by Liao and Pierce (1971). Moreover, studies have shown that combination of TSH-β with either LH-*a* or TSH-*a* produces a hormone with TSH activity or conversely, LH-β plus either TSH-*a* or LH-*a* produces a hormone with LH-type activity (Liao *et al.*, 1970). The foregoing information should be advantageous to studies on the correlation of hormonal structure with hormonal function in mammalian tissues.

The sequence of the LH-*a* subunit, the sequence which is identical to that for TSH-*a* reported by Liao *et al.* (1971), appears in Figure 3. Even the N-terminal heterogeneity is shared with TSH-*a*. The amino-acid sequence of LH-β is presented in Figure 4. This sequence represents the "hormone-specific" subunit. Since this subunit binds non-covalently to the alpha subunit just as does TSH-β, it follows that the homologous areas of the two sequences (TSH-β and LH-β) must be that portion of the molecule involved in this binding. A bar identifies these areas of homology (Figure 4). Then the other part or the molecule remaining must be involved in the interaction with the "discriminator" portion of the target-organ cells, namely Graafian follicle or corpora lutea in the female or interstitial cell of the testis in the male.

If the presumptions made are correct, something of the chemistry of the discriminator site has been defined. Probably future studies of correlations between hormonal structure and function will progress from the chemistry of the hormone to the chemistry of the "discriminator," then to the chemistry of the "transducer," and onward to the chemistry of the "amplifier," *etc.* This remains for the future to disclose.

THE AMINO-ACID SEQUENCE OF THE S - AMINOETHYLATED OVINE
LUTEINIZING HORMONE S - SUBUNIT (LH - α)

[R]$^+$ - Gln - Gly - CysAE - Pro - Gln - CysAE - Lys - Leu - Lys - Glu - Asn - Lys - Tyr - Phe - Ser - Lys - Pro
           10   15   20   25

Asp - Ala - Pro - Ile - Tyr - Gln - CysAE - Met - Gly - CysAE - CysAE - Phe - Ser - Arg - Ala - Tyr - Pro - Thr -
              30   35   40

Pro - Ala - Arg - Ser - Lys - Lys - Thr - Met - Leu - Val - Pro - Lys - Asn (CHO$_{S\alpha}$) - Ile - Thr - Ser - Glu -
       45   50   55   60

Ala - Thr - CysAE - CysAE - Val - Ala - Lys - Ala - Phe - Thr - Lys - Ala - Thr - Val - Met - Gly - Asn - Val--
                     65   70

Arg - Val - Glu - Asn (CHO$_{S\beta}$) - His - Thr - Glu - CysAE - His - CysAE - Ser - Thr - CysAE - Tyr - Tyr - His
       80   .   85   90

Lys - Ser ··OH   †[R] = H· Phe - Pro - Asn - Gly - Gln - Phe - Thr - Met -
                                                            1   5

Figure 3.

Amino-acid sequence of the LH-α subunit of ovine luteinizing hormone (Liu *et al.*, 1971). The [R] designates amino acids involved in N-terminal heterogeneity. The Met residues are points of cleavage by cyanogen bromide; CHO designates carbohydrate moieties Sα and Sβ.

THE AMINO ACID SEQUENCE OF S-CARBOXYMETHYLATED A-SUBUNIT
OF OVINE LH (LH–β)

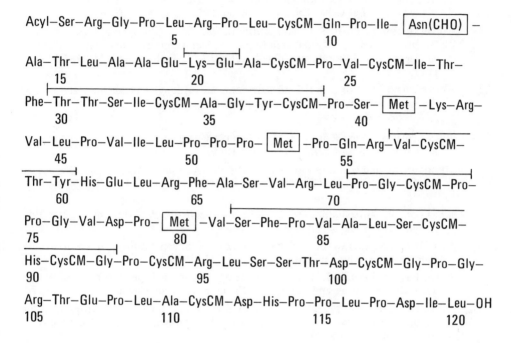

Figure 4.

The amino-acid sequence of the LH-β subunit of ovine luteinizing hormone. The carbohydrate moiety is on residue 13. Those amino acids with a bar overline are the areas of identical homology with TSH-β (or nearly identical homology in the case of the long runs). These areas must be involved in binding to the α-subunit (see text). The areas of interaction with the discriminator would not be limited to the areas not overlined.

References

1.   BAR, H. P. and HECHTER, O.: Adenyl Cyclase and Hormone Action. I. Effects of Adrenocorticotropic Hormone, Glucagon, and Epinephrine on the Plasma Membrane of Rat Fat Cells. Proc. Natl. Acad. Sci., U. S., *63*:350, 1969.

3.   BIRNBAUMER, L., POHL, S. L., and RODBELL, M.: The Glucagon-sensitive Adenyl Cyclase System in Plasma Membranes of Rat Liver. II. Comparison between Glucagon- and Fluoride-stimulated Activities. J. Biol. Chem., *246*:1857-1860, 1971.

2.   BIRNBAUMER, L., POHL, S. L., and RODBELL, M.: Adenyl Cyclase in Fat Cells. I. Properties and the Effects of Adrenocorticotropin and Fluoride. J. Biol. Chem., *244*:3468, 1969.

4.   BIRNBAUMER, L. and RODBELL, M.: Adenyl Cyclase in Fat Cells. II. Hormone Receptors. J. Biol. Chem., *244*:3477, 1969.

5.   HECHTER, O. and HALKERSTON, D. K.: On the Action of Mammalian Hormones. *In*: G. Pincus, K. V. Thiman, and E. B. Astwood (ed.), The Hormones, *5*:697, 1964.

6.   KARLSON, P.: Introduction to Modern Biochemistry. *In*: Hormones, 2nd Ed., p. 334. New York: Academic Press, 1965.

7.   LI, C. H. and STARMAN, B.: Molecular Weight of Sheep Pituitary Interstitial Cell-Stimulating Hormone. Nature, *202*:291-292, 1964.

8.   LIAO, T-H. and PIERCE, J. G.: The Presence of a Common Type of Subunit in Bovine Thyroid-stimulating and Luteinizing Hormones. J. Biol. Chem., *245*:3275, 1970.

9.   LIAO, T-H. and PIERCE, J. G.: The Primary Structure of Bovine Thyrotropin. II. The Amino Acid Sequences of the Reduced, S-carboxymethyl a and β Chains. J. Biol. Chem., *246*:850-865, 1971.

10. LIU, W-K., NAHM, H. S., SWEENEY, C. M., BAKER, H. N., LAMKIN, W. M., and WARD. D. N.: The Amino Acid Sequence of the S-aminoethylated Ovine Luteinizing Hormone S-subunit (LH-*a*). Res. Commun. Chem. Path. Pharmacol., *2*:168,1971.

11. LIU, W-K., SWEENEY, C. M., NAHM, H. S., HOLCOMB, G. N., and WARD, D. N.: The Amino Acid Sequence of the S-Carboxymethylated Ovine Luteinizing Hormone A-subunit (LH-*β*). Res. Commun. Chem. Path. Pharmacol., *1*:463, 1970.

12. POHL, S. L., BIRNBAUMER, L., and RODBELL, M.: The Glucagon-sensitive Adenyl Cyclase System in Plasma Membranes of Rat Liver. I. Properties. J. Biol. Chem., *246*:1849, 1971.

13. ROBISON, G. A., BUTCHER, R. W., and SUTHERLAND, E. W.: Cyclic AMP. Ann. Rev. Biochem., *37*:149-174, 1968.

14. RODBELL, M., BIRNBAUMER, L., POHL, S. L., and KRANS, H. M. J.: The Glucagon-sensitive Adenyl Cyclase System in Plasma Membranes of Rat Liver. V. An Obligatory Role of Guanyl Nucleotides in Glucagon Action. J. Biol. Chem., *246*:1877-1882, 1971.

15. RODBELL, M., KRANS, H. M. J., POHL, S. L., and BIRNBAUMER, L.,: The Glucagon-sensitive Adenyl Cyclase System in Plasma Membranes of Rat Liver. III. Binding of Glucagon: Method of Assay and Specificity. J. Biol. Chem., *246*:1861-1871, 1971.

16. RODBELL,M., KRANS, H. M. J., POHL, S. L., and BIRNBAUMER, L.: The Glucagon-sensitive Adenyl Cyclase System in Plasma Membranes of Rat Liver. IV. Effects of Guanyl Nucleotides on Binding of ^{125}I-glucagon. J. Biol. Chem., *246*:1872-1876, 1971.

17. SUTHERLAND, E. W. and ROBISON, G. A.: The Role of Cyclic-3´, .5´-AMP in Responses to Catecholamines and Other Hormones. Pharmacol. Rev., *18*:145-161, 1966.

18. WARD, D. N., FUJINO, M., and LAMKIN, W. M.: Evidence for Two Carbohydrate Moieties in Ovine Luteinizing Hormone (LH). Fed. Proc., *25*:348, 1966.

19. WARD, D. N., REICHERT, L. E., Jr., LIU, W.-K., NAHM, H. S., and LAMKIN, W. M.: Comparative Studies of Ovine, Bovine, and Human Luteinizing Hormone. *In*: B. B. Saxena, C. G. Beling, and H. M. Gandy (ed.), Gonadotropins, pp. 132-143. New York: John Wiley & Sons, 1972.

PART IV
HORMONAL HETEROPHYLLY

The Concept

THE CONCEPT of
HORMONAL HETEROPHYLLY

Walter J. Burdette

The idea that hormones elaborated in invertebrates have measurable effects on the function and appearance of tissues in vertebrates originated during the time when crude extracts containing invertebrate hormones were first available. The extractions of active material were made possible through identification of fractions by a number of respective bioassays. Much of the original work was directed toward understanding hormonal involvement in the development of the successive chitinous exoskeletal coats necessary to accommodate growth and differential shape characteristic of each stage in the life cycle of invertebrates. As time has elapsed, this has been extended to metabolic and molecular events underlying these and other phenotypic alterations. At first information was acquired chiefly through ablation and transplantation of endocrine organs. It was soon determined that the onset of development following neurosecretion emanating from brain and tropic for target organs was mediated by corpora allata secreting juvenile hormone and by prothoracic glands secreting molting hormone. As a result of a long series of studies by many investigators, the current orthodox or classical concept of endocrine control of metamorphosis ensued (Figure 1).

Hormonal Control of Metamorphosis

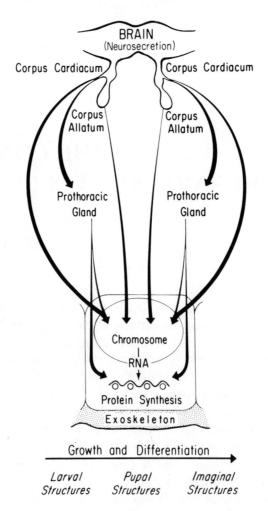

Figure 1

Classical Concept for Hormonal Control of Metamorphosis. This simplistic diagram out-
lines general interrelationships between endocrine glands, hormones, and stages in the life
cycle. Many variations between species are known, and alterations in the concept occur as
additional data are acquired. Much of this information is discussed throughout this volume.

The source of the hormones, mechanism for initiating and terminating their secretion, and interaction with other hormones, endocrine glands, and target tissues is currently in a state of transition with many questions unsettled. On the other hand, much information has been acquired; and, although the structure of brain hormone is unknown, crystalline zooecdysones, phytohormones, and analogs with chemical structures known are now available. Many analogs are known to have biological activities similar to those of native hormones. Juvenile hormone I and II, variations of them between species, and active analogs also are available in quantity; and the stage is set to determine their activity in a wide range of biological tissues. Because both ecdysones and juvenile hormones and their analogs are regarded as possible insecticides more desirable than those that persist in the environment, it is of particular interest to determine the pharmacology of these compounds for mammalian tissues before they are released in the biosphere in large quantities. In addition, evidence was first obtained a decade ago that ecdysones may elicit metabolic responses in vertebrates (Burdette, 1964).

The idea that invertebrate hormones might have some effect on mammalian cells evolved from our original observation that melanotic tumors appearing in Drosophila were inhibited by the presence of ecdysones (Burdette, 1954b). When we ligated Drosophila larvae posterior to the ring gland, the number with tumors was increased. In the tu^{wps} strain which develops tumors spontaneously, 142 out of 311 individuals ligated posterior to the ring gland had tumors, whereas only 27 out of 181 without ligatures were tumor-bearing (P<.05). In order to eliminate the effect of trauma on the appearance of tumors, a gene causing a defect in the ring gland, $l(2)gl$, was introduced into tu^{wps} and tu^{49h} inbred strains of Drosophila with heritable tumors (Burdette, 1954a). There were 21.4 per cent of 973 individuals with tumors in tu^{wps} individuals with defective ring glands compared to 11.4 per cent in 1,196 controls (P<.05); and 5.9 per cent of 425 tu^{49h} with defective glands had tumors compared to 0.7 per cent in 3,878 controls (P<.05). These melanotic tumors consist of aggregates of cells rather than a proliferating mass and none of them appear to be malignant, although viability may be altered by their presence. Many of these tumors consist of aggregates of blood cells and may have a fusiform stroma. Their site of origin may be related to pericardial cells, lymph gland, and fat body. They regress with metamorphosis and leave a pigmented residue in the imago. Despite the obvious dissimilarities between these tumors and benign and malignant neoplasms in mammals, these results suggested that it would be worthwhile to determine whether invertebrate hormones alter growth and metabolism of normal and neoplastic mammalian tissues and whether they occur in the cells of vertebrates.

Samples of fresh human tissues obtained at operation or autopsy were extracted immediately in a manner identical to that yielding extracts from *Bombyx mori* containing active hormone. When 1140 to 7000 G. from each tissue were extracted (Burdette, 1962), no active material was detected in liver, brain, skeletal muscle, small intestine, lung, colon, or kidney. Similar extractions of 2000 G. of Bombyx pupae yielded extracts in which activity for molting hormone was easily demonstrated when bioassayed by the Calliphora test (1 γ = 1 unit). Respective quantities of spleen, testis, cardiac muscle, stomach, pancreas, thyroid, and uterus weighing 703 G. or less also failed to yield positive bioassays. Although this does not rule out the presence of extremely small amounts of molting hormone in human tissues, no positive evidence has been obtained so far that these hormones do appear in them. Positive bioassays for juvenile hormone and brain hormone in material originating from mammals have been reported by Gilbert and Schneiderman (1958), Kobayashi *et al.* (1965), and others. However, the assays for these hormones appear to be somewhat less specific than that for ecdysone, and substances such as sterols not identical with JH that occur in mammals yield positive results.

Two types of experiments were performed to determine the effect of ecdysones on protein metabolism in mammalian tissues (Burdette and Coda, 1963; Burdette, 1964). In the first, the uptake of radioactive leucine into protein was determined for the macrosomal fraction of murine liver with and without crude ecdysones. An increased uptake was found, roughly proportional to the concentration of hormone. From 100 to 1,000 Calliphora units per ml. were tested, and the uptake was increased significantly when 250 Calliphora units or more were added. Later, cultures of HeLa cells were treated with 100 to 2,000 Calliphora units on the third day of growth. Aliquots counted with a Coulter counter showed the inhibition of proliferation with higher doses. When 600 Calliphora units/ml. were added and the mean amount of DNA and RNA in the cells determined subsequently, both were found to be increased, DNA from 20.0 to 87.8 μg./ml. and RNA from 70.1 to 167.6 μg./ mg. We detected no effect of ecdysone on the tensile strength of healing murine wounds (Burdette and Price, unpublished).

Since these studies were carried out with crude ecdysone, they could have been due, at least in part, to the presence of material other than the active ecdysone(s) known to be present. Nevertheless, a significant increase in RNA, DNA, and protein synthesis was recorded in this group of experiments. Variations in results between samples made the data on protein synthesis more open to question than those in the experiment with HeLa cells. This work, done at a time before crystalline material was available in large enough quantities for experimentation on mammalian tissues, represents the first indication that RNA, DNA, and protein synthesis in vertebrates can be altered by ecdysones.

A tissue known to respire aerobically and to have a very large number of mitochondria then was selected for testing the effect of ecdysones on carbohydrate metabolism. The Q_{O_2} of cardiac muscle from the rat was determined with and without the addition of crude ecdysone extract to medium in which slices were incubated. The ecdysones did not change the Q_{O_2} without exogenous substrate; but when substrate was added, there was a suggestive increment in Q_{O_2} within the first hours of incubation after the addition of the hormone. This suggested that additional inquiry about the effect of ecdysones on utilization of substrate by mammalian tissue would be worthwhile, although the differences found were not significant ($P > .05$) at the end of 3 hours (Table 1).

TABLE 1

THE EFFECT OF ECDYSONE ON RESPIRATION
OF MAMMALIAN CARDIAC MUSCLE

No. of Determinations	Substrate	30	60	90	120	150	180
63	0.02 M. Na Lactate	1.92*	3.29	4.45	5.55	6.30	7.15
63	Ecdysone + 0.02 M. Na Lactate	2.17	3.57	4.85	5.53	6.95	7.75
57	0.02 M. Na Succinate	4.94	9.71	14.17	18.75	20.77	26.21
57	Ecdysone + 0.02 M. Na Succinate	5.51	10.28	14.81	19.45	23.56	27.28

*   Mean cu. mm. O_2 consumed per mg. dry weight of tissue.

Burdette and Ashford (Burdette, 1964) perfused the livers of rats with active crude extract of ecdysone from Bombyx and studied the fine structure of the hepatic tissue at intervals subsequently. Although it is difficult to quantitate results in such studies, it appeared that there was alignment and prominence of rough endoplasmic reticulum in cells exposed to the hormone. Vacuoles and possible increase in pinocytosis were also observed.

These early studies could not be extended until crystalline hormones and analogs became available. However, they did provide a foundation for later work and established the basis for the idea that tissues in vertebrates may respond as well as those of invertebrates to this group of compounds. Of greatest interest, perhaps, is the response of mammalian tissues to hormones elaborated in invertebrates and plants and their synthetic analogs. The term, hormonal heterophylly, implies the response of tissues in one phylum to hormones that occur naturally in another. It does not connote the necessity either for a specific new target mechanism of sophisticated responses or the retention of one superseded in phylogeny and no longer used in the alien host. Pharmacological effects are of interest as well.

Although this discussion and much of the investigative work primarily have been concerned with ecdysones, possible action of juvenile hormones and analogs on vertebrate tissues should be explored with comparable enthusiasm. Inquiries into effects on reproduction and fetal development as well as interactions with ecdysones are of special interest.

It is clear from the results presented and those that will follow in subsequent chapters that both morphologic and metabolic responses occur when invertebrate hormones, analogs, and phytohormones are administered to mammals. Whether these effects are specific and whether transphylar target mechanisms exist in tissues removed by evolutionary epochs remain to be determined. However, there now seems to be sufficient evidence to warrant a broader view of the usefulness of this group of hormones, so that they possibly may unravel some of the secrets of molecular biology for mammalian tissues as well as for those tissues exposed to the hormones in the normal course of events.

Acknowledgement:

Aided by a grant from the National Cancer Institute U.S.P.H.S. CA 10037.

References

1. BURDETTE, W. J.: Effect of Defective Ring Gland on Incidence of Tumors in *Drosophila*. J. Nat. Cancer Institute, *15*:367-376, 1954a.
2. BURDETTE, W. J.: Effect of Ligation of *Drosophila* Larvae on Tumor Incidence. Cancer Research, *14*:780-782, 1954b.
3. BURDETTE, W. J.: Bioassay of Human Tissue for Ecdysone. Proc. Soc. Exptl. Biol. and Med *110*:730-731, 1962.
4. BURDETTE, W. J.: The Significance of Invertebrate Hormones in Relation to Differentiation. Cancer Research, *24*:526-536, 1964.
5. BURDETTE, W. J. and CODA, R. L.: Effect of Ecdysone Incorporation of ^{14}C - Leucine into Hepatic Protein *in Vitro*. Proc. Soc. Exper. Biol. Med., *112:* 216-217, 1963.
6. GILBERT, L. I. and SCHNEIDERMAN, H. A.: Occurrence of Substances with Juvenile Hormone Activity in Adrenal Cortex of Vertebrates. Science, *128*:844, 1958.
7. KOBAYASHI, M., SAITO, M., ISHITOYA, Y., and IKEKAWA, N.: Brain Hormone Activity in *Bombyx mori* of Sterols and Physiologically Vital Active Substances. Proc. Soc. Exptl. Biol. and Med., *114*:316-318, 1963.

Pharmacology

PHARMACOLOGY of ECDYSONES
in VERTEBRATES

Shuntaro Ogawa, Nobushige Nishimoto,
and Hiroyuki Matsuda

There are many reports of ecdysones related to invertebrates, but studies applied to mammals are relatively few. We examined some pharmacological effects of ecdysterone and inokosterone (Matsuda *et al.*, 1970) and found acute toxicities of both compounds to be very low. Oral administration of both compounds in a maximum permissible dose, 9.0 G./kg., in male mice did not give any fatal results. Therefore, the LD_{50} was not observed in practice. After intraperitoneal administration, the LD_{50} of ecdysterone is 6.4 G./kg. and that of inokosterone is 7.8 G./kg. respectively. Therefore, inokosterone has a somewhat lower toxicity than ecdysterone.

The administration of 200, 400, or 600 mg./kg. of ecdysterone or inokosterone in the lymph sinus of the bullfrog did not show any remarkable effect. Also these compounds failed to show any effect on the isolated heart of the bullfrog when applied in saturated solution.

Respective intravenous administration of 1.0, 10.0, and 100.0 mg./kg. of these compounds in the rabbit resulted in no effect on respiration and blood pressure. The Magnus method was used to study possible effects of these compounds on the smooth muscle of guinea pigs, and no direct effect, anti-acetylcholinergic effect, antibarium effect, or antihistaminic effect of these compounds were observed at the concentrations of $2 \times 10^{-6} - 2 \times 10^{-4}$ G./ml.

341

The molting hormones with steroidal skeleton suggest that they might have sexual hormonal, anabolic, and anti-inflammatory effects similar to those of steroidal compounds in general. However, 0.1, 0.5, and 5.0 mg./day/kg. of ecdysterone or inokosterone administered to castrated rats for 7 days failed to alter weight of prostate, seminal vesicles, or the levator ani when compared to similar measurements in animals not treated. Also the administration of 0.1, 1.0, 10.0, and 100.0 mg./day/kg. of both compounds for 3 days gave no effect on the uterine weight. Therefore, sex-hormonal and anabolic effects of these compounds were not demonstrated. When carrageenin edema of the foot and cotton-pellet granulomas in rats were observed after administration of these hormones, suppressive effects were not recognized, so effects on inflammatory response by these compounds were not observed.

Stimulation of protein synthesis of the phytoecdysones in rat liver has been known since the work of Burdette (1964). Therefore, it was thought that ecdysterone might accelerate regeneration of the corneal epithelium of the eye. However, no effect was observed when ecdysterone in concentrations of 0.1, 1.0, 10.0, and 100.0 mg. per cent was given to rabbits. Also inokosterone had no effect on the oxygen consumption of the whole cornea and the iris-ciliary body of rabbits in concentrations of 0.1, 1.0, 10.0, and 100.0 mg. per cent either.

Ecdysterone and inokosterone were not effective in altering the normal blood-sugar level in the rat, but these compounds showed the interesting property of suppressing the hyperglycemia appearing after glucagon (Tables 1 and 2). A mixture of half inokosterone and half ecdysterone was used to test the subacute toxicity of phytoecdysones. Male and female rats received orally 200—2000 mg./day/kg. of the sample for 35 days. During this period, the body weight and the feeding weight were recorded, and at the end of this period values for certain components of the blood (erythrocytes, hemoblogin, protein, cholesterol, and transaminase activity), bromosulphalein-excretion test, and the weights of various organs (pituitary, thyroid, thymus, lung, heart, liver, spleen, kidney, adrenal, prostate, testicle, epididymis, seminal vesicle, uterus, and ovary) were examined. There were no remarkable differences between animals treated and those used as controls and no toxicoses occurred.

These pharmacological experiments with ecdysterone and inokosterone suggest their toxicity to be exceedingly low for mammals. However, interesting effects on mammalian liver, blood lipids (Yoshida and Uchiyama, 1971), and blood sugar have been reported. In any event, these compounds not only stimulate metamorphosis in invertebrates, but also are interesting compounds possibly important for mankind as well.

TABLE 1

EFFECT OF INTRAPERITONEAL ADMINISTRATION OF ECDYSTERONE
AND INOKOSTERONE ON HYPERGLYCEMIA
IN RATS AFTER ADMINISTRATION OF GLUCAGON

Substance	Dose (Mg./Kg.)	Per Cent Change of Hyperglycemia after Glucagon	
		Administration 1 Day	Administration 7 Days
Control	0	100.0	100.0
Ecdysterone	0.1	54.3	60.6
Ecdysterone	0.5	53.0	59.1
Ecdysterone	1.0	61.8	52.5
Ecdysterone	10.0	62.5	60.5
Inokosterone	0.1	78.3	80.8
Inokosterone	0.5	68.2	81.0
Inokosterone	1.0	62.5	67.4
Inokosterone	10.0	60.4	69.3

TABLE 2

EFFECT OF ORAL ADMINISTRATION OF ECDYSTERONE AND INOKOSTERONE ON
HYPERGLYCEMIA IN RATS AFTER ADMINISTRATION OF GLUCAGON

Substance	Dose (Mg./Kg.)	Per Cent Change of Hyperglycemia after Glucagon	
		Administration 1 Day	Administration 7 Days
Control	0	100.0	100.0
Ecdysterone	1	84.3	76.0
Ecdysterone	5	74.0	55.0
Ecdysterone	10	73.0	51.0
Ecdysterone	100	54.9	46.0
Inokosterone	1	95.5	84.8
Inokosterone	5	91.9	76.5
Inokosterone	10	77.0	68.5
Inokosterone	100	69.0	55.0

References

1. BURDETTE, W. J.: The Significance of Invertebrate Hormones in Relation to Differentiation. Cancer Research, *24*:520-536, 1964.
2. MATSUDA, H., KAWABA, T., and YAMAMOTO, Y.: Pharmacological Studies of Insect Metamorphosing Steroids from *Achyranthis radix*. Folia Pharmacological Japonica, *66*:551-563, 1970.
3. YOSHIDA, T. and UCHIYAMA, M.: Effect of Ecdysterone on Lipid Metabolism. Pharm. Soc. of Japan, 91st Annual Meeting, Fukuoka, 240, 1971.

TESTS for
TOXICITY of JUVENILE
HORMONE and ANALOGS
in MAMMALIAN SYSTEMS

John B. Siddall and Michael Slade

S ince both natural juvenile hormones (Meyer *et al.*, 1970; Röller and
Dahm, 1968) and analogs may possibly be used extensively in the control of insect pests (Williams, 1956), it is important to determine possible
effects of these substances on animals and the human population. Although
testing has not been extensive so far, something is already known about the
results of exposure of mice, rabbits, and fish to the natural juvenile hormones I and II of *Hyalophora cecropia* (Figures 1 and 2) and two analogs
(Figures 3 and 4). The *trans, trans, cis* Cecropia hormone I in oral dosage
of 5000 mg./kg. of body weight produced no signs of toxicity in Swiss
Webster mice and the *trans, trans* hormone II was also found to be in-
nocuous in dosage of 5000 mg./kg. orally when administered in similar
fashion (Siddall and Slade, 1971). In these experiments, groups of five
males and five females were kept in the laboratory for one week and then
given the hormone synthesized stereoselectively (Siddall, 1970) as a single

345

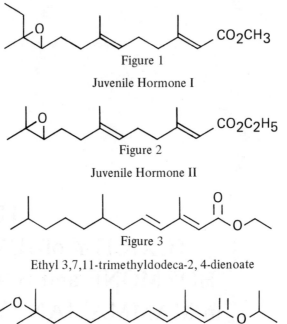

Figure 1

Juvenile Hormone I

Figure 2

Juvenile Hormone II

Figure 3

Ethyl 3,7,11-trimethyldodeca-2, 4-dienoate

Figure 4

Isopropyl 11-methoxy-3,7,11-trimethyldodeca-2, 4-dienoate

gastric lavage of 5000 mg./kg. in fasting mice weighing approximately 20 grams. The vehicle used for administration of the hormone was vegetable oil. Consumption of food and water was recorded; and after 21 days samples of blood were obtained, the animals were killed, and the organs examined. Gross examination of the lungs and heart, endocrine organs, liver, kidneys, and spleen revealed no lesions; and no abnormalities were found in the levels of glucose and urea nitrogen, sodium, or alkaline phosphatase in the blood or in the hemoglobin, hematocrit, total leucocytes, or differential blood counts. Intake of water and food were not affected, none of the animals died, and curves for gain in weight were not unusual.

The insect-hormone analog, ethyl 3, 7, 11-trimethyl dodeca, 2, 4-dienoate (Zoecon, 1971) has particularly high activity against aphids as well as several other economically important pests. The material gave minimal eye irritation when applied to the rabbit conjunctiva and mild skin irritation in rabbits. No adverse effects were found when up to 100 parts per million were added to the water containing both blue gills and trout or when 34,600 mg./kg. was administered orally to rats.

Another insect hormone analog, isopropyl, 11-methoxy, 3, 7, 11-tri-methyl dodeca-2, 4-dienoate (Zoecon, 1971), is of possible use in eliminating a number of important diptera and other insects affecting the economy as a result of morphogenetic effects rather than direct toxic activity. No deleterious effects were found in rats when this analog was administered orally in dosages of 10,200 mg./kg. No irritating effect on the conjunctiva of rabbits appeared, and neither blue gills nor trout exhibited any adverse effects when the water in which they were maintained contained 100 parts per million of this analog.

Male Swiss-Webster mice were given 3.0 μg of 2 - ^{14}C - JH in dimethyl-sulfoxide *via* gastric tube, and excretion of radiocarbon measured in urine and feces (Slade and Zibitt, 1972). Approximately 30 percent was excreted in the urine within 24 hours and negligible amounts thereafter. Only traces were found in the feces. Expired CO_2 was not collected. The possibility of storage of JH in mammals follows from these results and requires additional investigation to compare metabolic routes in vertebrates and those in insects.

In summary, the parameters tested for possible adverse effects of natural juvenile hormones I and II and two additional analogs showed no toxic effects either in the fish or mammals tested except for very mild skin irritation and conjunctival irritation in rabbits for one of the analogs. Although these acute toxicity tests are only preliminary in nature and not extensive, it is encouraging that large doses of juvenile hormones and at least one analog apparently can be tolerated respectively in large doses without harmful effects. Additional more extensive studies on acute and chronic toxicity of these compounds will be required to conclude that there is complete absence of toxicity in mammals, particularly since the question of storage of JH in vertebrates has been raised by preliminary experiments.

References

1. MEYER, A. S., HANZMANN, E., SCHNEIDERMAN, H. A., GILBERT, L. I., and BOY-ETTE, M.: The Isolation and Identification of the Two Juvenile Hormones from the Cecropia Silk Moth. Arch. Biochem., *137*:190-213, 1970.
2. RÖLLER, H. and DAHM, K. H.: The Chemistry and Biology of Juvenile Hormone. Recent Prog. Hormone Res., *24*:651-680, 1968.
3. SIDDALL, J. B.: Chemical Aspects of Hormonal Interactions. *In*: E. Sondheimer and J. B. Simeone (ed.), Chemical Ecology, pp. 281-306. New York: Academic Press, 1970.
4. SIDDALL, J. B. and SLADE, M.: Absence of Acute Oral Toxicity of *Hyalophora cecropia* Juvenile Hormone in Mice. Nature New Biology, *229*:158, 1971.
5. SLADE, M. and ZIBITT, C. H.: Metabolism of Cecropia Juvenile Hormone in Insects and in Mammals. *In:* J. J. Menn and M. Beroza (ed.), Insect Juvenile Hormones, pp. 155-176. New York: Academic Press, 1972.
6. WILLIAMS, C. M.: The Juvenile Hormone of Insects. Nature, *178*:212-213, 1956.
7. Zoecon Chemical Bulletin, November 4, 1971.

*Effect of Invertebrate Hormones
and Analogs on Tumors*

INVERTEBRATE
HORMONES and TUMORS

Walter J. Burdette

TUMORS IN DROSOPHILA

Hereditary, melanotic tumors in Drosophila have attracted the attention of research workers since the report of Bridges (1916) that a gene, *1(1)7,* causes melanotic tumors associated with the presence of clusters of larval cells that become pigmented. Stark (1935) viewed these tumors as possibly analogous to lymphosarcoma in vertebrates. Subsequent observers (Burdette, 1959) have studied many mutant strains of these tumors that originate spontaneously and also have noted tumors sporadically in populations of Drosophila in which they are observed only on rare occasions. Both susceptibility of these strains to the tumors and their pathogenesis have been reported Three types of tumors have been encountered in Drosophila, tumorous head *(tu^h)* and ovarian tumors, transplanted tumors originating in *l(2)gl^4* mutants, and the melanotic tumors which appear chiefly in the abdomen but may be found in the head and extremities as well.

In strains with genes for melanotic tumors, clusters of the cellular components appear early in larval life and consist of polygonal cells with which fusiform cells may be associated. The latter represent the stroma observed in cultures of tumors reported by Ghelelovitch (1959) or other hemocytes of the type(s) described by Jones (1969) and others (Scharrer and Lochhead, 1950; Strunge *et al.,* 1951). The tumors appear often to arise in the region of the lymph glands, fat body, and pericardium. When they become detached in the circulation their mobility gives them a bizarre appearance. Lamello-cytes may encapsulate other tissues to produce the appearance of tumors according to Rizki (1957). The tumors represent aggregates of cells rather than proliferating masses characteristic of benign and malignant neoplasms in mammals. Melanization begins at the periphery quite early, and pigment is visible grossly in the later instars, in pupae, and in the imaginal stages. Cel-lular elements finally disappear, leaving residual pigment as mute evidence of their prior existence. Recently we (Burdette, 1973) have found that the im-mune mechanism against infection by *Aerobacter cloacae* is impaired in the $tu^{48a}vg\ bw$ strain when results are compared to those with the Oregon R strain in which melanotic tumors are found very rarely. This would fit in with the hypothesis that the cells forming tumors are derived from those in-volved in cellular defenses, but additional study is required for confirmation. Melanotic tumors are, of course, not all necessarily composed of hemocytes.

In 1952 we were able to show that ligation of larvae behind the ring gland at the appropriate larval stage (Burdette, 1954b), impeding the flow of hor-mone to posterior segment, increased the number with these tumors. The role of hormones was confirmed in two strains of Drosophila with heredi-tary, melanotic tumors by showing that the numbers of tumors was increased when the ring gland was defective after introducing the gene, *l(2)gl,* into the tu^{wps} and *se* $e^{11}\ tu^{49h}$ tumor strains of *Drosophila melanogaster* (Burdette, 1954a). Recently Madhavan (1972) has reported the induction of these tu-mors with juvenile hormone. Earlier, Bryant and Sang (1969) reported that mimics of JH such as farnesol methyl ether also lead to an increased inci-dence of tumors in Drosophila. One problem encountered in studying these tumors is the fact that similar disposition of hemocytes and pigmentation occurs following injury. These tumors are usually not considered to be malig-nant although Hartung (1948), El Shatoury (1954), Ardashnikov (1941), and others have reported reduced viability of individuals bearing them. The leth-ality associated with the *lethal (1)7* stock is a result of obstruction in the alimentary tract and is not the direct result of the presence of tumors (Russell, 1940).

The incidence of tumors in the large number of strains of melanotic tu-mors varies from a penetrance of less than 1 to more than 99 per cent (Bur-dette, 1951, 1954e, 1959). We obtained isogenic strains of Drosophila with-out increasing the incidence to 100 per cent (Burdette, 1952b) and found that the number with tumors is related to environmental factors such as temperature and nutrition. For example, the tu^g strain has a high incidence at 20° C., but this may be reduced to a tenth of that at 25° C., whereas in other strains there may be little change with alterations in temperature, although extremes of temperature have a greater effect on penetrance than those in the intermediate range, as a rule. Herskowitz and Burdette (1951) reported an inverse relationship between the size of the population and incidence of tumors. Possibly this is related to the nutritional state of larvae, since the reduction in the amount of yeast available has resulted in concomitant diminution in the number of tumors observed. Many other reports emphasizing the effect of environment and nutrition on penetrance also have appeared (Harnly *et al.,* 1951; Sang, 1969; Scharrer and Lochhead, 1950).

Over the years, a comparison of incidence shows that the penetrance for some of the strains changes (Table 1), perhaps due to the acquisition of modifying mutants. The number of genes involved in susceptibility is usually multiple, and the genes may be located on all four chromosomes, on three, on

TABLE 1

Stock	1951			1968		
	No. With Tumors	Total No. Observed	Per Cent With Tumors	No. With Tumors	Total No. Observed	Per Cent With Tumors
tu^{36a} st sr e^s ro ca	182	3394	5.4	48	600	8.0
$f^{257\text{-}19}$/In (1) AM	415	2449	17.0	49	700	7.0
tu^{wps}	1423	8077	17.6	0	550	0.0
$_w$bf $_f$257-5	715	2827	25.3	196	670	29.2
tu^{50d}	1901	7144	26.6	62	480	12.9
tu^{bw}	2434	8614	28.3	100	100	100.0
tu^h	6616	12236	54.1	128	350	36.6
vg mt^A bw	5944	10069	59.0	637	740	86.1
y $_B$263-43	2274	3120	72.9	47	580	8.1
tu^g	9113	11967	76.2	306	600	51.0
tu^{48a} vg bw	10540	10555	99.7	315	350	90.0

two, but infrequently on one alone (Burdette, 1959). Usually there is a main gene accompanied by enhancer and/or suppressor modifiers. Some of these genes have been localized, and for some reason more appear on the second chromosome than elsewhere. In view of the multiplicity of these genes, it is surprising that very few of them are alleles (Burdette and Olivier, 1952). Also few chromosomal abnormalities have been noted in these strains, and there is no reason to believe that the mutants for susceptibility to these tumors are necessarily associated with chromosomal aberrations. By adding heterochromatin in the form of multiple Y chromosomes, we found that there was no consistent alteration in incidence of tumors either to increase or decrease them related to amount of heterochromatin present (Burdette, 1954d, 1959).

When mutators from the Florida stocks were introduced into tumor strains (Burdette, 1954c), there was no consistent alteration in incidence of tumors related to fluctuations in mutation rate. The $tu^{48a}vg\ bw$ strain was used to determine whether the main tumor gene was a deletion or a true genic mutant by determining whether a reverse mutation could be induced. When males were exposed to 2,000 r of X-irradiation and appropriately tested for reverse mutations, two reversals were found in 76,483 tests, thus ruling out the possibility that a deletion was responsible for the mutant tumor phenotype (Burdette, 1959). Both nitrogen mustard and 20-methylcholanthrene have increased the incidence of tumors when tumor strains were exposed to these agents (Burdette, 1952a, 1952c). Introduction of the genoid for CO_2 sensitivity resulted in diminished incidence of tumors in the $tu^{48a}vg\ bw$ strain (Burdette, 1958). The *forte, faible,* and *Tr* strains of the genoid were used in the studies. Later investigations (Burdette, 1968, 1969; Burdette and Yoon, 1967) showed a rather inconstant increase in tumor incidence when both RNA and DNA viruses oncogenic for mammals were administered either in the food or by injection. The effect was noted both in strains developing tumors spontaneously and in those in which they are rarely encountered. Quantitatively, results varied with the strain of virus and the specific virion tested as well as with the strain of Drosophila used for scoring results. A summary of some of these results is contained in Table 2. The fact that all viruses were not effective and not all strains of Drosophila responsive suggests that a more refined analysis will be required to determine the reason(s) for these differences.

The tu^h strain develops excrescences about the head consisting of enlargements characteristic of tissue in the local area. A maternal effect has been reported by Gardner and Wolff (1949) and others. King (1969) and colleagues have reported that ovarian tumors appear in the presence of two recessive mutations causing sterility in females *fused (fu)* and *female sterile (fes).* The tumors do not invade nonovarian tissue and have no effect on viability of the donor when transplanted, although division of cells may continue. These divisions of supernumerary ovarian cystocytes continue to produce cells of the same type, and inhibitory mechanisms ordinarily operative are absent.

TABLE 2

TUMOR INCIDENCE IN DROSOPHILA FOLLOWING
TREATMENT WITH ONCOGENIC VIRUS

Strain	Virus Administered	Dilution	Tumors	
			Per cent With Tumors	Total No. Observed
Multipurpose	Control		2.3	2,230
	Rous Virus (Bryan)	1:1	5.2	852*
	Simian Virus 40	1:1	8.5	1,396*
	Rous-associated Virus I	1:1	4.2	1,702*
	Rous Virus (Bryan)	1:50	7.9	1,846*
	Simian Virus 40	1:50	7.8	742*
	Rous-associated Virus I	1:50	8.1	1,530*
	Control		0.3	9,303
	Feline Picorna Virus	1:1	0.4	9,510
Oregon R	Control		0.3	1,320
	Rous Virus (Bryan)	1:1	2.6	760*
	Simian Virus 40	1:1	0.9	1,337
	Rous Virus (Bryan)	1:50	3.2	801*
	Simian Virus 40	1:50	1.0	314
	Control		0.5	1,774
	Feline Picorna Virus	1:1	1.1	58,211*
	Control		0.1	24,026
	Moloney Leukemia Virus	1:1	0.1	9,325
	Control		0.0	649
	Sendai Virus	1:1	0.1	2,043
	Control		0.5	16,531
	Feline Herpes Virus	1:1	0.7	26,091

Gateff and Schneiderman (1969) have reported that neuroblastomas of
the larval brain occur in *Drosophila melanogaster* and have transplanted them
serially into adults for numerous generations. The tumor appears to be invasive, lethal, and truly neoplastic. They were found to occur in flies when

the *lethal giant* mutant, $l(2)gl^4$, produced disorganization of brain and aberrant shapes of imaginal structures. Although many of the larval tissues undergo dissolution, the brain and imaginal discs in the larvae with this mutant expression are transplantable, the former giving rise to the malignant neoplasms described, and the latter to growths that are not invasive or lethal. The atypical cell lines derived from larval imaginal discs are transplantable but do not metamorphose in autotypic fashion (Hadorn, 1969).

NORMAL AND NEOPLASTIC MAMMALIAN TISSUES

Since the ecdysones and juvenile hormones do alter the incidence of tumors in Drosophila and hormonal imbalance plays a role in the origin of a transplantable malignant neoplasm, it is logical to investigate possible effects of invertebrate hormones in vertebrate neoplastic tissues. These studies were started when only crude extracts tested by bioassay were available for this purpose. More recently crystalline hormones and analogs have become available and have been used in this work as well.

Crude extracts of *Bombyx mori* showing activity of ecdysone(s) was administered (Burdette, 1954f, 1960, 1962) to both the Gardner tumor and sarcoma 180. Three complete regressions occurred in 12 transplantable Gardner tumors after injection of 400 Calliphora units of crude ecdysone. (Occasional regressions occurring spontaneously were noted in other experiments using the same tumor.) However, when crystalline hormone in amounts from 1,000 to 5,700 Calliphora units was injected into 8 mice bearing the Gardner tumor, no regressions occurred. Three regressions occurred in 14 mice bearing sarcoma 180 when 500 Calliphora units of this extract was inoculated, but none were observed in 4 receiving 400 Calliphora units. Three regressions occurred in 10 with transplantable sarcoma 180 receiving 2,400 Calliphora units, and one additional tumor was noted to regress temporarily. Tumors in none of 25 animals with sarcoma 180 used as controls were noted to regress. No regressions occurred in 6 mice with transplantable sarcoma 180 when they were inoculated with the brain hormone originally extracted by Dr. Kobayashi and colleagues. No experiments have been done with proteinic brain hormone.

When 0.1 to 0.2 ml. of farnesol was administered subcutaneously in from 1 to 5 doses respectively into mice bearing sarcoma 180, complete regression of the tumors occurred in 25 mice and partial regression in 21 mice (Burdette, 1964). In 35 additional animals, early death occurred as a result of the growth of the neoplasm. Three complete and two partial regressions occurred in the group of 53 animals used as control without inoculation of crude extract showing ecdysone activity when bioassayed or farnesol.

The effect of farnesol on fetal development was tested in Ajax and Swiss mice by inoculating nonparous females with 2 ml. of farnesol subcutaneously at the time of fertilization and 14 days later determining preimplantation loss (discrepancy between corpora lutea and implantations), early postimplantation deaths (deciduomata), late deaths (embryos dying between implantation at 5 days and dissection on the fourteenth day), and abnormalities in the offspring of mice living to term. The results are tabulated in Table 3 for fetal development. No remarkable difference was found when

TABLE 3

EFFECT OF FARNESOL* ON FETAL DEVELOPMENT IN MICE

	Control		Treated	
	No.	Per cent	No.	Per cent
Corpora lutea	417		442	
Viable fetuses	364	87.3	375	85.0
Preimplantation loss	24	5.8	39	8.6
Early postimplantation deaths	28	6.7	22	5.0
Late postimplantation deaths	1	0.2	6	1.4
Total Lethality	53	13.0	67	15.0

* 0.2 ml. subcutaneously at time of fertilization

control and treated groups were compared, and no anomalies were encountered either in viable fetuses at 14 days or in offspring at term. Therefore no terotogenic effects were found when the dosage of farnesol used was administered.

CRUDE ECDYSONES AND GROWTH OF TISSUES *IN VITRO*

When HeLa cells were grown in a medium containing concentrations of ecdysone from 100 to 2,000 Calliphora units per ml., the numbers of cells surviving was reduced roughly proportional to the concentration of crude hormone. In amounts of 15,000 Calliphora units per ml. or greater, all cells were dead within 48 hours (Burdette, 1964). Additional experiments utilizing sarcoma 180 and embryonic murine fibroblasts were carried out by culturing very small explants of tumor 1 mm. or less in diameter by the double coverslip method in chick plasma clot with Eagle's basal medium, minimal essential medium, and chick-embryo extract (Burdette and Richards, 1961). The results are given in Table 4. There was rapid initial growth of cells treated

TABLE 4

EFFECT OF ACTIVE CRUDE ECDYSONE ON EMBRYONIC
AND NEOPLASTIC CELLS *IN VITRO*

Embryonic Fibroblasts			Sarcoma 180		
No. of Cultures	Concentration of Ecdysone (Calliphora Units)	Results Day Growth Begins	No. of Cultures	Concentration of Ecdysone (Calliphora Units)	Results Day Inhibition Begins
12	6	2	5	1	No Inhibition
14	12	3	29	12	2
12	22	4	17	25	1
15	40	Total Inhibition	5	62	Almost Complete Suppression

with the extract and then subsequent inhibition, but initial growth was not as easy to substantiate as the inhibition given in the table. The criteria for inhibition was the time required for maximum growth, death of the cells, and the number of cells in cultures. In these early experiments crystalline material was not available, and results must be interpreted in this context. Experiments with bacteria failed to suggest that the ecdysones in these extracts caused any appreciable alteration in the rate of proliferation (Table 5).

TABLE 5

MEAN NUMBER OF BACTERIA IN MEDIUM CONTAINING CRUDE ECDYSONES

Organism	Time (Hr.)	Concentration (Calliphora Units/20 ml.)					
		1		100		500	
		Control	Hormone	Control	Hormone	Control	Hormone
S. aureus	0	1.43×10^3	1.61×10^3	1.43×10^3	1.43×10^3	1.40×10^3	1.60×10^3
S. aureus	3	7.50×10^3	7.70×10^3	7.50×10^3	7.80×10^3	2.05×10^3	2.25×10^3
S. aureus	6	7.23×10^5	5.90×10^5	7.23×10^5	6.45×10^5	1.68×10^6	1.75×10^6
E. coli	0	3.47×10^3	3.68×10^3	3.47×10^3	3.16×10^3	1.20×10^3	1.45×10^3
E. coli	3	1.06×10^5	1.06×10^5	1.06×10^5	1.36×10^5	8.20×10^4	7.55×10^4
E. coli	6	4.49×10^7	4.43×10^7	4.49×10^7	4.12×10^7	2.75×10^7	2.50×10^7

EFFECT OF ECDYSTERONE ON SARCOMA 180 *IN VITRO*

The effect of crystalline ecdysterone on sarcoma 180 cells *in vitro* was carried out in Falcon flasks of 39 ml. capacity. The neoplastic cells were cultured from a transplanted ascites tumor growing in HAICR mice. Approximately four weeks were required to establish the cells in culture. Waymouth's medium with 20 per cent fetal calf serum and 50 units per ml. each of penicillin, streptomycin, and anti-PPLO were used to receive the inoculum. Each flask contained 0.1 to 0.4 x 10^6 cells in 5 ml. total volume. Amounts of ecdysterone tested were 2, 4, 8, 25, 50, 100, 200, 400, 500, and 800 μg. respectively. For each concentration, 10 test flasks and two to six control flasks were set up.

Control studies indicated that a maximum rate of growth was usually achieved in 3 days. The cultures of cells and respective amounts of ecdysterone were placed in the flasks simultaneously, and multiple cultures were harvested on the successive days indicated in Table 6. The number of cells contained in each culture was determined by computing the total number of cells multiplied by the ratio of viable cells to this total. (The vital stain used to determine viability was trypan blue.) Except in the experiment in which the dosage was 800 μg., ecdysterone was not added on days when medium in the cultures was changed.

The number of viable cells after treatment of sarcoma 180 *in vitro* with various concentrations of crystalline ecdysterone seems to be increased with the lower concentration of hormone after medium containing ecdysterone had been replaced. Definite inhibition appears in higher concentration, although this is not very impressive with a dosage of 200 μg. When no hormone was added at the time the medium was changed after an initial dosage of 500 μg., inhibition was not sustained. However, when ecdysterone was added with the medium, inhibition was continued, illustrated in the experiment with a dosage of 800 μg.

EFFECTS OF CRYSTALLINE ECDYSONES AND CYASTERONE ON ASCITES TUMORS *IN VIVO*

Three types of tumors were used to test the effect of crystalline ecdysones on the growth of mammalian tumors. Neoplasms utilized were the TA 3 mammary tumor carried in HAICR Swiss mice and L1210 leukemia and sarcoma 180 both carried in BDF_1 mice. Approximately equal numbers of male and female mice weighing 25 to 30 grams and five to six weeks old were injected intraperitoneally with suspensions of ascites cells at 9:00 A.M. About

TABLE 6

EFFECT OF CRYSTALLINE ECDYSTERONE ON GROWTH OF SARCOMA 180 *IN VITRO*

Amount of Ecdysterone (μg.)	Inoculations (No. of Cells)	Number of Viable Cells x 10^6					
		Day 1	2	3	4	5	6
2	$0.10^†$	0.026	—	0.42*	0.89 (2)	1.90*	7.20
Control		0.030		0.65*	0.82 (1)	1.70*	2.50
4	$0.10^†$	0.058	—	0.33*	1.03 (2)	2.90*	12.50
Control		0.030		0.65*	0.82 (1)	1.70*	2.50
8	$0.10^†$	0.045	—	0.49*	1.10 (1)	3.20*	3.00
Control		0.030		0.65*	0.82 (1)	1.70*	2.50
25	$0.38^†$	0.390	1.60	1.80*	1.70	—	—
Control		0.378	1.09	1.58*	2.70		
50	$0.38^†$	0.440	.85	1.55*	1.85	—	—
Control		0.378	1.09	1.58*	2.70		
100	$0.38^†$	0.420	.79	1.35*	1.40	—	—
Control		0.378	1.09	1.58*	2.70		
200	$0.32^†$	0.510	—	1.35	—	*	2.20
Control		0.500		1.63		*	2.29
400	$0.32^†$	0.510	—	0.63	—	*	0.94
Control		0.500		1.63		*	2.29
500	$0.33^†$	0.396	—	1.70*	*	*	6.52
Control		0.520		4.20*	*	*	7.03
800	$1.40^†$	0.190	*e	0.79	*e		1.67
Control		0.290	*	2.14	*		5.95

† Initial Inoculation of Cells and Ecdysterone
* Medium changed
e Ecdysterone added

400,000 TA 3 cells, approximately 200,000 L1210 leukemia cells, and approximately 400,000 sarcoma-180 cells were used for respective inoculations. Twenty-four hours after the malignant cells were introduced into the peritoneal cavity, 0.5 to 30 µg./G. of crystalline hormone in saline was injected intraperitoneally respectively. Animals used as controls received a similar number of cells, and saline without hormone was introduced into the peritoneal cavity in the same volume (6.25 µl./G.). Five days after injection of the hormone the animals were sacrificed, the peritoneal cavity opened, and cells removed after injection of 2 ml. of saline into the abdominal cavity to insure that most of the cells were removed when the fluid was withdrawn. Then they were counted visually in a hemocytometer and with a Coulter counter. The packed volume was also determined. Crystalline hormones tested were ecdysterone, inokosterone, and cyasterone. Conclusions were not altered when results with all three methods were reviewed; and therefore only the data for counts with hemocytometer are presented in the tables, since they appeared to be somewhat more consistent when duplicates were compared.

The effect of ecdysterone on the TA 3, L1210, and sarcoma-180 ascites tumors failed to show any dramatic inhibition of growth after a single inoculation in any of the dosages used, but in some determinations there was a suggestive effect when higher concentrations of hormone were used (Tables 7-10). Actually in the concentrations of cyasterone used with the TA 3 and L1210 tumors there is a suggestion of enhancement of cellular proliferation (Table 7), reminiscent of the initial proliferation of sarcoma-180 cells *in vitro* after explants were treated with crude ecdysone. In the case of inokosterone, the highest concentration failed to yield smaller numbers of TA 3 cells than the controls, although the opposite was true for lower concentrations (Table 8). A smaller number of cells was found with only the intermediate concentrations of inokosterone when L1210 cells were tested. In Table 10 there is as much reason to imply that ecdysterone enhances proliferation of TA 3 and L1210 ascites cells as to postulate any inhibition, since only the two lowest concentrations of hormone yielded lower mean numbers of cells than control preparation. In Table 9 only one out of three tests showed smaller numbers of cells when hormone was administered to mice with either TA 3 or L1210 neoplasms. On the other hand, the three concentrations of ecdysterone used resulted in a reduction in the mean numbers of sarcoma-180 cells (Table 10). The results with sarcoma 180 *in vitro* coupled with the suggestive results *in vivo* interdict the conclusion that ecdysones do not inhibit the growth of mammalian neoplasms and other tissues. It should be noted that the results reported have been carried out with a single dose of hormone; the effect of continuing the dosage should be tested adequately. No doubt unknown inhibitory substances were present when the original crude extracts which also contained ecdysones were tested. However, this does not necessarily mean that atypical growth of mammalian tissues may not be altered by ecdysone or analogs under certain conditions, even though Hoffmeister and Lang (1964) and Hirono *et al.* (1969) reported negative results with crystalline ecdysones similar to those recorded above.

TABLE 7

EFFECT OF CYASTERONE ON PROLIFERATION OF ASCITES TUMORS

Dosage (μg./G.)	Neoplasm			
	TA 3		L1210	
	No. of Mice	Mean No. Cells x 10^6	No. of Mice	Mean No. Cells x 10^6
5.0	4	146	4	86
Control	4	114	4	73
10.0	4	163	3	112
Control	4	110	4	90

TABLE 8

EFFECT OF INOKOSTERONE ON PROLIFERATION OF ASCITES TUMORS

Dosage (μg./G.)	Neoplasm			
	TA 3		L1210	
	No. of Mice	Mean No. Cells x 10^6	No. of Mice	Mean No. Cells x 10^6
5.0	4	43	4	60
Control	4	93	4	45
10.0	4	69	4	36
Control	4	93	4	45
20.0	11	49	11	53
Control	11	82	11	62
30.0	2	118	2	124
Control	2	112	2	69

TABLE 9

EFFECT OF ECDYSTERONE ON PROLIFERATION OF ASCITES TUMORS

Dosage (μg.)	Type of Neoplasm			
	TA 3		L1210	
	No. of Mice	Mean No. Cells x 10^6	No. of Mice	Mean No. Cells x 10^6
0.5	4	62	4	113
Control	1	98	2	163
1.0	4	244	4	69
Control	2	95	3	49
2.5	14	190	11	64
Control	6	92	7	14
5.0	12	161	8	68
Control	11	102	7	19

TABLE 10

EFFECT OF ECDYSTERONE ON PROLIFERATION OF ASCITES TUMORS

Dosage (μg.)	Type of Neoplasm					
	TA 3		L1210		Sarcoma 180	
	No. of Mice	Mean No. Cells x 10^6	No. of Mice	Mean No. Cells x 10^6	No. of Mice	Mean No. Cells x 10^6
10.0	4	69	4	48	12	221
Control	3	57	3	64	14	273
20.0	7	49	7	62	6	209
Control	7	81	7	57	7	234
30.0	2	181	2	89	45	115
Control	2	112	2	69	15	154

SUMMARY

The incidence of melanotic tumors and the origin of transplantable malignant neuroblastomas in Drosophila both are related to the balance of invertebrate hormone. The melanotic tumors are hereditary; they are increased in numbers by oncogenic mammalian viruses and juvenile hormones; and they are inhibited by ecdysones. The system of melanotic tumors is a labile one and the tumors bear little similarity to mammalian neoplasms. On the other hand, the transplantable neuroblastomas originating when ring gland is deficient as a result of the action of the $l(2)gl^4$ gene fulfills the criteria for malignancy when transplanted.

Although inhibition of mammalian neoplasms was suggested by early work with crude ecdysones from Bombyx assayed by the Calliphora test, subsequent testing with crystalline hormones has failed to substantiate the results in a number of studies. There is some suggestive evidence, however, both from tests *in vivo* and *in vitro* that the proliferation of sarcoma 180 is inhibited by ecdysterone, and altering the dosage schedule may yield definite evidence for inhibition of this neoplasm. There is also some evidence that the rate of proliferation of mammalian cells may be increased by ecdysones under appropriate conditions. One mimic of juvenile hormone inhibits the growth of mammalian neoplasms, but the preparation used proved highly toxic. It seems clear that the possible usefulness of invertebrate hormones, phytohormones, and analogs in controlling growth of mammalian neoplastic tissue has not yet been investigated in sufficient depth to draw any definitive conclusion. It is likely that refined and penetrating analyses will be required to unlock the useful information which is suggested by past experimentation but is still beyond reach.

Acknowledgement:

This work was aided by grants from U. S. Department of Health, Education and Welfare National Cancer Institute CA 10089, CA 10037, and CA 10043. Professors T. Takemoto and H. Hikino kindly supplied the cyasterone used in these studies.

References

1. ARDASHNIKOV, S. N.: Malignant Tumors in *Drosophila melanogaster*. Influence of the Left End of the Sex Chromosome on the Development of Tumors. C. R. Acad. Sci., U. S. S. R., *30*:344-346, 1941.

2. BRIDGES, C. G.: Non-disjunction as Proof of the Chromosome Theory of Heredity. Genetics, *1*:107-163, 1916.

3. BRYANT, P. J. and SANG, J. H.: Physiological Genetics of Melanotic Tumors in *Drosophila melanogaster*. VI. The Tumorigenic Effects of Juvenile Hormone-like Substances. Genetics, *62*:321-336, 1969.

4. BURDETTE, W. J.: Incidence of Tumors in Different Strains of Drosophila. Drosophila Information Service, *25*:101-102, 1951.

5. BURDETTE, W. J.: Effect of Nitrogen Mustard on Tumor Incidence and Lethal Mutation Rate in Drosophila. Cancer Research, *12*:366-368, 1952a.

6. BURDETTE, W. J.: Incidence of Tumors in Isogenic Strains. J. Nat. Cancer Inst., *12*:709-714, 1952b.

7. BURDETTE, W. J.: Tumor Incidence and Lethal Mutation Rate in Drosophila Treated with 20-Methylcholanthrene. Cancer Research, *12*:201-205, 1952c.

8. BURDETTE, W. J.: Effect of Defective Ring Gland on Incidence of Tumors in Drosophila. J. Nat. Cancer Inst., *15*:367-376, 1954a.

9. BURDETTE, W. J.: Effect of Ligation of Drosophila Larvae on Tumor Incidence. Cancer Research, *14*:780-782, 1954b.

10. BURDETTE, W. J.: Effect of Mutator, *HIGH*, on Tumor Incidence in Drosophila. Cancer Research, *14*:149-153, 1954c.

11. BURDETTE, W. J.: Heterochromatin and Tumor Incidence. Drosophila Information Service, *28*:110-111, 1954d.

12. BURDETTE, W. J.: Penetrance of Tumors in Drosophila. Drosophila Information Service, *28*:109-110, 1954e.

13. BURDETTE, W. J.: The Effect of Larval Hormone on Tumors. Caryologia, *6*:1160-1163, 1954f.

14. BURDETTE, W. J.: Cellular Aspects of Tumorigenesis. Ann. N. Y. Acad. Sci., *71*:1068-1071, 1958.

15. BURDETTE, W. J.: Tumors in Drosophila. Biological Contributions, The University of Texas, Austin, Publication No. 5914, pp. 57-68, 1959.

16. BURDETTE, W. J.: Invertebrate Hormones and Cancer. ACTA Unio Internationale contre le Cancrum, *16*:157-159, 1960.

17. BURDETTE, W. J.: Effect of Invertebrate Hormones on Vertebrate Tissues. Science, *139*:987, 1962.

18. BURDETTE, W. J.: The Significance of Invertebrate Hormones in Relation to Differentiation. Cancer Research, *24*:521-536, 1964.

19. BURDETTE, W. J.: Visible Alterations in Gene Activation Caused by Hormone and Oncogenic Viruses. *In:* Exploitable Molecular Mechanisms and Neoplasia, pp. 507-520. Baltimore: Williams & Wilkins Co., 1968.

20. BURDETTE, W. J.: Tumors, Hormones, and Viruses in Drosophila. *In:* Smithsonian Institution Symposium on Neoplasia of Invertebrate Animals. U. S. Government Printing Office, Washington, D. C., pp. 303-321, 1969.

21. BURDETTE, W. J.: Tumors in Drosophila and Antibacterial Immunity. J. Invert. Path., in press, 1973.

22. BURDETTE, W. J. and OLIVIER, H. R.: Tumor Incidence in F_1 Progeny of Tumor Strains. Drosophila Information Service, *26*:94-95, 1952.

23. BURDETTE, W. J. and RICHARDS, R. C.: Alteration of the Growth of Mammalian Cells *in Vitro* by Ecdysone Extract. Nature, *189*:666-668, 1961.

24. BURDETTE, W. J. and YOON, J. S.: Mutations, Chromosomal Aberrations, and Tumors in Insects Treated with Oncogenic Virus. Science, *155*:340-341, 1967.

25. EL SHATOURY, H. H.: A Malignant Tumor in Drosophila. Drosophila Information Service, *28*:114, 1954.

26. GARDNER, E. J. and WOOLF, C. M.: Maternal Effect Involved in the Inheritance of Abnormal Growth in the Head Region of *Drosophila melanogaster.* Genetics, *34*:573-585, 1949.

27. GATEFF, E. and SCHNEIDERMAN, H. A.: Neoplasms in Mutant and Cultured Wildtype Tissues of Drosophila. *In*: Smithsonian Institution Symposium on Neoplasia of Invertebrate Animals. U. S. pp. 365-397, 1969.

28. GHELELOVITCH, S.: Une Tumeur Hereditaire de la Drosophile (*Drosophila melanogaster* Meig.) Etude Genetique, Physiologique, et Histologique, Maruice Declum, Paris, pp. 153, 1959.

29. HADORN, E.: Proliferation and Dynamics of Cell Hereditary in Blastema Cultures of Drosophila. *In*: Smithsonian Institution Symposium on Neoplasia of Invertebrate Animals. U. S. 363, 1969.

30. HARNLY, M. H., FREIDMAN, F., EMERY, G. C., and GLASSMAN, E.: Nutritional and Temperature Effects on the Frequency of an Hereditary Melanoma in *Drosophila melanogaster.* Cancer Research, *11*:254, 1951.

31. HARTUNG, E. W.: Some Observations on the Larval Growth Rate and Viability of Two Tumor Strains of *Drosophila melanogaster.* Science, *107*:296-297, 1948.

32. HERSKOWITZ, I. H. and BURDETTE, W. J.: Some Genetic and Environmental Influences on the Incidence of a Melanotic Tumor in Drosophila. J. Exp. Zool., *117*:499-522, 1951.

33. HIRONO, I., SASAOKA, I., and SHIMIZU, M.: Effect of Insect-molting Hormones, Ecdysterone and Inokosterone, on Tumor Cells. Gann, *60*:341-342, 1969.

34. HOFFMEISTER, H. and LANG, N.: Zum Einfluss des Ecdysons auf des Wachstum von Wirbeltiergewebe. Naturwiss., *51*:112, 1964.

35. JONES, J. C.: Hemocytes and the Problem of Tumors in Insects. *In*: Smithsonian Institution Symposium on Neoplasia of Invertebrate Animals. U. S. Government Printing Office, Washington, D. C., pp. 481-485, 1969.

36. KING, R. C.: Hereditary Ovarian Tumors of *Drosophila melanogaster. In*: Smithsonian Institution Symposium on Neoplasia of Invertebrate Animals. U. S. Government Printing Office, Washington, D. C., pp. 323-345, 1969.

37. MADHAVEN, K.: Induction of Melanotic Pseudotumors in *Drosophila melanogaster* by Juvenile Hormone. Wilhelm Roux' Archiv., *169*:345-349, 1972.

38. RIZKI, M. T. M.: Tumor Formation in Relation to Metamorphosis in *Drosophila melanogaster.* J. Morph., *100*:459-472, 1957.

39. RUSSELL, E. S.: A Comparison of Bening and "Malignant" Tumors in *Drosophila melanogaster.* J. Exp. Zool., *84*:363-379, 1940.

40. SANG, J. H.: Biochemical Basis of Hereditary Melanotic Tumors in Drosophila. *In*: Smithsonian Institution Symposium on Neoplasia of Invertebrate Animals. U. S. Government Printing Office, Washington, D. C., pp. 291-301, 1969.

41. SCHARRER, B. and LOCHHEAD, M. S.: Tumors in the Invertebrates: A Review. Cancer Research, *10*:403-419, 1950.

42. STRUNGE, T., GIGANTE, D., and BERNHARD, W.:Hemopathie de Type Leucemique Chez la Larve de Drosophila. Etudiee au Microscope Ordinaire, au Microscope Electronique et au Microscope a Contraste de Phase. C. R. 3^e Congr. Soc. Internat. de' Hematol., Rome, pp. 607-617, 1951.

43. STARK, M. B.: An Hereditary Lymphosarcoma in Drosophila. Collected Papers N. Y. Med. Coll. and Flower Hospital, *1*:397-400, 1935.

Action of Invertebrate Hormones on Vertebrate Tissues

NUMBERS of
CHROMOSOMES in
HUMAN LEUCOCYTES
EXPOSED to ECDYSTERONE

Walter J. Burdette

All chromosomes could not be identified with certainty until relatively recently even with radiolabeling. Differential patterns in staining heterochromatin were then obtained by Gall and Pardue (1971) and others (Gagne' *et al.*,1971). In addition,Caspersson and colleagues (Caspersson and Zech, 1972) and others have used fluorescent banding that appears with ultra-violet illumination of chromosomes stained with quinacrine mustard to characterize each chromosome uniquely. This has clarified quickly some confusion in karyotyping syndromes of clinical significance. For example, trisomic chromosome 21 (newer terminology) in Down's disease proved to be distinct from the Philadelphia chromosome now known to be chromosome 22 with a portion deleted. Previously the postulate that the same chromosome was involved in both abnormalities was attractive, since both are associated with neoplastic disease. Quinacrine mustard was selected on the basis of the supposition that it would bind to one of the nitrogen atoms in the guanine base of the nucleotide (Casperson *et al.,* 1967). However, the bands that fluoresce do not correspond to the distribution of DNA determined spectrophotometrically, and the reason for differential regional affinity is not entirely clear at the present time.

It also has been possible to obtain a somewhat different pattern of banding by pretreatment with heat, sodium hydroxide, acetic acid, saline, trypsin, etc. before applying Giemsa stain (Sumner *et al.,* 1971; Evans *et al.,* 1971). These preparations may be retained permanently for study in contrast to the evanescent pattern seen when quinacrine mustard is used, although resolution and quantitative measurements of intensity may be inferior (Casperson and Zech, 1972; Evans *et al.,* 1971). These developments and the possibilities of additional resolution of the banded pattern with the electron microscope offer more than variations in numbers of chromosomes as criteria for testing possible response of mammalian chromosomes to invertebrate hormones already known to have a profound effect on chromosomal puffing in insects (Ashburner, 1970; Burdette and Carver, this volume). As part of a study on possible inhibitory effects of ecdysones on proliferation of mammalian neoplastic cells, Hirono *et al.* (1969) reported that the hormones tested did not alter the mitotic index, but no full-scale investigation of possible effects of invertebrate hormones and analogs on karyotype of mammalian chromosomes has been reported previously.

A beginning has been made to study human chromosomes after exposure to invertebrate hormones with a pilot investigation in which metaphase chromosomes were observed after culturing with ecdysterone, and the numbers of chromosomes tabulated can be reported at this time. Leucocytes from four young, healthy individuals (one female and three males) were cultured in Waymouth's medium with 20 per cent fetal-calf serum, heparin, and phytohemagglutinin at 37° C. Ecdysterone in final respective concentrations of 5 ng.–55 μg./ml. was added to three-fourths of the cultures during the last 24 of the 96 hours they were cultured. The remainder were used as controls. Then the cells were placed on slides, stained with Giemsa and/or quinacrine mustard, and the number of chromosomes was determined for 158 preparations exposed to ecdysterone and 47 without addition of hormone (Table 1). Photographs were made of metaphase plates of good quality and these were used to determine the numbers of chromosomes present.

Among the controls, 75 per cent of the karyotype were euploid, 17 per cent hypodiploid (n < 46), 4 per cent hyperdiploid (n = 47, n = 48), and 4 per cent were in the tetraploid range (n = 86, n = 89). After treatment with ecdysterone, 70 per cent were euploid, 15 per cent were hypodiploid (n < 46), 4 per cent were hyperdiploid (n = 47 or 48), and 11 per cent had

60 or more chromosomes. Aside from counts of 60, 64, 67, and 76, the number of chromosomes were in the tetraploid range or greater (n > 81) in 14 of the karyotypes. Large numbers of chromosomes were found in cultures from 3 of the 4 patients tested for ecdysterone. Higher concentrations of hormone were not associated with a greater number of metaphases with 60 or more chromosomes. An additional 280 cells were scanned for the presence of numbers of chromosomes greater than 60. Among the new total of 485 metaphases, 5 per cent (6/119) of control cultures and 8 per cent (29/366) of those treated with ecdysterone were hyperploid, a less impressive difference (P=.26) than that in the table when only those with more detailed scoring were evaluated (P=.14).

EFFECT OF EXPOSURE OF HUMAN
LEUCOCYTES TO ECDYSTERONE

Treatment		Number of Chromosomes				Total
		< 46	46	47 - 48	≥ 60	
None	No.	8	35	2	2	47
	%	17	75	4	4	100
Ecdysterone*	No.	23	110	7	18	158
* 5 mg. – 55μg./ml.	%	15	70	4	11	100

No definitive conclusion seems justified on the basis of this preliminary experiment. Perhaps the only comment warranted about the polyploidy encountered when ecdysterone was added to the culture medium is that the results are interesting and encourage additional exploration. Data are not yet sufficiently extensive for any remarks about morphology of individual chromosomes and the pattern of banding after exposure to ecdysterone. Should any consistent alterations in banding, numbers of chromosomes, or characteristics of any individual pair be found in the future, the potential usefulness of this information in exploiting the study of chromosomes in relation to human disease easily warrants continued effort to determine the response, if any, of human chromosomes to ecdysterone, juvenile hormones, and analogs alone and in combination. It also would require careful evaluation in relation to the exposure of the population to pesticides of this type. Should no effects be detected, it would lend assurance to the innocuousness to man of this means for controlling insect pests.

Aided by a grant from the National Cancer Institute, U. S. P. H. S. CA 05831 and a grant from the National Science Foundation GF 28889 as a part of the U. S. Japan Cooperative Science Program.

References

1.   ASHBURNER, M. : Function and Structure of Polytene Chromosomes during Insect Development. *In:* Advances in Insect Physiology, *7*:1-95, 1970.
2.   BURDETTE, W. J. and CARVER, J. E. : Effect of Invertebrate Hormones and Oncogenic Viruses on Chromosomes. This volume.
3.   CASPERSSON, T., FARBER, S., FOLEY, G. E., KUDYNOWSKI, J., MODEST, E. J., SIMONSSON, E., WAGH, U., and ZECH, L.: Chemical Differentiation along Metaphase Chromosomes. Exper. Cell Res., *49*:219-222, 1967.
4.   CASPERSSON, T. and ZECH, L. : Chromosome Identification by Fluorescence. Hospital Practice, *7*:51-62, 1972.
5.   GALL, J. G. and PARDUE, M. L. : Nucleic Acid Hybridization in Cytological Preparations. *In*: Grossman, L. and Moldave, K. (ed.), Methods in Enzymology , *Nucleic Acid Part D, 21*:470-480, 1971.
6.   EVANS, H. J., BUCKTON, K. G., and SUMNER, A. T.: Cytological Mapping of Human Chromosomes: Results Obtained with Quinacrine Fluorescence and the Acetic-saline-Giemsa Techniques. Chromosoma, *35*:310-325, 1971.
7.   GAGNÉ, R., TANGUAY, R., and LABERGE, C. : Differential Staining Patterns of Heterochromatin in Man. Nature New Biology, *232*:29-30, 1971.
8.   HIRONO, I., SASAOKA, I., and SHIMIZU, M.: Effect of Insect-molting Hormones, Ecdysterone and Inokosterone, on Tumor Cells. Gann, *60*:341-342, 1969.
9.   SUMNER, A. T., EVANS, H. J., and BUCKLAND, R. A.: New Techniques for Distinguishing between Human Chromosomes. Nature New Biology, *232*:31-32, 1971.

PHYTOECDYSONES and PROTEIN METABOLISM in MAMMALIA

Mitsuru Uchiyama and Tadahiko Otaka

I t has become generally recognized that metamorphosing hormones of insects are distributed widely in the plant kingdom, and isolation and chemical characterization of several kinds of these substances, the phytoecdysones, have been reported (Hikino *et al.*, 1970). Since these phytoecdysones have a steroidal skeleton such as that of adrenal corticoids, sex hormones, *etc.* and since the plants containing these steroids are generally used in oriental medicine and are dietary sources for mammals, it seemed of interest to investigate the effect of these steroids on mammalian metabolic systems.

In this report the mode of action of ecdysterone, the representative phytoecdysone, on protein synthesis (Okui *et al.*, 1968; Otaka *et al.*, 1969; Otaka and Uchiyama, 1969) in murine liver will be described, comparing it to that of 4-chlorotestosterone, a potent anabolic steroid. Then, the structure-activity relationship will be described and illustrated, using several kinds of phytoecdysones (Otaka *et al.*, 1968; Otaka and Uchiyama, 1969).

METHODS

Animals and Treatment

Male mice (18-22G.) of the dd strain were used with no restriction on their intake of food throughout the experiments. Each steroid was dissolved in 0.9 per cent saline and injected intraperitoneally in a dose of 0.05 mg./100G. body weight at 9:00 A.M. For oral administration ecdysterone dissolved in water was administered in a dose of 0.5 mg./100G. body weight. 4-Chlorotestosterone was also suspended in saline and injected in a dose of 1 mg./100G. body weight at 9:00 A.M. Actinomycin-D dissolved in ethanol-saline solution was injected intraperitoneally in a dose of 40 μg./mouse.

Assay of Protein Synthetic Activity *in Vivo*

One μCi. of ^{14}C-chlorella hydrolysate was injected into mice pretreated with a steroid 15 minutes before sacrifice. The liver was homogenized in 3 volumes of medium-I (Koike *et al.*, 1966) (0.25 M. sucrose; 0.01 M. MgSO$_4$; 0.025 M. KCl; 0.05 M. *tris*-HCl, pH 7.6) and fractionated as described in the legend for Figure 1.

Preparation of Cell-free Fraction for Protein Synthesis *in Vitro*

After the mice were decapitated at the indicated time after treatment, the liver was removed rapidly and rinsed in ice-cold 1.15 per cent KCl, weighed, and homogenized with 1.5 volumes of medium-I by means of a Potter-Elvehjem teflon homogenizer. The homogenate was centrifuged at 20,000 x g. for 15 minutes at 0° C. to remove mitochondria, nuclei, and cellular debris, and this supernatant fluid was designated as S-20 fluid. The microsomal fraction was prepared by centrifuging S-20 fluid; 3 volumes of the medium was used in this case, centrifuged for 60 minutes at 105,000 x g. in an Hitachi ultracentrifuge and the pellets suspended in medium-II (0.01 M. MgSO$_4$; 0.025 M. KCl; 0.05 M. tris-HCl, pH 7.6) for use.

Preparation of polysomes was performed by the method of Wettstein *et al.* (1963) as follows: The S-20 fluid was treated with one-seventh its volume with an ice-cold 10 per cent (w./v.) solution of sodium deoxycholate. Five ml. of deoxycholate-treated S-20 fluid was layered over 2 ml. of 0.5 M. sucrose solution in medium-II, which was layered over 3 ml. of 2.0 M. sucrose solution in medium-II. After centrifuging for 3 hours at 105,000 x g., the supernatant fluid was removed, and the sides of the centrifuge tube were cleaned and wiped to dryness with a filter paper. The pellet was rinsed in medium-II by gentle agitation. The resultant fluid was used as the polysome fluid. When necessary, the supernatant after separation of microsomes described above was treated with Sephadex G-25 to remove low molecules, and this fraction was used as the source of enzyme and designated as S-105 fluid.

Assay for Template Activity of RNA

The reaction mixture for the incorporation of amino acid into protein was the same as described above. RNA prepared from control and animals treated with ecdysterone was dissolved in 0.1 ml. of water as indicated in Table 10 and added to the reaction mixture. Incubation was carried out in air for 30 minutes at 37° C. Procedures for the preparation of acid-insoluble protein and the measurement of radioactivity were the same as described above. Protein was determined by the Biuret method (Gornall and Bardawill, 1949).

RESULTS

Effect of Ecdysterone and 4-Chlorotestosterone on Amino-acid Incorporation into Hepatic Protein *in Vivo*

In view of the stimulatory effect of ecdysterone and 4-chlorotestosterone on protein synthesis in murine liver, experiments were designed to determine which component in the cell responded to treatment with these steroids. Results presented in Figure 1 show the incorporation of ^{14}C-amino acids into protein of the hepatic subfractions in normal and treated mice that were given a single injection of 10 µg. of ecdysterone 1, 2, and 4 hours before death or of 200 µg. of 4-chlorotestosterone 4 hours before death. Incorporation of ^{14}C-amino acids into protein *in vivo* was obviously enhanced by the treatment with the steroid in all subcellular fractions. The degree of stimulation by these steroids was almost the same in all three fractions, nuclei, mitochondria, and microsomes. The amount of ^{14}C-amino acids incorporated into protein in the liver of the mouse treated with ecdysterone increased with time and was about the same as that with a 20-fold dose of 4-chlorotestosterone.

Incorporation of Amino Acids into Protein *in Vitro* with S-20 Fluid from the Liver of Normal and Steroid - treated Mice.

Table 1A shows that the S-20 fluid obtained from the liver of mice treated with ecdysterone or 4-chlorotestosterone is more active in incorporating amino acids than that obtained from the normal liver. The incorporation increased significantly at 2 and 4 hours after treatment with ecdysterone. The magnitude of the increment was almost equal to that with 4-chlorotestosterone treatment. When ^{14}C-alanine was used instead of ^{14}C-chlorella hydrolysate, a similar result was obtained (Table 1B). These results are consistent with that of amino-acid incorporation *in vivo* (Figure 1). The elevated dose of the steroid above 0.05 mg./100G. body weight prolonged the duration of enhanced protein synthesis but did not alter the absolute ratio of increment when protein synthesis was maximal (Figure 2). Ecdysterone stimulated protein synthesis not only when introduced by intraperitonial injec-

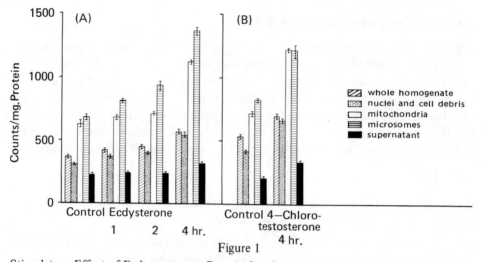

Figure 1

Stimulatory Effect of Ecdysterone on Protein Synthetic Activity in Murine Liver *in Vitro*

Ecdysterone or 4-chlorotestosterone was injected intraperitoneally in a dose of 0.05 and 1 mg. per 100 g. body weight, respectively, and 1 μCi. of ^{14}C-chlorella hydrolysate was also injected intraperitoneally 15 min. before sacrifice. The livers were homogenized in 3 volumes of medium-I (see text). Nuclei and cellular debris were sedimented at 600 x. g. for 10 min., mitochondria at 9,000 x. g. for 10 min., microsomes at 85,000 x. g. for 90 min., and supernatant was taken as the postmicrosomal fluid. The treatment of protein samples is given in the experimental section.

TABLE 1

STIMULATORY EFFECT OF ECDYSTERONE AND 4–CHLORO-
TESTOSTERONE ON THE *IN-VITRO* INCORPORATION OF AMINO
ACIDS INTO HOT-ACID INSOLUBLE PROTEIN FRACTION

Treatment		c.p.m./mg. Protein	Stimulation %
(A) Control		307 ± 1	100
Ecdysterone	1 hr.	400 ± 62	130
	2 hr.	553 ± 31	180
	4 hr.	603 ± 12	196
4-Chlorotesterone	1 hr.	398 ± 8	130
	2 hr.	580 ± 16	189
	4 hr.	610 ± 20	199
(B) Control		118 ± 4	100
Ecdysterone	2 hr.	153 ± 6	130

(A) ^{14}C-Chlorella hydrolysate was used as labeled amino acids. Each result is the mean ± standard error for 10 mice used.

(B) ^{14}C-L-Alanine was used as a labeled amino acid. Each result is the mean ± standard error for 4 mice used.

tion, but also by oral administration (Otaka *et al.*, 1968; Hikino *et al.*, 1969). Although all the above results were obtained using male mice, stimulation of protein synthesis by ecdysterone was also effective on female mice (Table 3).

System of Incubation

The reaction mixture consisted of 50 μmoles of sucrose, 25 μmoles of tris-HCl (pH 7.6), 5 μmoles of $MgSO_4$, 12.5 μmoles of KCl, 2.0 μmoles of ATP, 0.2 μmole of GTP, 10 μmoles of phosphocreatine, 10 μG. of creatine phos-phokinase [EC 2.7.3.2.], 0.1 μCi. of ^{14}C-labeled chlorella hydrolysate or 0.2 μCi. of ^{14}C-alanine, 0.1 ml. of polysome fluid or 0.1 ml. of microsomal fluid, 0.1 ml. of S-105 fluid (approximately 2.5 mg. of protein) as the polysomal or microsomal system, and 0.2 ml. of S-20 fluid (approximately 10 mg. of pro-tein) as the S-20 system in a total of 0.5 ml. Incubation was carried out in test tubes in air at 37° C. for 25 minutes for the S-20 system and for 40 min-utes for the microsomal or polysomal system.

Preparation and Counting of Radioactive Protein

After incubation, the reaction was stopped by adding 4 ml. of 6 per cent perchloric acid. The precipitate was separated by centrifugation, washed three times with 6 per cent perchloric acid, treated with the same reagent at 90° C. for 15 minutes and finally extracted twice with ether-ethanol-chloro-form (2:2:1). The resulting labeled protein was dissolved in 90 per cent (v./v.) formic acid, plated on planchets, and dried under an infrared lamp. The pro-tein synthetic activity *in vivo* was also measured by the procedure mentioned above. A 2π gas-flow counter was used for the counting. Protein content was determined by a slight modification of the method of Gornall and Bardawill (1949) or by gravimetric analysis. The incorporation of ^{14}C-amino acids was calibrated after correction for self-absorption.

Gradient Analysis of Products in the S-20 System of Incubation

The products in the S-20 system of incubation were analyzed by sucrose density-gradient centrifugation by layering 0.3 ml. on a linear 5-20 per cent sucrose gradient set up with medium-II. A cushion of 0.6 ml. of 2 M. sucrose solution in medium-II was placed at the bottom of the tube. After centrifuga-tion for 3.5 hours at 39,000 r.p.m. in the ultracentrifuge, 4-drop fractions were collected from the bottom of the tube. Two mg. of albumin were added to each tube as a carrier, and the protein was precipitated by the addition of 4 ml. of 6 per cent perchloric acid. The subsequent procedures were the same as described in the preparation for protein counting.

Preparation of Cell-free Fraction for Preparation of RNA

The liver was homogenized in 4 volumes of medium-III (0.05 M. *tris*-HCl, pH 7.4; 10^{-4} M. $MgSO_4$; 10^{-4} M. EDTA: 4 mg./ml. of polyvinyl sulfate). The cytoplasmic fraction used was prepared by centrifugation of the homogenate at 600 x g. for 10 minutes or at 12,000 x g. for 10 minutes depending on the experiment. Ribosomes used for assay of template activity were isolated as follows: The livers obtained from mice fasted for 24 hours were homogenized. After removal of mitochondria, nuclei, and debris by centrifugation at 20,000 x g. for 15 minutes at 0° C., the supernatant was treated with one-ninth its volume of ice-cold 10 per cent (w./v.) sodium deoxycholate freshly dissolved in deionized water. The resulting mixture was laid on top of a centrifugation tube containing medium-I in 1 M. sucrose to prepare the total ribonucleoprotein particles by centrifugation at 105,000 x g. for 3 hours. Cellular sap was prepared by centrifugation of the 20,000 x g. supernatant (without the addition of deoxycholate) at 105,000 x g. for 3 hours.

Preparation and Analysis of Ribonucleic Acid

Cytoplasm and nuclei were treated at room temperature and at 60° C., respectively, by shaking with an equal volume of water-saturated phenol containing 0.5 per cent sodium dodecyl sulfate. After repeated treatment with phenol, RNA in the aqueous layer was precipitated with 2 per cent (final concentration) sodium acetate and 2 volumes of ethanol. The resulting precipitate was again dissolved in water and reprecipitated with ethanol. Finally, RNA was dissolved in water and analyzed by centrifugation for 3 or 3.5 hours at 39,000 r.p.m. on a linear 5-20 per cent sucrose gradient containing tris-HCl, pH 7.6 (0.05 M.) and KCl (0.025 M.), with the RPS-40 rotor of the Hitachi ultracentrifuge. Following centrifugation, the bottom of the tube was punctured with an hypodermic needle, and successive three-drop samples were collected. From each fraction 0.1 ml. was separated for determination of radioactivity by subsequent addition of albumin (2 mg.) as carrier and precipitation with 6 per cent perchloric acid. The radioactive precipitate was dissolved in 90 per cent (v./v.) formic acid, plated in planchettes, dried under an infrared lamp, and radioactivity measured with a 2π gas-flow counter. Each of the remaining fractions was diluted with 3 ml. of water, and the content of RNA was calculated from absorbance at 260 nm. (1 mg. RNA = 21.6 A_{260} units.) RNA with alkali extracted was prepared by the procedure of Hadjivassiliou and Brawerman (1967). High molecular RNA was prepared according to the LiCl method: An equal volume of 4 M. LiCl solution was added to the total RNA solution to make a final concentration of 2 M. The solution was kept at 0° C., and the white flocculant precipitate was used as the high molecular RNA.

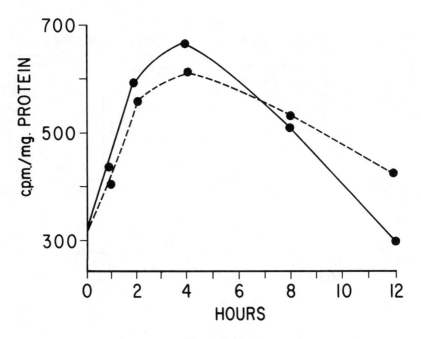

Figure 2

The Time Course of the Stimulation of Amino- acid Incorporation after the Injection of Ecdysterone. ———— ecdysterone 0.05 mg./100G. body weight, – – – – ecdysterone 0.5 mg./100G. body weight.

TABLE 2

EFFECT OF ECDYSTERONE ON PROTEIN SYNTHESIS BY ORAL ADMINISTRATION

Treatment	c.p.m./mg. Protein
Control	386 ± 5
Ecdysterone 4 hr.	584 ± 14

Dose: 0.5 mg./100G. body weight. Each result is the mean ± standard error for six mice used.

Kinetics of Amino-acid Incorporation in the S-20 System

As illustrated in Figure 3, a similar temporal course of amino-acid incorporation in the S-20 system was obtained in both normal and steroid-treated liver, and the incorporation of amino acids already was increased significantly 5 minutes after incubation. These facts indicate that the increment of amino-acid incorporating activity by the steroids may not be due to stabilization of protein synthetic machine but augmentation of its capacity.

TABLE 3

EFFECT OF ECDYSTERONE ON PROTEIN SYNTHESIS IN FEMALE-MICE LIVER

Treatment	Time after Injection (Hr.)	cpm/mg Protein	Stimulation (%)
Control	2	123 ± 2	100
Ecdysterone	2	182 ± 5	148
	4	200 ± 7	163

Dose: 0.05 mg./100 G. body weight. Each result is the mean ± standard error for six mice used.

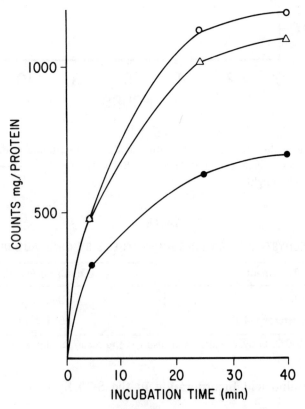

Figure 3

Time Course of Incorporation of ^{14}C-Chlorella Hydrolysate into Hot Acid-insoluble Proteins in *in Vitro* System Consisting of S-20 Fluid from Normal and Steroid-treated Murine Liver. Ecdysterone or 4-chlorotestosterone was administered by intraperitoneal injection 2 hr. prior to sacrifice. —●— normal, —○— ecdysterone-treated, —△— 4-chlorotestosterone-treated.

Sucrose Density-gradient Analysis of Protein Produced in the S-20 System

Figure 4 illustrates a typical result of sucrose-gradient centrifugation for the distribution of protein produced in the S-20 system of normal, ecdysterone-treated, and 4-chlorotestosterone-treated liver. It is clear that the incorporation of amino acids into protein increased equally in interface, membranes and ribosomes, and supernatant (free protein).

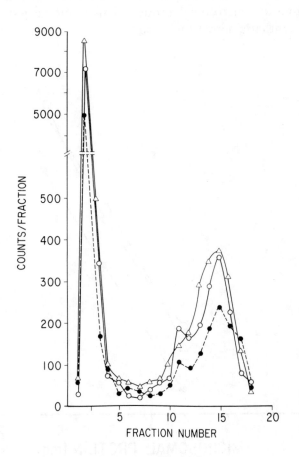

Figure 4

Sucrose Density-gradient Analysis of Proteins Produced in the S-20 System. Experimental details are described in the text. Mice were injected with ecdysterone or 4-chlorotestosterone 2 hr. prior to sacrifice. The position of the interface is between 2 and 20 per cent (w./v.) sucrose layers. Normal 628 c.p.m./mg. protein, Ecdysterone 1012 c.p.m./mg. protein, 4-Chlorotestosterone 1256 c.p.m./mg. protein.   —●— normal,   —○— ecdysterone,   −△− 4-chlorotestosterone-treated.

Alteration of Protein Synthesis in Microsomes after the Administration of Ecdysterone or 4-Chlorotestosterone

Results presented in Figure 5 show the incorporation of amino acids into protein in the systems consisting of microsomes from treated murine liver plus S-105 fluid (without Sephadex G-25 treatment) from normal liver. When the activity of microsomal fractions from normal and steroid-treated liver was compared, it was apparent that the microsomal particles from the steroid-treated liver are more active than those from normal liver, especially in the case of lower amounts of microsomal protein. This result suggests that increment of protein synthetic activity may be due to a change in the protein synthetic machine.

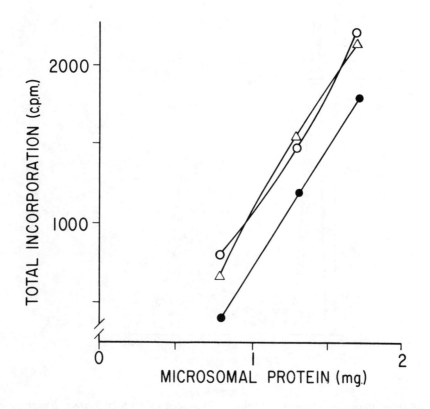

Figure 5

Incorporation of ^{14}C-Chlorella Hydrolysate into Hot Acid-insoluble Proteins with a Fixed Quantity of Cell Sap from Normal Liver and Increasing Amount of Microsomal Proteins. Mice were injected with ecdysterone or 4-chlorotestosterone 2 hr. prior to sacrifice. —●— normal, —○— ecdysterone-treated, —△— 4-chlorotestosterone-treated.

Alteration of Protein Synthesis in Polysomes after Administration of Ecdysterone or 4-Chlorotestosterone

Polysomes are aggregates of ribosomes held together by RNA, consisting of functional units for protein biosynthesis according to Wettstein *et al.* (1963) and Noll *et al.* (1963). This viewpoint is also supported by other workers (Goodman and Rich, 1963). Results presented in Table 4 show the incorporation of ^{14}C-amino acids into protein in the systems consisting of polysomes from normal or steroid-treated murine liver plus S-105 fluid from normal or steroid-treated liver. It is evident from Table 4A that protein synthetic activity of polysomes from steroid-treated mice was higher than that from normal mice.

TABLE 4

EFFECT OF ECDYSTERONE OF 4–CHLOROTESTOSTERONE
ON THE INCORPORATION OF ^{14}C-CHLORELLA HYDROLYSATE
INTO PROTEIN IN THE POLYSOMAL SYSTEM

	Polysomes from	S−105	Total Counts
(A)	Normal	Normal	3679 ± 87
	Ecdysterone−Treated	Normal	4352 ± 25
	4-Chlorotestosterone−Treated	Normal	4395 ± 44
(B)	Normal	Normal [a]	9388 ± 58
	Normal	Ecdysterone−Treated [a]	9694 ± 150
	Normal	4-Chlorotestosterone−Treated [a]	9790 ± 176

(A) ^{14}C-Chlorella hydrolysate was used as labeled amino acids. Each result is the mean ± standard error for ten mice used. (B) ^{14}C-L-Alanine was used as a labeled amino acid. Each result is the mean ± standard error for four mice used.

Addition of Ecdysterone to the Reaction Mixture for Protein Synthesis

Burdette and Coda (1963) have reported that when the extracts of silkworm that contains ecdysone activity was added to the postmitochondrial

TABLE 5

EFFECT OF ECDYSTERONE ADDED IN VITRO ON THE INCORPORATION
OF AMINO ACIDS INTO PROTEIN

Addition	c.p.m./mg.Protein	Addition	c.p.m./mg.Protein
None	173 ± 20	Ecdysterone 0.1 mg	182 ± 16
Ecdysterone 0.005 mg	176 ± 28	0.5 mg	163 ± 23
0.01 mg	186 ± 24		

supernatant, the rate of hepatic protein synthesis *in vitro* was enhanced. However, ecdysterone solution did not enhance the rate of protein synthesis when added *in vitro* (Table 5) in our studies. Burdette (1964) also reported that the amount of both DNA and RNA was increased in HeLa cells cultured with extracts containing ecdysones.

Effect of Actinomycin on Stimulation of Protein Synthetic Activity by Ecdysterone or 4-Chlorotestosterone

Since the above results suggested that stimulation of protein synthetic activity by ecdysterone or 4-chlorotestosterone was associated with newly synthesized RNA, at least partly, the effect of actinomycin, an inhibitor of DNA-dependent RNA synthesis (Reich *et al.*, 1961), on its stimulation was investigated. As shown in Table 6, the two steroids employed differed in inhibition of protein synthesis by Actinomycin; ecdysterone can partly stimulate the protein synthetic activity even in the presence of Actinomycin, but Actinomycin completely repressed the activation of 4-chlorotestosterone. These results indicate that stimulation of protein synthetic activity by 4-chlorotestosterone must be due solely to the newly synthesized RNA.

TABLE 6

EFFECT OF ACTINOMYCIN ON STIMULATION OF PROTEIN SYNTHETIC ACTIVITY IN S–20 SYSTEM BY ECDYSTERONE OR 4–CHLOROTESTOSTERONE

Treatment	c.p.m./mg. Protein	Treatment	c.p.m./mg. Protein
Normal	1220 ± 20	Actinomycin D	1196 ± 15
Ecdysterone	2271 ± 43	Act. D + Ecdysterone	1655 ± 20
4-Chlorotestosterone	2538 ± 30	Act. D + 4-Chlorotestosterone	1016 ± 12

Mice were injected simultaneously with ecdysterone or 4-chlorotestosterone and/or actinomycin D 2 hr. prior to sacrifice. Each result is the mean ± standard error for ten mice used.

Stimulatory Effect of Ecdysterone on Incorporation of Orotic Acid into RNA *in Vivo*

Table 7 summarizes the labeling of nuclear and cytoplasmic RNA in normal and ecdysterone-treated murine liver with ^{14}C-orotic acid. A single injection of ecdysterone into normal mice remarkably enhanced the incorporation of radioactivity into both nuclear RNA and cytoplasmic RNA. The increment was rather great at an early period after administration. As shown in Table 8, the label in high molecular RNA obtained from nuclear and cytoplasmic RNA was also significantly elevated 2 hours after administration, by optical extinction. Treatment of normal mice with ecdysterone resulted as well as low-molecule RNA. Actinomycin treatment of the mice produced

TABLE 7

INCORPORATION OF ^{14}C–OROTIC ACID INTO LIVER NUCLEAR
AND CYTOPLASMIC RNA OF NORMAL MICE GIVEN ECDYSTERONE

Treatment		c.p.m./mg. RNA	%
(A) Cytoplasm			
Control		121 ± 10	100
Ecdysterone	2.0 hr. [a]	364 ± 13	301
	2.5 hr.	261 ± 12	216
	3.5 hr.	235 ± 11	194
(B) Nuclei			
Control		491 ± 15	100
Ecdysterone	2.0 hr.	1243 ± 17	253
	2.5 hr.	1017 ± 11	207
	3.5 hr.	998 ± 18	203

Ecdysterone (10 μg. per mouse) was administered to normal mice. In this experiment, cytoplasmic fraction is 12,000 x g. supernatant. Values are the mean ± standard error for six mice used.

a) ^{14}C-orotic acid (1 μCi.per mouse) was injected 1.5 , 2 and 3 hr.after ecdysterone administration and 30 min. later the animals were killed and livers removed.

TABLE 8

EFFECT OF ECDYSTERONE ADMINISTRATION ON ^{14}C–OROTIC ACID
INCORPORATION INTO HIGH–MOLECULAR RNA OF CYTOPLASMIC
AND NUCLEAR RNA FROM LIVER

Treatment		c.p.m./mg. RNA	%
(A) Cytoplasm			
Control		71 ± 3	100
Ecdysterone	2 hr.	205 ± 12	289
(B) Nuclei			
Control		276 ± 16	100
Ecdysterone	2 hr.	768 ± 20	278

Experimental details are given in the experimental section. Values are the mean ± standard error for six mice used.

the expected (Meritz, 1963; Reich *et al.*, 1961) inhibition of RNA synthesis either with or without ecdysterone (Table 9).

Sucrose Density-gradient Analysis of RNA

The result of density-gradient analysis of labeled cytoplasmic RNA obtained from normal and ecdysterone-treated mice is given in Figure 6. The distribution of radioactivity in cytoplasmic RNA after pulse-labeling with orotic acid was heterogeneous and not associated with major peaks drawn

TABLE 9

EFFECT OF ACTINOMYCIN D ON STIMULATION OF ^{14}C–OROTIC–
ACID INCORPORATION INTO CYTOPLASMIC AND NUCLEAR RNA BY ECDYSTERONE

Treatment		c.p.m./mg. RNA	%
(A)	Cytoplasm		
	Normal	124 ± 2	100
	Actinomycin D	56 ± 5	45
	Act. D + Ecdysterone	59 ± 4	48
(B)	Nuclei		
	Normal	877 ± 3	100
	Actinomycin D	269 ± 17	31
	Act. D + Ecdysterone	211 ± 21	24

Actinomycin D (40 µg. per mouse) and/or ecdysterone was administered to normal mice. ^{14}C-Orotic acid (1 µCi. per mouse) was injected after 1.5 hr., and the animals were killed 30 min. later. Values are the mean ± standard error for six mice used.

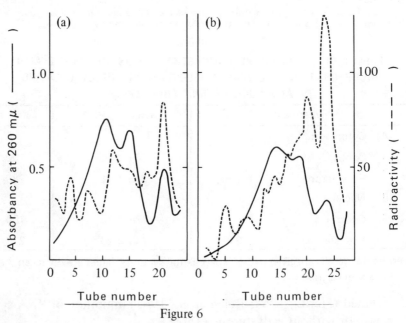

Figure 6

Labeling Pattern of Cytoplasmic RNA Influenced by Ecdysterone. Ecdysterone was administered to normal mice 2 hr. before the animals were killed (b). Saline was administered to the controls (a). ^{14}C-Orotic acid was injected 30 min. prior to sacrificing the animals. The hepatic cytoplasmic fraction (600 x g. supernatant) was isolated, the RNA extracted and centrifuged at 39,000 r.p.m. for 3.5 hr. on a linear sucrose density gradient (5-20 per cent) in an Hitachi RPS 40 rotor.

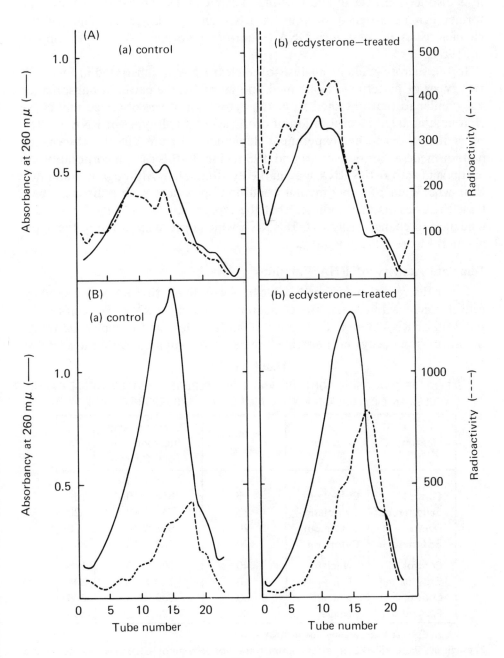

Figure 7

Labeling Pattern of Nuclear RNA Influenced by Ecdysterone. Experimental conditions are the same as that in Figure 6. (A) and (B) are results of different experiments.

in a distinct increase in the labeling of RNA in 4S and 6-18S regions. The former can be assigned to transfer RNA, and the latter has some of the characteristics of messenger RNA (Munro and Korner, 1962; Traketellio *et al.*, 1964).

In the sucrose-gradient analysis of nuclear RNA, as illustrated in Figure 7, two types of pattern were obtained. In Figure 7A, the pattern of absorbance was similar to that obtained from the cytoplasm. It was observed that ecdysterone stimulated incorporation of orotic acid into all types of RNA. On the other hand, in another experiment depicted in Figure 7B, the absorbance pattern made a single peak around 19S region. In this case, incorporation of orotic acid into 6-18S RNA was markedly stimulated. Although it is still not clear what kind of experimental conditions produces such a different pattern, these results may indicate that the rapidly labeled nuclear RNA has a tendency to change easily to 6-18S RNA which in turn appeared in the cytoplasm as Figure 6 demonstrates.

Template Activity of RNA Fractions

From the results mentioned above, it is very likely that RNA increased by ecdysterone treatment has the character of messenger RNA. To confirm the function of RNA, template activity of both nuclear and cytoplasmic RNAs obtained from ecdysterone-treated mice was compared with those RNAs

TABLE 10

EFFECT OF RNA FROM CONTROL AND ECDYSTERONE–TREATED MOUSE–LIVER
NUCLEI AND CYTOPLASM ON AN AMINO–ACID INCORPORATION *IN VITRO*

Treatment	Fraction	Amount (μg.)	^{14}C-Amino Acids Incorporated (Total Counts)	Δ a)
—	—	—	414 ± 11	
Control	Cytoplasm	35	574 ± 10	160
Ecdysterone	Cytoplasm	35	746 ± 12	322
Control	Cytoplasm	70	536 ± 6	122
Ecdysterone	Cytoplasm	70	666 ± 10	252
Control	Nuclei	40	590 ± 5	176
Ecdysterone	Nuclei	40	718 ± 6	304
Control	Nuclei	80	692 ± 3	278
Ecdysterone	Nuclei	80	794 ± 2	380

a) Δ = net incorporation due to RNA added

The animals were killed 3 hr. after administration of ecdysterone. Nuclear or cytoplasmic (600 x g. supernatant) RNA was added, in the amounts indicated, to the ribosomal amino acid-incorporating system. Incubation procedure is given in the experimental section. Values are the mean ± standard error for six mice used.

from normal mice. Table 10 shows the significantly higher template activity produced by ecdysterone.

It is also interesting that template activity of cytoplasmic RNA declined at higher concentrations, whereas that of nuclear RNA did not. It has been reported that RNA having template activity can be extracted with alkaline solution (Hadjivassiliou and Brawerman, 1967). As shown in Table 11, incorporation of orotic acid into alkali-extracted RNA was markedly stimulated by administration of ecdysterone, which is compatible with the fact that the RNA formed by administration of ecdysterone has a higher template activity.

TABLE 11

EFFECT OF ECDYSTERONE ON ^{14}C–OROTIC ACID INCORPORATION INTO
ALKALI–EXTRACTED RIBONUCLEIC ACIDS

Treatment	c.p.m./mg. RNA	%
(A) Cytoplasm		
Control	136 ± 13	100
Ecdysterone	205 ± 11	152
(B) Nuclei		
Control	114 ± 7	100
Ecdysterone	487 ± 20	427

The animals were killed 2 hr. after administration of ecdysterone. Values are the mean ± standard error for mice used.

Stimulatory Effect of Various Phytoecdysones on Protein Synthesis in Mice

Takemoto, Hikino, and co-workers (Hikino and Hikino, 1970) isolated the metamorphosing substances, ecdysterone and inokosterone, first from *Achyranthes fauriei* Leveille *et* Vaniot (Amaranthaceae) and later from a number of Achyranthes species. They also reported the isolation of the unique analogs, cyasterone and rubrosterone, from *Cyathula capitata* Moquin-Tandon (Amaranthaceae) and *Achyranthes rubrofusca* Wight, respectively. They also found that the crude extract of ferns show insect-metamorphosing activity in high frequency and have isolated from them a number of active substances, ecdysone, ponasterone A, pterosterone, ecdysterone, lemmasterone, shidasterone, and ponasteroside A. Among these steroids, ecdysone and ecdysterone are the genuine insect-metamorphosing hormones originally isolated from the silkworm (*Bombyx mori*) and other arthropods. Meanwhile, Jizba *et al.* have isolated an insect-metamorphosing substance, polypodine B, from a fern (Goldberg and Rabinowitz, 1962).

It has been demonstrated that all of these steroids exhibit substantial insect-metamorphosing activity except rubrosterone which shows little activity

TABLE 12

EFFECT OF INSECT–METAMORPHOSING STEROIDS ON PROTEIN SYNTHESIS

Treatment	Time after Injection (Hr)	c.p.m./mg. Protein	Stimulation %
(A) Control		307 ± 4	100
Ecdysterone	1	400 ± 62	130
	2	553 ± 31	180
	4	603 ± 12	196
Inokosterone	1	327 ± 4	107
	2	522 ± 10	170
	4	625 ± 13	206
Cyasterone	1	350 ± 10	114
	2	540 ± 9	176
	4	632 ± 21	206
(B) Control		202 ± 2	100
Rubrosterone	1	201 ± 4	100
	2	249 ± 6	123
	3	316 ± 3	156
Ecdysterone	3	271 ± 3	134
(C) Control		307 ± 4	100
Ponasterone A	1	290 ± 10	95
	2	582 ± 15	190
Pterosterone	1	328 ± 20	107
	2	571 ± 16	186
Ecdysterone1q	1	400 ± 62	130
	2	553 ± 31	180
(D) Control		257 ± 9	100
Shidasterone	1	241 ± 16	94
	2	401 ± 6	156
Lemmasterone	1	273 ± 8	107
	2	468 ± 12	182
Ponasteroside A	1	271 ± 5	106
	2	356 ± 6	139
Ecdysone	1	270 ± 4	105
	2	279 ± 5	108
(E) Control		195 ± 10	100
Ecdysterone	2	348 ± 7	178
Polypodine B	2	233 ± 4	120

The experiments of (A), (B), (C), (D), and (E) were done at different periods. Dose: 0.05 mg./100 G. body weight. Numbers of mice employed: A-10; B-6; C-10; D-6; D-4.

in the Sarcophaga test. Therefore, it seemed of interest to assay their ability to stimulate protein synthesis in murine liver. As summarized in Table 12, all the steroids except ecdysone stimulated protein synthesis in the liver of the mouse. Thus, though no pronounced effect was observed 1 hour after administration, a significant increase in protein anabolic activity was found after 2 hours. On the other hand, ecdysone showed little stimulation of protein synthesis. When the dose of each steroid was lowered to 0.005 mg./100G. body weight, only cyasterone showed anabolic activity among four phytoecdysones tested as indicated in Table 13.

TABLE 13

EFFECT OF INSECT–METAMORPHOSING STEROIDS
(0.005 MG./100 G. BODY WEIGHT) ON PROTEIN SYNTHESIS

Treatment	c.p.m./mg. Protein	%
Control	435 ± 10	100
Ecdysterone	412 ± 21	95
Inokosterone	380 ± 25	87
Cyasterone	541 ± 31	124
Rubrosterone	465 ± 32	107

The mice were sacrificed 2 hr. after the administration. Each result is the mean ± standard error for eight mice used.

DISCUSSION

Mode of Action of Ecdysterone on Protein Synthesis in Mice

The effect of insect-molting steroids, especially ecdysone, on larval epidermis of *Calliphora erythrocephala* Meig has been investigated in detail. Our results suggested that these steroids also can stimulate protein synthetic activity in the liver of the mouse, as does 4-chlorotestosterone, a potent anabolic steroid.

Enhancement of incorporation of amino acids into protein in all subcellular components *in vivo* suggests that these steroids can stimulate the protein synthetic activity not only in microsomes, but also in nuclei and mitochondria. In the present experiment, stimulatory effect of ecdysterone on protein synthesis in microsomes was examined in detail.

The absolute increment was about the same both in doses of 0.05 and 0.5 mg. of ecdysterone *per* 100G. body weight. This indicates that the degree of stimulation of protein synthesis is maximum in 0.05-mg. dose. The observation of ecdysterone was effective even by oral administration suggests that it is absorbable and not completely degraded in digestive organs. A sex difference was not observed in the response to ecdysterone.

These stimulatory effects must be the result of accelerated detachment of newly synthesized polypeptides from ribosomes or microsomes, based on the ratio of increment of amino-acid incorporation into microsomes and cell-sap proteins in both *in-vivo* and *in-vitro* systems (Figure 1).

The temporal course of amino-acid incorporation into proteins in the S-20 system suggests that these stimulatory effects may not be the result of stability of the protein synthetic machine, but augmentation of its capacity.

The reaction using microsomes from the steroid-treated liver plus S-105 fluid from normal liver suggested that the stimulatory factor is associated with microsomes (Figure 5). A preliminary study demonstrated that the RNA/protein ratio of the microsomes was slightly higher in steroid-treated liver. Thus the enhanced rate of protein synthesis by microsomes from steroid-treated liver may result from the presence of a greater amount of RNA, including messenger RNA.

In the system consisting of microsomes plus S-105 fluid, a slight stimulation of protein synthesis by S-105 fluid from steroid-treated liver was observed (Table 14). On the other hand, no stimulation by S-105 fluid was observed (Table 4) in the system consisting of polysomes plus S-105 fluid. These results suggest that the microsomal membrane plays a certain role in the stimulation by S-105 fluid.

TABLE 14

EFFECT OF S–105 FLUID ON THE INCORPORATION OF ^{14}C–CHLORELLA
HYDROLYSATE INTO PROTEIN IN THE MICROSOMAL SYSTEM

Microsome	S–105	Total Counts
Normal	Normal	1900 ± 82
Normal	Ecdysterone	2312 ± 75
Normal	4–Chlorotestosterone	2439 ± 96

The experimental conditions are described in the text. Mice were injected with ecdysterone or 4-chlorotestosterone 2 hr. prior to sacrifice. Each result is the mean ± standard error for eight mice used.

In the system consisting of polysomes plus S-105 fluid, an enhanced rate of protein synthesis by polysomes from steroid-treated liver was observed, but it was not increased by S-105 fluid, enzyme for protein synthesis and tRNA, whether treated with Sephadex G-15 or not, which was different from the microsomal system. An increment of protein synthetic activity by steroid-treated polysomes may be associated with its structural change from inactive to active form (Koike *et al.*, 1967), and, at the same time, an increment of polysomal content itself cannot be ruled out, because the polysomal fraction may be contaminated with free ribosomes. Therefore, the increment of protein synthetic activity by the steroid-treated polysome may be the result both of an increment in content of polysomes and a functional change.

There was a significant difference in the effect of actinomycin on the enhanced incorporation of amino acids into protein in the S-20 system from the liver of mice treated with two kinds of steroid. A part of the enhancement by ecdysterone was insensitive to actinomycin, but the stimulation by 4-chlorotestosterone was repressed completely. This result suggests that the stimulation of protein synthetic activity by ecdysterone is not dependent entirely on newly-synthesized RNA.

From the results obtained in the present experiments, it is clear that the administration of ecdysterone to mice was attended by an increase in the incorporation of a precursor into both cytoplasmic and nuclear RNA of the liver. The stimulatory effect of ecdysterone on RNA synthesis was completely abolished by actinomycin which has been known to exert its effect on RNA synthesis by masking the guanine bases of the primer DNA (Goldberg and Rabinowitz, 1962) and thus stopping the polymerization of all DNA-primed RNAs.

Although Hiatt (1962) failed to detect any rapidly labeled RNA around the 6-18S region in the cytoplasm of hepatic cells, Munro and Korner (1962) and Trakatellio *et al.* (1964) reported the detection of rapidly labeled 6-18S RNA and presumed that it is the messenger RNA. In the present experiments also the labeling pattern of cytoplasmic RNA obtained by means of sucrose density-gradient analysis indicated that ecdysterone enhanced the incorporation of orotic acid not only into structural RNA of ribosomes and 4-5S RNA, but also into 6-18S RNA.

Moreover, the extinction and labeling patterns obtained from nuclear RNA showed two distinct types, depending on the experimental condition; one was the spread labeling throughout the gradient and the other was a single labeling at about 6-18S. This phenomenon is likely to suggest that high-density nuclear RNA may be unstable and easily degraded to 6-18S RNA, which may be transported into cytoplasm and show the characteristics of messenger RNA.

Most of RNA of nuclei became labeled shortly after the injection of orotic acid, and it is not easy to assign the name, messenger RNA, to any of the nuclear RNA fractions. It is clear, however, that the amount of RNA active as template *in vitro* was increased by ecdysterone. This could be a relative increase of template RNA per cytoplasmic or nuclear bulk RNA.

More likely, judging from RNA labeling and the stimulatory incorporation of orotic acid into alkali-extracted RNA, the above facts can be interpreted as a true increase of messenger RNA by hormonal (ecdysterone) stimulation.

The resultant new messenger RNA may elevate the synthesis *de novo* of proteins as reported here. In fact, long-term administration of ecdysterone to mice brought histological changes in the liver, consisting of evidence for stimulated metabolism and active regeneration of cells (Hikino *et al.*, 1969).

The present findings give a reasonable explanation for the effective activation of protein synthesis in mammalian cells introduced by insect-molting steroids derived from the plant kingdom. It remains obscure what kind of proteins are produced and what is the actual role of such proteins in physiological functions.

Structural Difference of Phytoecdysones and Their Anabolic Activities

Ecdysterone, inokosterone, cyasterone, ponasterone A, pterosterone, and lemmasterone have the common feature of the 2β, 3β, $14a$, 2-(R), 22(R)-pentahydroxy-7-en-6-one system in their 5(H)-steroid skeleton. Therefore, some part of this structure must be indispensable for exhibition of stimulatory effect on protein synthesis. Shidasterone, which is a stereoisomer of ecdysterone, exhibits high activity, indicating that some alteration in stereochemistry does not seem to affect anabolic activity. The observation that polypodine B, 5β-hydroxyecdysterone, was much less active in stimulating protein synthesis, suggests that 5β-hydroxyls in ecdysterols participate less potently than 5β-hydrogens in elevating anabolic activity. Ponasteroside A, ponasterone A 3-β-D-glucopyranoside, still shows this activity; but the effect is less than that of its aglycone, ponasterone A. In this case, however, the possibility cannot be excluded that ponasteroside A reveals the activity only enzymic hydrolysis in the mouse. If this were the case, the apparent anabolic activity must depend on the rate of its hydrolysis in animals.

It is interesting to note that rubrosterone exhibits little metamorphosing activity in the Sarcophaga test, although it exhibits anabolic activity. Therefore, it seems that a certain side-chain structure may be required for the metamorphosis of insects, but no side-chain may be necessary for the stimulation of protein synthesis in murine liver.

On the other hand, ecdysone, different from all the steroids mentioned above, showed little anabolic activity. This result may agree with the observation of Lukacs and Sekeris that ecdysone exhibited no effect on RNA polymerase activity in hepatic nuclei of the rat (1967). The difference in activities among these steroids may be explained by the following difference in their structures; ecdysone has an hydroxyl group at C-22 but not at C-20, whereas the other steroids that show anabolic activity have hydroxyl groups at C-20 and C-22. However, for complete understanding of the structure-activity relationship, additional study is required. It is of interest to note that ecdysone is highly effective in causing metamorphosis in insects, but it does not stimulate protein synthesis in mammalian cells. This fact, as in the case of rubrosterone, also indicates that the structural component of hormones responsible for metamorphosing activity in insects is not always the same as that for anabolic activity in the mouse.

SUMMARY

The effect of ecdysterone, representative phytoecdysone, on protein and RNA syntheses in murine liver was studied, and the structure-activity relationship of various phytoecdysones examined.

The administration of ecdysterone caused early stimulation of protein synthesis, as indicated by pronounced increase in the incorporation of ^{14}C-chlorella hydrolysate into hot acid-insoluble protein as early as 2 hours after treatment as does 4-chlorotestosterone.

Oral administration of ecdysterone produced a similar activation and the hormone stimulated protein synthesis not only in male mice but also in female mice.

Ecdysterone was able to exert its stimulatory effect on the protein synthetic ability of microsomes or polysomes, but not the 105,000 x g. supernatant.

The stimulation induced by ecdysterone was partly insensitive to actinomycin, an inhibitor of DNA-dependent RNA synthesis, whereas the stimulation of 4-chlorotestosterone was completely repressed by it.

The administration of ecdysterone to mice is accompanied by the elevated incorporation of orotic acid into ribonucleic acids in the liver. This effect was completely repressed by actinomycin-D.

Judging from the template activity of RNA in an amino-acid-incorporating system and the results of sucrose-gradient analysis, it is obvious that the rate of synthesis of messenger RNA is regulated by ecdysterone as well as other RNA in murine liver. The stimulating effect of ecdysterone on protein synthesis reported here can be explained, at least partially, in terms of its influence on synthesis of messenger RNA.

Various phytoecdysones isolated from Achyranthes and Cyathula (Amaranthaceae) (ecdysterone, inokosterone, and cyasterone) and ferns (ponasterone A, pterosterone, ecdysterone, ecdysone, shidasterone, lemmasterone, and polypodine B), and related substance (rubrosterone) were assayed in terms of their ability to stimulate protein synthesis in the liver of the mouse. Among them, polypodine B (5β-hydroxyecdysterone) was much less active in accelerating protein synthesis. Ponasteroside A (ponasterone A 3-β-D-glucopyranoside) also revealed anabolic activity. Ecdysone, having an hydroxyl at C-22 but not at C-20, exhibited little stimulation. Great stimulation of protein anabolic activity in murine liver was produced by all other phytoecdysones including rubrosterone which does not affect molting in insects.

Acknowledgement

Among the phytoecdysones employed in this work, ecdysterone and inokosterone were kindly given by Dr. S. Ogawa, the Research Laboratories of Rhoto Pharmaceutical Co., Osaka, and the others were kindly supplied by Drs. T. Takemoto and H. Hikino, Pharmaceutical Institute, Tohoku University. ^{14}C-labeled compounds were obtained from the Daiichi Pure Chemical Co., Tokyo.

References

1. BURDETTE, W. J. and CODA, R. C.: Effect of Ecdysone on Incorporation of C^{14}-Leucine into Hepatic Protein *in Vitro*. Proc. Soc. Exptl. Biol. Med., *112*:216, 1963.
2. BURDETTE, W. J.: The Significance of Invertebrate Hormones in Relation to Differentiation. Cancer Research, *24*:521-536, 1964.
3. GOLDBERG, L. H. and RABINOWITZ, M.: Actinomycin-D Inhibition of Deoxyribonucleic Acid-dependent Synthesis of Ribonucleic Acid. Science, *136*:315-316, 1962.
4. GOODMAN, H. M. and RICH, A.: Mechanism of Polyribosome Action During Protein Synthesis. Nature, *199*:318-322, 1963.
5. GORNALL, A. G., BARDAWILL, C. J., and HERMAN, M.: Determination of Serum Proteins by Means of Biuret Reaction. J. Biol. Chem., *177*:751-766, 1949.
6. FRANKLIN, R. M.: The Inhibition of Ribonucleic Acid Synthesis in Mammalian Cells by Actinomycin D. Biochem. Biophys. Acta, *72*:555-565, 1963.
7. HADJIVASSILIOU, A. and BRAWERMAN, G.: Template and Ribosomal Ribonucleic Acid Components in the Nucleus and the Cytoplasm of Rat Liver. Biochemistry, *6*:1934, 1967.
8. HIATT, H. H.: A Rapidly Labeled RNA in Rat Liver Nuclei. J. Mol. Biol., *5*:217-229, 1962.
9. HIKINO, H. and HIKINO, Y.: Arthropod Molting Hormones. Fortschr. Chem. Org. Naturstoffe, *28*:256, 1970.
10. HIKINO, H., NABETANI, S., NOMOTO, K., ARAI, T., TAKEMOTO, T., OTAKA, T., and UCHIYAMA, M.: Effect of Long Term Administration of Insect-metamorphosing Substances on Higher Animals. Yakugaku Zasshi, *89*:235, 1969.
11. KOIKE, K., OTAKA, T., and OKUI, S.: Regulation of Protein Synthesis in Mouse Liver by Steroid Hormones. J. Biochem. (Tokyo), *61*:679, 1967.
12. KOIKE, K., OTAKA, T., and OKUI, S.: Induction of Heme-protein Enzyme in Animal Cells IV. Relationship Between Rapidly Labeled RNA and Induced Synthesis of Tryptophan Oxygenase *in Vivo*. J. Biochem. (Tokyo), *59*:201, 1966.
13. LUKÁCS, I. and SEKERIS, C. E.: On the Mechanism of Human Action IX. Stimulation of RNA Polymerase Activity of Rat Liver Nuclei by Cortisol *in Vitro*. Biochim. Biophys. Acta, *134*:85, 1967.
14. MERITZ, I.: Actinomycin Inhibition of RNA Synthesis in Rat Liver. Biochem. Biophys. Res. Commun., *10*:254, 1963.
15. MUNRO, A. J. and KORNER, A.: Determination of a Rapidly Labeled Ribonucleic Acid in the Cytoplasm of Rat Liver. Biochem. J., *85*:37P, 1962.
16. NOLL, H., STAEHELIN, T., and WETTSTEIN, F. O.: Ribosomal Aggregates Engaged in Protein Synthesis; Ergosome Breakdown and Messenger Ribonucleic Acid Transport. Nature, *198*:632-638, 1963.
17. OKUI, S., OTAKA, T., UCHIYAMA, M., TAKEMOTO, T., HIKINO, H., OGAWA, S., and NISHIMOTO, N.: Stimulation of Protein Synthesis in Mouse Liver by Insect-moulting Steroids. Chem. Pharm. Bull., *16*:384, 1968.
18. OTAKA, T., OKUI, S., and UCHIYAMA, M.: Stimulation of Protein Synthesis in Mouse Liver by Ecdysterone. Chem. Pharm. Bull., *17*:75, 1969.
19. OTAKA, T. and UCHIYAMA, M.: Stimulatory Effect of Ecdysterone on RNA Synthesis in Mouse Liver. Chem. Pharm. Bull., *17*:1883, 1969.

20. OTAKA, T. and UCHIYAMA, M. : Stimulatory Effect of Insect-metamorphosing Steroids from Ferns on Protein Synthesis in Mouse Liver. Chem. Pharm. Bull., *17*:1352, 1969.

21. OTAKA, T., UCHIYAMA, M., and OKUI, S. : Stimulatory Effects of Insect-metamorphosing Steroids from *Achyranthes* and *Cyathula* on Protein Synthesis in Mouse Liver. Chem. Pharm. Bull., *16*:2426, 1968.

22. REICH, E., FRANKLIN, R. M., SHATKIN, A. J., and TATUM, E.L. : Effect of Actinomycin D on Cellular Nucleic Acid Synthesis and Virus Production. Science, *134*:556-557, 1961.

23. TRAKATELLIS, A. C., AXELROD, A. E., and MONTJAR, M.: Actinomycin D and Messenger RNA Turnover. Nature, *203*:1134-1136, 1964.

24. WETTSTEIN, F. O., STAEHELIN, T., and NOLL, H.: Ribosomal Aggregate Engaged in Protein Synthesis: Characterization of the Ergosome. Nature, *197*:430-435, 1963.

EFFECT of ECDYSTERONE
on CARBOHYDRATE
and LIPID METABOLISM

Mitsuru Uchiyama and Takemi Yoshida

In the preceding chapter, it was reported that ecdysterone and many other phyto-ecdysones show high protein-anabolic activity in murine liver. Since some of the steroids are effective in regulating carbohydrate and lipid metabolism in clinical and experimental applications, it became of interest to know whether ecdysterone also can influence carbohydrate and lipid metabolism. Therefore studies were carried out on the effect of ecdysterone on high blood-glucose levels induced by the administration of glucagon, alloxan, or anti-insulin serum (AIS) in rats and mice. The alteration of enzymatic activity concerned with carbohydrate metabolism was tested preliminarily, and changes of lipid component in rats treated with ecdysterone were determined as well.

MATERIALS AND METHODS

Animals and Treatment Male Donryu rats weighing 200 G. and male ddy mice weighing 20G. maintained on standard laboratory chow were used.

Figure 1

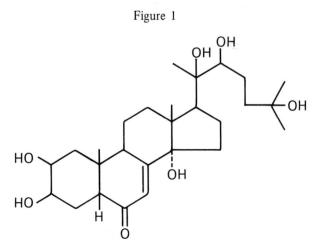

Structure of Ecdysterone

Glucagon was injected intraperitoneally in a dose of 0.2 mg./kg. body weight into animals starved for 3 or 6 hours before injection. Alloxan diabetes was induced by a single intravenous injection of alloxan monohydrate in a dose of 70 mg./kg. body weight into animals starved for 24 hours. Five to 7 days after the injection, animals were used for experiments after confirmation of high blood-glucose levels.

Anti-insulin serum was injected into mice intravenously in a dose of 100 or 350 mg./kg. body weight. Ecdysterone was injected intraperitoneally by the various techniques mentioned in each experiment.

Chemicals ^{14}C-Labeled glucose, acetate, and cholesterol were purchased from the Daiichi Pure Chemical Company, Tokyo; glucagon was obtained from Eli Lilly and Company; and alloxan monohydrate from Wako Pure Chemical Industries, Tokyo. AIS was harvested from guinea pigs treated with repeated injections of crystalline bovine insulin with bacillus Calmette-Guerin (BCG) as adjuvant (Kitagawa *et al.*, 1960). The serum obtained was lyophilized. One mg. of AIS neutralized the activity of 2 mu. of bovine insulin.

Analyses Blood was sampled by orbital puncture and cardiac puncture in the mouse and rat, respectively. Blood-glucose levels were determined by glucose oxidase (Oser, 1965) and by 3, 6-dinitrophthalic acid (Momose *et al.*, 1960) in the rat and mouse, respectively. Incorporation of ^{14}C into hot acid-insoluble protein was assayed as described in the preceding chapter. Incorporation of ^{14}C-glucose was determined according to the method of Hassid and Abraham (1957). Serum triglyceride was determined by the method of Van Handel and Zilversmit (1961). Free fatty acids in serum was analyzed by the method of Itaya and Ui (1965).

Cholesterol Biosynthesis In the experiment on cholesterol biosynthesis *in vivo,* rats were starved 20 hours and injected intraperitoneally with 0.5 ml. of aqueous solution containing 10 μCi. of ^{14}C-acetate (Wood and Migicovsky, 1958). The animals were killed 2 hours after treatment for estimation of cholesterol content and ^{14}C-incorporation into cholesterol; cholesterol in serum and liver was extracted with isopropanol (Ferro and Ham, 1960) and hexane, respectively, and precipitated with digitonin. The digitonide was determined by colorimetry with anthrone reagent.

Measurement of Enzymatic Activity Effect of ecdysterone treatment on several enzymes *in vivo* was examined by the measurement of changes in glycogen synthetase (Leloir and Goldenberg,(1960), glucokinase (Vinuela *et al.,* 1963), glucose-6-phosphate dehydrogenase (Glock and McLean, 1954), pyruvate kinase (Kackmar and Boyer, 1953), UDP-glucose dehydrogenase (Strominger *et al.,* 1957) and glucose-6-phosphatase (Swanson, 1950).

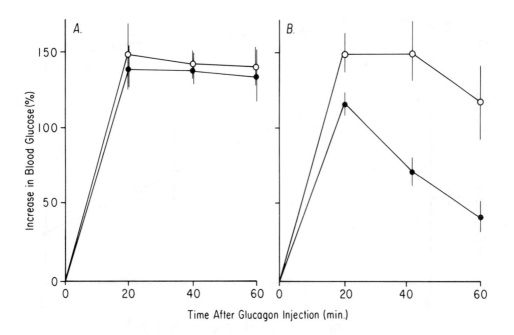

Figure 2
Effect of A Single Dose of Ecdysterone on Hyperglycemia Induced with Glucagon in Mice. Ecdysterone was given in the following ways: (a) Simultaneously with glucagon and (b) 1 hr. before injection of glucagon. ○——○ : Control, ●——● : Ecdysterone.

RESULTS

Effect of Ecdysterone on Hyperglycemia Evoked by Glucagon Figure 2
demonstrates the effect of ecdysterone on glucagon-induced hyperglycemia
in mice. The administration of glucagon elevated blood-glucose levels, but
hypoglycemic action was not observed when ecdysterone was injected
simultaneously with glucagon. The elevation of blood glucose tended to
be suppressed by the injection of ecdysterone 1 or 2 hours prior to the
administration of glucagon.

Ecdysterone also shortened the period required for the restoration of
blood-glucose to normal levels, as well as the depression of maximum
glucose content in blood induced by glucagon. Such modification of
blood glucose was not demonstrated in normal animals either fasted or not
fasted.

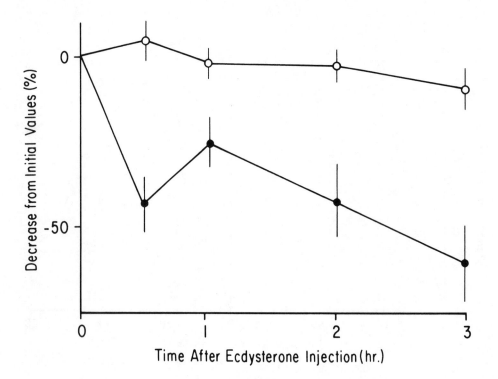

Figure 3
Effect of A Single Dose of Ecdysterone on Hyperglycemia Induced with Alloxan in Mice.
○——○ : Control, ●——● : Ecdysterone.

TABLE 1

EFFECT OF SINGLE ADMINISTRATION OF ECDYSTERONE ON HYPERGLYCEMIA WITH ALLOXAN IN RATS

Treatment	Within 400 mg. (per cent)			More than 400 mg. (per cent)		
	Before	After	Change	Before	After	Change (per cent)
Ecdysterone (0.1 mg./kg.)	316 ± 14	278 ± 16	-12.1 ± 1.3 (5)	558 ± 27	569 ± 38	+2.1 (3)
Ecdysterone (0.5 mg./kg.)	307 ± 27	249 ± 24	-18.9 ± 3.2 (6)	547 ± 44	565 ± 45	+3.4 (3)
Ecdysterone (1 mg./kg.)	344 ± 16	280 ± 17	-18.4 ± 3.4 (5)	568 ± 46	588 ± 16	+4.5 (3)
Ecdysterone (10 mg./kg.)	362 ± 14	298 ± 14	-17.7 ± 2.4 (5)	552 ± 45	561 ± 44	+1.9 (5)

Seven days after the administration of alloxan, rats were given an injection of ecdysterone 2 hours before death. Values recorded are means ± standard error. Figures in parentheses indicate the number of observations in each group.

Effect of Ecdysterone on Hyperglycemia Induced by Alloxan After the injection of ecdysterone, as shown in Figure 3, mice recovered from alloxan-induced hyperglycemia. Approximately 3 hours after the administration of ecdysterone the glucose level was reduced by about 60 per cent from the initial hyperglycemic value. In alloxan-diabetic rats (blood-glucose <400 mg. per cent), a significant decrease in blood glucose was observed 2 hours after the administration of ecdysterone. However, rats with severe alloxan diabetes (blood glucose >400 mg. per cent) were not responsive to ecdysterone (Table 1).

Effect of Ecdysterone on Hyperglycemia Caused by AIS   At about 30 minutes after injection of AIS, the blood glucose of mice reached the maximum. When ecdysterone was injected 1 to 3 hours before AIS injection in a dose of 100 mg./kg. the hyperglycemic response to AIS was supressed, whereas the hyperglycemia caused by the injection of higher dose of AIS (350 mg./kg.) exhibited a diminished response to ecdysterone (Figures 4 and 5).

Incorporation of ^{14}C from Glucose into Protein and Glycogen The ability of ecdysterone to stimulate glucose-carbon incorporation into protein and glycogen fractions of murine liver was employed as one of the indices to estimate the utilization of glucose *in vivo*. As shown in Table 2, stimulation of the incorporation of ^{14}C into protein was observed 2 and 4 hours after the administration of ecdysterone. This stimulation was about the same magnitude as the effect of the steroid on the incorporation of amino acids into protein reported in the preceding chapter. The incorporation of ^{14}C into protein was observed 2 and 4 hours after the administration of ecdysterone both in normal and diabetic animals(Table 3).

TABLE 2

EFFECT OF ECDYSTERONE ON ^{14}C-GLUCOSE INCORPORATION
INTO HEPATIC PROTEIN OF THE MOUSE

Treatment	c.p.m./mg. Protein	Stimulation (per cent)
Control	120 ± 2	100
Ecdysterone 2 hr.	160 ± 7	133
4 hr.	180 ± 3	150

Mice were killed 1 hour after the injection of ^{14}C-glucose (2 μCi./0.1 ml.).
The results are the mean $\pm$ S.D. of 6 mice per group.

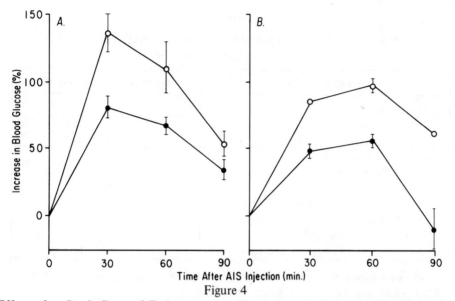

Figure 4

Effect of a Single Dose of Ecdysterone on Hyperglycemia Induced with AIS in Mice. Ecdysterone was administered in the following ways: (a) 1 hr. before injection of AIS and (b) 3 hr. before injection of AIS. ○—○ : Control, ●—● : Ecdysterone.

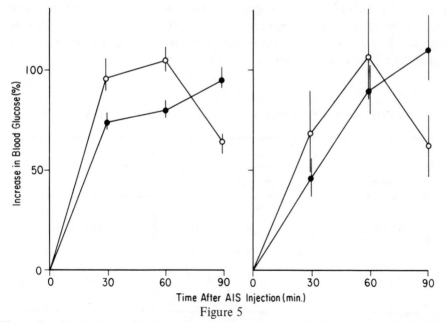

Figure 5

Effect of A Single Dose of Ecdysterone on Hyperglycemia Induced with a Higher Dose of AIS in Mice. Ecdysterone was administered in the following ways: (a) 1 hr. before injection of AIS and (b) 3 hr. before injection of AIS. ○—○ : Control, ●—● : Ecdysterone.

TABLE 3

EFFECT OF ECDYSTERONE ON ^{14}C-GLUCOSE INCORPORATION
INTO HEPATIC GLYCOGEN OF THE MOUSE

Treatment	c.p.m./G. Wet Weight Liver
Normal Mice	
Control	3660 ± 384
Ecdysterone 1 hr.	5750 ± 820
Alloxan-Diabetic Mice	
Experiment 1	
Control	1230 ± 120
Ecdysterone 1 hr.	2060 ± 180
Experiment 2	
Control	660 ± 50
Ecdysterone 3 hr.	1140 ± 170

Mice were killed 30 minutes after the injection of ^{14}C-glucoxe (2 μCi./0.1 ml.).
The results are the mean ± S. D. of 6 mice per group.

Activity of Glycogen Synthetase after Treatment with Ecdysterone Administration of ecdysterone in normal rats resulted in the elevation of glycogen synthetase. Two glycogen synthetases, *i. e.*, glucose-6-phosphate (G-6-P) dependent and independent types, were both activated as shown in Table 4. In diabetic rats, pronounced activation of glucose-6-phosphate - independent glycogen synthetase was recognized.

TABLE 4

EFFECT OF ECDYSTERONE ON GLYCOGEN—SYNTHETASE ACTIVITY

Treatment	Normal Mice	
	+G6P	-G6P
Control	5.17 ± 0.10	0.05 ± 0.04
Ecdysterone	7.55 ± 0.42	1.03 ± 0.10
(Insulin)	(8.84 ± 0.60)	(1.82 ± 0.22)

Glycogen synthetase activity is expressed as mμ moles UDP formed per mg. protein per minute.

TABLE 5

EFFECT OF ECDYSTERONE ON VARIOUS ENZYMES IN THE LIVER

Enzymes	Normal Mice		Diabetic Mice	
	Control	Ecdysterone	Control	Ecdysterone
G6P—ase	58.33 ± 4.40	37.59 ± 4.42	196.82 ± 19.35	144.60 ± 12.85
Glucokinase	3.39 ± 0.17	3.81 ± 0.46	1.52 ± 0.15	2.37 ± 0.16
G6P—Dehydrogenase	2.14 ± 0.23	3.81 ± 0.46	1.53 ± 0.31	3.40 ± 0.36
Pyruvate Kinase	326.46 ± 32.32	307.12 ± 34.12	273.65 ± 18.31	297.69 ± 29.25
UDpG—Dehydrogenase	0.54 ± 0.14	0.86 ± 0.15	0.64 ± 0.08	1.23 ± 0.11

G6P—ase activity is expressed as $m\mu$ moles of liberated Pi *per* mg. protein *per* 15 minutes. Other enzymatic activities are expressed as $m\mu$ moles of product formed *per* mg. protein *per* minutes.

Effect of Ecdysterone in Vivo on Some Key Enzymes in Glucose Metabolism Glucose-6-phosphatase, which is in the final stage of gluconeogenesis, was suppressed by the administration of ecdysterone, both in normal and and diabetic rats. On the other hand, some of the enzymes contributing to utilization of glucose were activated to a significant extent as indicated in Table 5. The specific activities of glucokinase, glucose-6-phosphate dehydrogenase, and UDP-glucose dehydrogenase of liver from normal and diabetic rats were elevated by the injection of ecdysterone, whereas the activity of pyruvate kinase remained unchanged.

Serum Triglycerides and Free Fatty Acids As the first step in examining the effect of ecdysterone on lipid metabolism, its influence on the amount of lipid in serum was assayed. It was found that the content of triglyceride was not influenced by the administration of ecdysterone.

Serum free fatty acid in normal rats was unchanged by the injection of ecdysterone, but ecdysterone lowered the elevated level of free fatty acid produced by lipolysis when animals were starved for 48 hours prior to experiments. A similar phenomenon was observed on the high content of free fatty acid induced by alloxan diabetes (Table 6).

TABLE 6

EFFECT OF ECDYSTERONE ON SERUM FREE FATTY ACID IN THE RAT

Treatment	FFA (μeq./ml.)
Normal	
Control	0.334 ± 0.071
Ecdysterone	0.334 ± 0.032
Starved	
Control	1.299 ± 0.136
Ecdysterone 30 min.	0.929 ± 0.103
3 hr.	0.980 ± 0.073
6 hr.	0.971 ± 0.076
Alloxan Diabetes	
Control	2.119 ± 0.176
Ecdysterone 6 hr.	1.440 ± 0.115

TABLE 7

EFFECT OF ECDYSTERONE ON CHOLESTEROL IN LIVER AND SERUM OF THE RAT

| Time after Treatment (Hr.) | | Cholesterol | | | |
| | | Levels | | Biosynthesis (d.p.m./mg. Cholesterol) | |
		Liver (mg./G.)	Serum (mg. per cent)	Liver	Serum
Control		2.42 ± 0.25	76.5 ± 2.47	1315 ± 167	508 ± 139
Ecdysterone	4	2.25 ± 0.21	75.9 ± 2.50	918 ± 93	453 ± 54
Control		2.36 ± 0.11	77.2 ± 3.05	1819 ± 303	855 ± 41
Ecdysterone	8	2.24 ± 0.15	76.0 ± 4.05	1281 ± 174	511 ± 85

Rats were starved for 20 hours. ^{14}C—Acetate was injected intraperitoneally. Rats were sacrificed 2 hours after treatment with ^{14}C—Acetate. Each value represents the mean ±S. D.

TABLE 8

EFFECT OF REPEATED DOSES OF ECDYSTERONE ON CHOLESTEROL IN LIVER AND SERUM

| Days | | Cholesterol | | | |
| | | Levels | | Biosynthesis (d.p.m./mg. Cholesterol) | |
		Liver (mg./G.)	Serum (mg. per cent)	Liver	Serum
Control		2.41 ± 0.27	76.3 ± 5.05	3331 ± 463	1285 ± 234
Ecdysterone	7	2.07 ± 0.12	67.1 ± 3.01	1699 ± 88	659 ± 111

Rats were treated with ecdysterone for 7 days. Each value represents the mean ±S. D.

Effect of Ecdysterone on Cholesterol Metabolism   Recently, Lupien *et al.* (1969) reported the influence of ecdysone on cholesterol biosynthesis in rats. Ecdysterone, which is different from ecdysone in terms of anabolic action in mammals, was employed for the test on cholesterol metabolism. A single injection of ecdysterone in a dose of 100 μg./ rat did not alter the content of cholesterol either in liver or serum. The incorporation of ^{14}C-acetate *in vivo* into cholesterol in liver was decreased by about 30 per cent at 4 and 8 hours after treatment with ecdysterone. Such inhibition of incorporation was also demonstrated for serum cholesterol (Table 7). Further, repeated administration of ecdysterone exhibited a more significant influence than a single injection; the cholesterol content in liver and serum was reduced a little, and the incorporation of ^{14}C-acetate into cholesterol was significantly inhibited both in liver and serum as indicated in Table 8.

On the other hand, the disappearance of ^{14}C-cholesterol from the blood was tested after its intravenous injection in normal rats and those with multiple doses of ecdysterone. As demonstrated in Table 9, specific activity in the blood of ecdysterone-treated animals was somewhat lower than that of normal rats. The difference in rate of disappearance in the two groups apparently was not remarkable when estimated only from Figure 6.

TABLE 9

DISAPPEARANCE OF ^{14}C-CHOLESTEROL FROM THE BLOODSTREAM

	4 Hr.	12 Hr.	24 Hr.	48 Hr.	
Control	46855	36304	29858	17807	d.p.m./mg.
Ecdysterone	38190	29298	24198	12819	

Each value is the mean for 4 rats.

DISCUSSION

A depressive effect of ecdysterone on the effect of hyperglycemic agents was demonstrated in the present series of experiments. Ecdysterone had no effect on normal blood-glucose levels but apparently reversed the hyperglycemia induced by glucagon. The fact that such modification can take place only when ecdysterone is given prior to the administration of glucagon indicates that this effect is not produced by direct action of ecdysterone on glucagon but is coupled with some changes in the level of a certain mediator or metabolic system. Ecdysterone was also found to be effective

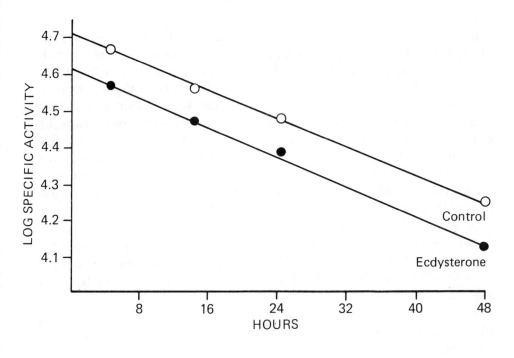

Figure 6

Disappearance of ^{14}C-Cholesterol From the Bloodstream

in modifying the hyperglycemic response to AIS. In this case, however, ecdysterone did not reduce the hyperglycemic response caused by an overdosage of AIS. In alloxan diabetic mice, a pronounced decrease in blood glucose was induced by the administration of ecdysterone. However, the application of ecdysterone could not reduce hyperglycemia when the alloxan-diabetes was severe in rats. These facts reveal that ecdysterone may require the availability of a certain amount of insulin or at least minimal function of the pancreas for manifestation of its effect on hyperglycemia.

The hyperglycemic response to glucagon is usually interpreted as an index of hepatic glycogenolysis, but it has also been suggested that gluconeogenetic action of glucagon is most likely responsible for hyperglycemia (Adnitt, 1969). AIS is also known to stimulate gluconeogenesis (Wagel and Ashmore, 1963; Exton *et al.,* 1966). Hazelwood and O'Brien (1961) suggested that Norethandrolone acts by blocking gluconeogensis leading to diminished stores of hepatic glycogen.

Examination of the effect of ecdysterone on the activity of enzymes concerned in the metabolism of glucose is very important, of course. This has not yet been undertaken in detail, but the tendency for change in activity of some of the enzymes that were tested seemed to be in the direction of accelerating glucose utilization. Such changes may be one of the mechanisms involved in regulation of glucose and free fatty acid resulting from treatment with ecdysterone, but it is still obscure whether these phenomena are due to the direct (allosteric) effect of ecdysterone on enzymes, to the stimulation of enzyme synthesis, or to the change in the amount of some mediator such as insulin. Determination of insulin in the blood of animals under various experimental conditions is now under way.

Inhibition of cholesterol biosynthesis by treatment with ecdysterone was recognized *in vivo,* but its effect *in vitro* is still unknown. Judging from the dose of ecdysterone employed, it is hardly likely that the ecdysterone injected still remains accumulated in the hepatic cell and acts as a feedback inhibitor of cholesterol synthesis.

Therefore additional study will be needed to ascertain the detailed mechanism involved, although there are many possibilities to explain the results observed.

SUMMARY

Ecdysterone has been recognized to have a supressive effect on hyperglycemia induced by several hyperglycemic agents. Although the administration of ecdysterone did not alter the level of glucose in the blood of normal animals, treatment with ecdysterone before that with hyperglycemic agents supressed hyperglycemia induced by either glucagon or anti-insulin serum.

An effect of ecdysterone was also demonstrated when diabetes was brought about in the animals with alloxan. After the administration of ecdysterone to alloxan-diabetic mice, the level of glucose in the blood was reduced to about one-half the value observed before the administration of ecdysterone.

The incorporation of ^{14}C-glucose into glycogen and protein of murine liver was stimulated by treatment with ecdysterone.

Changes in the specific activities of some enzymes related to glucose metabolism seemed to be responsible for promoting glucose utilization.

The elevated level of free fatty acid induced by starvation or diabetes was reduced by the administration of ecdysterone. Incorporation of ^{14}C-acetate into cholesterol was inhibited, but the rate of disappearance of ^{14}C-cholesterol from the blood was apparently unchanged by treatment with ecdysterone.

References

1. ADNITT, P. I.: Hepatic Glycogen and Blood Glucose Control. Biochem. Pharmacol., *18:*2599, 1969.

2. EXTON, J. H., JEFFERSON, L. S., BUTCHER, R. W., and PARK, C. R.: Gluconeogenesis in the Perfused Liver. The Effects of Fasting, Alloxan Diabetes, Glucagon, Epinephrine, Adenosin 3′, 5′ - Monophosphate and Insulin. Amer. J. Med., *40:*709-715, 1966.

3. FERRO, P. V. and HAM, A. B.: Rapid Determination of Total and Free Cholesterol in Serum. Amer. J. Clin. Pathology, *33:*545, 1960.

4. GLOCK, G. E. and McLEAN, P.: Levels of Enzymes of Direct Oxidative Pathway of Carbohydrate Metabolism in Mammalin Tissues and Tumors. Biochem. J. *56:*171-175, 1954.

5. HANDEL, E. VAN and ZILVERSMIT, D. B.: Modification of the Microdetermination of Triglycerides. Clin. Chem., *7:*249, 1961.

6. HASSID, W. Z. and ABRAHAM, S.: Assay of ^{14}C-labeled Glycogen. In *Method in in Enzymology,* S. P. Colowick and N. O. Kaplan, ed. Academic Press, New York, *3:*37, 1957.

7. HAZELWOOD, R. L. and O'BRIEN, K.: Modification of Glucagon-induced Hyperglycemia in Rats by 17-ethyl-19-nortestosterone. Proc. Soc. Exptl. Biol. Med., *106:*851-854, 1961.

8. KACHMAR, J. F. and BOYER, P. D.: Kinetic Analysis of Enzyme Reactions II. The Potassium Activation and Calcium Inhibition of Potassium Activation and Calcium Inhibition of Pyruvic Phosphoferase. J. Biol. Chem., *200:*669, 1953.

9. ITAYA, K., and UI, M.: Colorimetric Determination of Free Fatty Acids in biological Fluids. J. Lipid Res., *6:*16-20, 1965.

10. KITAGAWA, M., ONOUE, K., OKAMURA, Y., YANAI, M., and YAMAMURA, Y.: Immunochemical Studies with Insulin. I. Enhancement of Neutralizing Antibody Formation Against Insulin by Lipid Substances Derived from Mycobacterium Tuberculosis. J. Biochem. (Tokyo), *48:*43, 1960.

11. LELOIR, L. F. and GOLDENBERG, S. H.: Synthesis of Glycogen from Uridinediphosphate Glucose in Liver. J. Biol. Chem., *235:*919, 1960.

12. LUPIEN, P. J., HINSE, C., and CHAUDHARY, K. D.: Ecdysone as a Hypocholesterolemic Agent. Arch. Internation. Physio. et Biochi., *77:*206, 1969.

13. MOMOSE, T., INABA, A., MUKAI, Y.. and SHINKAI, T.: Organic Analysis XXIV. Approximate Colorimetric Estimation of Blood Sugar and Urine Sugar with the Naked Eye. Chem. Pharm. Bull. (Tokyo), *8:*514, 1960.

14. OSER, B. L.: ed. McGraw-Hill, Hawk's Physiological Chemistry New York, p. 89 1965.

15. STOMINGER, J. L., MAXWELL, E. S., AXELORD, J., and KALCKAR, H. M.: Enzymatic Formation of Uridine Disphosphoglucuronic Acid. J. Biol. Chem. *224:*79,1957.

16. SWANSON, M. A.: Phosphatases of Liver; Glucose-6-phosphatase. J. Biol. Chem., *184:*647-659, 1950.

17. VINUELA, E., SALAS, M., and SOLS, A.: Glucokinase and Hexokinase in Liver in
     Relation to Glycogen Synthesis. J. Biol. Chem., *238:*   1175-1177, 1963.

18. WAGEL, S. R. and ASHMORE, J.: Studies on Experimental Diabetes II. Carbon
     Dioxide Fixation. J. Biol. Chem., *238:*17, 1963.

19. WOOD, J. D. and MIGICOVSKY, B. B.. The Effect of Dietary Oils and Fatty Acids
     on Cholesterol Metabolism in the Rat. Canad. J. Biochem. Physiol., *36:*
     433-438, 1958.

INDEX